Katarína Valčová, Michal Valčo (Eds.)

The Future of *Imago Dei* Theologies in the Context of the New Challenges of Transhumanism

Theology East – West
European Perspectives
Theologie Ost – West
Europäische Perspektiven

Founded by
Prof. Dr. Janez Juhant and Prof. Dr. Albert Franz (†)

edited by

Prof. Dr. Janez Juhant
(University of Ljubljana)

and

Prof. Dr. Margit Eckholt
(University of Osnabrück)

Volume 32

LIT

The Future of *Imago Dei* Theologies in the Context of the New Challenges of Transhumanism

Edited by

Katarína Valčová and Michal Valčo

LIT

Cover image:
 The images on the cover and back cover were created using DALL-E, an AI image generation tool developed by OpenAI. Used with permission.

This book was prepared and published with the support of the University of Oxford project 'New Horizons for Science and Religion in Central and Eastern Europe' funded by the John Templeton Foundation. The opinions expressed in the publication are those of the authors and do not necessarily reflect the view of the John Templeton Foundation.

This book is printed on acid-free paper.

Bibliographic information published by the Deutsche Nationalbibliothek
The Deutsche Nationalbibliothek lists this publication in the Deutsche Nationalbibliografie; detailed bibliographic data are available on the Internet at https://dnb.dnb.de.

ISBN 978-3-643-91625-9 (pb)
ISBm 978-3-643-96625-4 (PDF)

A catalogue record for this book is available from the British Library.

Contact:
Fresnostr. 2 D-48159 Münster
Tel. +49 (0) 2 51-62 03 20 Fax +49 (0) 2 51-23 19 72
e-Mail: lit@lit-verlag.de https://www.lit-verlag.de
Distribution:
In the UK: Global Book Marketing, e-mail: mo@centralbooks.com

Contents

Acknowledgments

This book was prepared and published with the support of the University of Oxford project 'New Horizons for Science and Religion in Central and Eastern Europe' funded by the John Templeton Foundation. The opinions expressed in the publication are those of the authors and do not necessarily reflect the view of the John Templeton Foundation.

We extend our sincere gratitude to the authors of this volume whose scholarly rigor and insightful contributions have been instrumental in shaping this volume into a beacon of intellectual inquiry. Our heartfelt thanks also go to the dedicated collaborators and reviewers whose meticulous efforts and unwavering commitment have significantly enriched the depth and breadth of this project, forging a path for meaningful discourse in the ever-evolving landscape of theology and transhumanism.

Katarína Valčová and Michal Valčo, the editors
Bratislava, December 2023

Introduction

This volume, "The Future of Imago Dei Theologies in the Context of the New Challenges of Transhumanism", seeks to navigate the intricate and often uncharted waters of theological discourse as it encounters the burgeoning field of transhumanism. Our endeavor is grounded in the recognition that the human pursuit of transcendence and the quest for enhanced existence have reached unprecedented dimensions in the era of technological innovation. The central premise of this book is the exploration of whether the traditional notions theological anthropology, relying heavily on the concept of 'Imago Dei', can be reconciled with the transhumanist aspirations. Our work wishes to examine the profound implications these advancements hold for our understanding of the self, society, and the divine.

We startby exploring the claim that human nature, particularly in its embodiment of the divine image (which is itself understood in diverse ways), is not merely a static biological entity but a dynamic construct that evolves within social, cultural, and technological contexts. Indeed, this volume addresses the fundamental anthropological question of what it means to be human in an age where the boundaries between the human and the technologically enhanced are increasingly blurred. It scrutinizes the ethical dimensions of transhumanism, weighing the potential benefits against the profound existential and moral dilemmas it poses.

The purpose of this collection is to present a thorough and multifaceted examination of the theological and ethical issues raised by transhumanism. We investigate alternate viewpoints on human enhancement, arguing for a comprehensive approach that stresses equal access to healthcare, education, and stable social environments. We believe that this method may be more favorable to reaching humanity's full potential than relying simply on genetic or technology augmentation.

Our book explores theological, philosophical, anthropological, and cultural traditions, as well as modern ideas and science. This volume features various Vietnamese authors who bring non-Western perspectives to the discussion. These new perspectives from a rich cultural background apart from the Western narrative help us grasp transhumanism. Through this diversity, we aim to deepen the ethical discourse on transhumanism, widen scientific and cultural knowledge, and lay a solid framework for resolving its tensions and conflicts. This addition deepens our investigation and emphasizes the need for a multi-cultural approach to transhumanist developments' worldwide challenges and opportunities.

One strength of this volume is its interdisciplinary nature. Philosophical, theological, bioethical, religious, and cultural studies are among the main approaches. Using humanities and social sciences, this method provides a deeper grasp of transhumanism's ethical issues.

"The Future of Imago Dei Theologies in the Context of the New Challenges of Transhumanism" is really an invitation to a deep conversation about humanity's destiny at the nexus of divine image and technological growth, rather than merely a compilation of academic pieces. To ensure that the quest of human improvement stays rooted in the values of human dignity, moral rectitude, and the common good, we aim to shed light on the ways in which theologies of Imago Dei can inform, critique, and direct the transhumanist vision. Beyond this goal, we also hope to support the encroachment of conventional theological anthropologies into a more expansive and critical discourse by bringing them into a lively dialogue with a variety of religious perspectives and secular ideologies.

Section 1: Philosophical and Theological Foundations

This section provides reflections that rigorously engage a dialectic between traditional knowledge and modern difficulties. The papers collected here provide a comprehensive examination of Imago Dei, not as a dated relic of theological thought but rather as a dynamic paradigm that is challenged by contemporary philosophical research and technological development. Imago Dei remains relevant because each participant, in their own scholarly way, rekindles the conversation between traditional theological ideas and the revolutionary possibilities of transhumanism.

Claudiu Marius Mesaroş commences our intellectual journey with a detailed examination of Gregory of Nyssa's 'De Hominis Opificio,' presenting a synthesis of philosophical, scientific, and theological perspectives.

Mesaroş' discourse probes into the intricate relationship between the soul and body, thus inviting a reassessment of the human entity in the context of Imago Dei.

Following Mesaroş, Wolfgang Palaver delves into the implications of Artificial Intelligence, articulating the anthropological and theological dimensions that intertwine with technology. Palaver's discourse is a clarion call to understand the desires and fears that AI engenders within the framework of the sacred and the secular.

Noemi Bravená's exploration into Dietrich Bonhoeffer's theological anthropology offers a poignant contrast between human limitations and divine perfection. Her analysis of Bonhoeffer's thoughts provides a critical lens through which to examine the ethical and existential dimensions that transhumanism unfurls.

In the vein of rigorous philosophical discourse, Piotr Orłowski embarks on a critique of transhumanist interpretations of Imago Dei, particularly in the context of Thomas Aquinas's thought. Orłowski's contribution is a testament to the depth and complexity of theological and philosophical interpretations in the face of emerging technologies.

Martin Kmec's study of Comenius's anthropological vision offers an enlightening exploration of the pedagogical and philosophical dimensions of human nature, skillfully interweaving historical insights with contemporary implications.

Concluding this section, Mendo Castro Henriques evaluates transhumanist objectives through Bruno Latour's analytical lens. Henriques' discourse is a thought-provoking exposition on the category mistakes inherent in transhumanist aspirations, challenging the reader to reconsider the boundaries between the human and the non-human.

Section 2: Cultural and Ideological Perspectives

In the realm of scholarly inquiry, the exploration of cultural and ideological perspectives provides a unique lens through which the complex nature of human thought and experience can be understood. This is particularly pertinent in the context of transhumanism, a movement that stands at the vanguard of contemporary debates on the evolution of humanity. Section 2 aspires to interweave the threads of diverse cultural beliefs and ideological doctrines with the transformative narrative of transhumanism.

This section commences with Dong Tai Nguyen's insightful juxtaposition of transhumanist ideology against the backdrop of Confucian philosophy and anthropology. His paper examines the intricate layers of Confucian thought, presenting an alternative viewpoint on human nature and ethics, thus complementing and challenging the predominant narratives of transhumanism.

Continuing this cultural dialogue, Hung Quang Nguyen's exploration delves into the Vietnamese experience of Confucianism in the face of the Fourth Industrial Revolution. Quang's analysis is a testament to the resilience and adaptability of traditional philosophies amidst the surge of technological advancements, offering a unique perspective on the interplay between ancient wisdom and modern innovation.

The paper by Hoa Thi Kim Do presents a comparative analysis of Ho Chi Minh's humanistic philosophy against the backdrop of transhumanism. Her work is a reflection on the divergent paths of human development and enhancement as envisaged through different ideological prisms.

Bojan Žalec's contribution further enriches this section by examining the intersection of New Age and Romanticism with transhumanism and Enlightenment thought. His work highlights the critical role of transcendence and authenticity in the modern Western social and political grammar, providing a philosophical lens to comprehend the implications of transhumanist endeavors.

Ha Thanh Pham and Hai Hoang Nguyen's analysis of transhumanism offer their reflections from the vantage point of Engaged Buddhism in Vietnam. Their paper serves as a bridge between traditional religious perspectives and contemporary scientific advancements, offering a nuanced view of the ethical and spiritual implications of transhumanist technologies.

Section 3: Practical Implications and Future Prospects

In the ever-evolving discourse on transhumanism, it becomes imperative to transcend theoretical reflections and delve into the tangible, real-world implications of this transformative ideology. Section 3embarks on this critical journey, presenting a collection of scholarly works that scrutinize the impact of transhumanism on various facets of human life and society.

This section opens with Hoa Thi Kim Do and Duc Hong Nguyen's comprehensive assessment of the Fourth Industrial Revolution's societal impacts, particularly in Vietnam. Their work is a significant contribution to understanding the multidimensional effects of Artificial Intelligence on human emotions, ethics, morality, and religious beliefs, thus offering invaluable insights for policymakers, educators, and AI developers.

Ion Cordoneanu's metaphysical interpretation of posthumanism further enriches this section, presenting a thought-provoking analysis of humanity's relationship with technology. His chapter delves into the philosophical and existential dimensions of technological advancement, raising critical questions about the future role of humanity in an increasingly digital world.

Jozef Jenčík's examination of the interplay between transhumanism, power dynamics, and anarchy offers a unique perspective on collective empowerment through technologies. His study challenges conventional notions of sovereignty and power, advocating for inclusive and participatory frameworks in the context of technological progress.

Martin Turčan's discussion on anarcho-transhumanism from a theological standpoint presents a critical evaluation of the values underpinning this ideology, drawing parallels with the biblical narrative of Genesis 6. His analysis serves as a cautionary tale, highlighting the potential pitfalls of unchecked transhumanist aspirations.

The section further includes Noemi Bravená and Helena Hejlová's paper on integrating transhumanism into primary education. This contribution is pivotal in shaping the future discourse, as it addresses the need for an inclusive educational framework that embraces technological, ethical, and transcendent aspects of human development.

Hang Thi Thu Vu presents a meticulous exploration of the impacts of technology on happiness and well-being in Vietnam. Her paper is a seminal contribution, examining the multifaceted influences of technological advancements on social interactions, leisure activities, and access to information. Vu's work is important in understanding the relationship between technology and human contentment, particularly in the Vietnamese context, offering broader implications for global discussions on technological impact and human welfare.

Winfried Löffler delves into the concept of 'human nature' and its inherent plasticities, navigating the intricate balance between existential concerns and transhumanist ideals. His critical examination begins with a philosophical analysis of defining human nature, addressing potential pitfalls of essentialism and authoritarianism. Löffler integrates insights from classical philosophy, particularly the Aristotelian-Scholastic tradition, and contemporary perspectives on human evolution and medical technologies. His work culminates in a thoughtful discourse on the ethical implications and potential risks of altering human nature through technological means, advocating for a balanced and ethical approach.

Michal Valčo and RadoslavHanus engage in a thought-provoking discussion on contingency, relationality, and narrativity as foundational elements in human identity. Their chapter posits a robust anthropological framework, integrating insights from philosophy, psychology, and theology. This multidisciplinary approach illuminates the dynamic interplay of these aspects in shaping human identity, providing critical insights into addressing the challenges posed by transhumanism. Their perspective underscores the intrinsic value and interconnectedness of human beings, countering the fragmented view often presented by transhumanist ideologies.

The following chapter by Michal Valčo offers an incisive analysis of transhumanism through the lens of techno-Gnosticism, examining the philosophical and theological underpinnings of this movement. His study draws parallels between transhumanist aspirations and the Gnostic pursuit of transcendence through knowledge and technological manipulation. Valčo's chapter raises essential questions about the relationship between technology and human flourishing, contending that while transhumanism presents intriguing possibilities for human enhancement, it also carries significant risks and challenges that necessitate careful consideration.

Katarína Valčová sets out on an exploration of the existential, spiritual, and practical dimensions of mortality. Her comprehensive study traverses existential thought, spiritual reflection, and practical discourse, addressing the emotional experiences of grieving, philosophical aspects of mortality, and practical approaches to discussing death. Valčová's work integrates psychological, pastoral, and existential perspectives, offering a holistic narrative on how individuals and communities confront and navigate the reality of death, especially in the context of transhumanism's quest for immortality.

Let us conclude by emphasizing once more that the three sections of this book aim to be more than just an assortment of scholarly articles; rather, they are meant to be a lively discussion forum where the real-world applications of transhumanism are scrutinized. They encourage readers to engage in a conversation that strikes a balance between the possibilities of transhumanism and the ethical, societal, and existential issues it raises as well as to reflect on the future of mankind in an era defined by rapid technological advancement. In addition to encouraging a careful and educated approach to navigating the unknown waters of our collective future, we seek to cultivate a nuanced understanding and spark a vibrant discourse about how transhumanist philosophies could transform the human experience.

Katarína Valčová and Michal Valčo, the editors

PHILOSOPHICAL AND THEOLOGICAL FOUNDATIONS

Explorations of Imago Dei and Human Nature in Historical and Contemporary Contexts

A PHILOSOPHICAL COMMENTARY ON THE IMAGO DEI IN GREGORY OF NYSSSA'S DE HOMINIS OPIFICIO

Claudiu Marius Mesaroş

1. An Aristotelian methodology for the philosophy of creation

Gregory of Nyssa's relation to his contemporary philosophical schools is for some time a classical problem: suggestions have been made to sustain Gregory's dependence on Platonism, on Posidonius, or eventually on Stoic and Neoplatonic sources. Still, recent critical investigations favor the less canonical evaluation of Gregory's links with the philosophical sources, showing that Gregory was rather accessing and using eclectic and polemical versions of different theories and vocabularies (Barnes 2020, 338–339). In *De Hominis Opificio* Gregory seems to be closer to the method of Nemesius of Emesa, an Aristotelian, albeit in other works the Platonic thinking is more apparent (Bell 1980). So, although *De Hominis Opificio* was intended to complete the Hexaëmeron of Saint Basil, it is still classified as a philosophical treaty. Along with other texts by Gregory, even those unanimously labeled as "ascetic", it is deeply linked to the scientific and psychological ideas of the time, some claim especially Stoic (Barnes 2002, 477) but not exclusively. This involves multiple conceptual connections open to Stoic, Platonist, Aristotelian, or Neoplatonist literature.

One of the first things that strike is the depiction of Creation as composition of opposites: heaven and earth are diametrically opposed and underlie nature as an interval or realm of motion and change. Thus, the creation of God was shaped as a realm of instability or movement between two extremes that are contrary to each other.

> "All things are offspring of rest and motion, brought into being by the Divine will. Now the heaven and the earth being diametrically opposed to each other in their

> operations, the creation which lies between the opposites, … acts as a mean between the extremes, so that there is manifestly a mutual contact of the opposites through the mean; for air in a manner imitates the perpetual motion and subtlety of the fiery substance, … yet it is not such as to be alienated from the solid substance, for it is no more in a state of continual flux and dispersion than in a permanent state of immobility, but becomes, in its affinity to each, a kind of borderland of the opposition between operations, at once uniting in itself and dividing things which are naturally distinct" (Schaff et al. 1892, 48; PG 44, 129a).[1]

A methodology of this kind is hard to spot as belonging to Platonic or Origenian or any other precise philosophical school. It is a sort of eclecticism avoiding falling into any commodity trap like dualism or idealism (Jeffrey 2000, 528). The fragment rather reminds of the Aristotelian theoretical grounds detailed in *Physics*, I, 1–6, where such a framework is built as methodology of investigation for the inquiry of nature, based on a critical evaluation of previous doctrines on Being with the aim of obtaining a rationally limited and complete list of axioms necessary and sufficient for the investigation of the nature: matter, form, and movement, that is, two opposite and one intermediary principles, "for first principles must not be derived from one another nor from anything else, while everything has to be derived from them". As the objects in nature are multiple, the universe is compound and therefore compatible with this system of two opposite and one intermediary principle that contain the ability to explain motion (see Barnes 1984, *Physics:* 185a 1–3; 188a27–188a31; 188b21–188b26). Apart from these contrary principles, that will eventually be identified as matter and form, there must be an intermediate principle, not contrary but continuous to them, compatible with both and underlying the change from one contrary to another. Aristotle also says that the principles of nature cannot be innumerable; if infinite, they will not be epistemologically accessible therefore unusable (Barnes 1984, *Physics:* 189a20–189a27). Motion is co-extensive with nature and so the opposites and the in-between interval are the fundamental constituents of the world, or that the world of the corporeal substances is forever in motion.

Gregory of Nyssa's *De hominis opificio* is relying on the Aristotelian methodology by saying that God as depicted in the *Genesis* created the

[1] The original version of the treatise can be found Migne J-P. (1863). *Patrologiae Graecae* (*PG*), pp.123–258. My chapter will refer to it as PG and rely on the English translation in Schaff & Wace (1892), accordingly refer to its pagination.

Universe as a *mean* between opposites, and that creation is understood through the properties of contrary natures which are harmonious and allow an interval of agreement: in *Genesis*, the earth and the water were "holding each other in" and "took the middle place of the universe" while "the Divine power and skill was implanted in the growth of things, guiding all things with the reins of a double operation" (Schaff et al. 1892, 48; PG 44, 127c).

The essence of nature is motion: "for it was by rest and motion that it devised the genesis of the things that were not, and the continuance of the things that are" (Schaff et al. 1892, 48; PG 44, 127d); the Biblical exegesis renders the intrinsic motion of nature as Divine power implanted into things that operates according to the Aristotelian dual principles which are not mentioned as matter and form but simply as contrariety *per se* as characteristic of a whirling universal revolution:

> "the Divine power and skill was implanted (*enapetethe*) in the growth of things, guiding all things with the reins of a double operation (...) driving around, about the heavy and changeless element contributed by the creation that does not move, as about some fixed path, the exceedingly rapid motion of the sphere, like a wheel, and preserving the indissolubility of both by their mutual action, as the circling substance by its rapid motion compresses the compact body of the earth round about, while that which is firm and unyielding, by reason of its unchanging fixedness, continually augments the whirling motion of those things which revolve round it" (Schaff et al. 1892, 48; PG 44, 127d).

The paragraph speculates on the aforementioned dual methodology but offers an original interpretation of the principle of contraries assumed in the context of Biblical creation: speculating on the Aristotelian typology of motions, Gregory introduces the *providence* saying that there is a "providential dispensation" or alteration that combines the unchangeable and the changeable in a reversed manner regarding the immovable respectively the movable nature.

This intervention of providence has at least two visible functions in the context: first, it acts as explanatory agent for the previously mentioned "implantation" of the Divine power and skill, and second, it develops a further Nyssenian idea, that of the universal harmony of contraries, expressed as a "mixture of properties" or participation. Now, the participationis a technical term in Nyssa: "participation in God is not a state, but an ongoing process of receiving more and more from God; μετουςία may express better the relationship envisaged between the (rational) creature and the Creator" (Mateo-Seco et al. 2010, 501). The philosophical term associated with it is *methexis*, coming from Plato's philosophy, meaning the relationship of the sensible things to the intelligible forms or ideas, but in Gregory's theology the same term (*vb. metousia*, also *metoche* or *koinonia* and also *metechein*) refers primarily to the "relationship of spiritual creatures (angels and human beings as having rational souls) to God". (Mateo-Seco et.al. 2010, 581). Less prominent but still important is the "horizontal" participation, which is "found on each level of reality and consists in sharing in the common nature of the species" (Mateo-Seco et.al. 2010, 582; 586–587). In the present fragment, the "mixture" as participation invokes the planning by divine providence of a harmonious nature in which a "mutual agreement" or union is manifest:

> "The very nature of the contraries themselves is not entirely without *mixture of properties*, each with the other, so that, as I think, all that we see in the world *mutually agree* (*mixis ton enantion kai synodos*), and the creation, though discovered in properties of contrary natures, is yet at union with itself. For as motion is not conceived merely as local shifting, but is also contemplated in change and alteration, and, on the other hand, the immovable nature does not admit motion by way of alteration, the wisdom of God has transposed these properties, and wrought unchangeableness in that which is ever moving, and change in that which is immovable" (Schaff et al. 1892, 48; PG 44, 130 c-d).

Not only does the Aristotelian concept of *genesis* or becoming receive the particular interpretation as harmonious mixture of movements that mutually agree, but on this very ground the Divine creation will be depicted as paradoxical: "the earth is stable without being immutable, while the heaven, on the contrary, as it has no mutability, so has not stability either". This kind of attributes alienation acts like a reasonable cause for the universal harmony of movements: the immovable nature gets changeability, and the moving nature receives unchangeability. The mixture must be taken without a connotation of chance or coincidence since it occurs because of Divine will. However, such a view does not entail any divine determination: Divine will creates harmony but not the detailed events of the contingency. To introduce a metaphysical convention for this, Nyssa considers that the stability of the physical earth should have been compensated by mutability, while the instability of heaven is compensated by its immutability. This way, the Creator operated a mixture of attributes so that neither nature nor Heaven could be too close to the Deity. This way the both are alien from the possibility to apprehend (*hypolepsin*) Deity in case of accidental move. In short, the creation is rather a harmony of mixtures between motion and rest so that accidental or mechanical approach to God is avoided.

> "The Divine power, by interweaving change in the stable nature and motion with that which is not subject to change, might, by the interchange of attributes, at once join them both closely to each other, and make them alien from the conception of Deity" (Schaff et al.1892, 48; PG44, 130 d).

2. Enjoyment as designed relation of man with the changing universe and nature

Within this world of opposition between movement and rest, the place of humans is that of a created inheritor of a kingdom. The universe and the whole nature that surrounds humanity were prepared by God so that humanity, the final created being, receives at its arrival the ready-made divine prepared environment "as one whom it behoved to be king over his subjects at his very birth" (Schaff et al. 1892, 49; PG44, 133 a). According to this scenario, the relation of man and nature is a relation of participation to one whole that is the universe; to this extent, human being is the final part or rather the purpose of the creation, so that, with the focus on the whole, humanity comes as the ending (*telos*) of the created realm. What is special about the divine design is not that the humanity needed the universe as an environment but on the contrary, the universe needed a finality, and for that purpose humanity was added as the reason of the whole. On this ground it is rather true that humanity can never be considered as separated from the whole universe but on the contrary only as an inseparable meaning of it. It is equally important that this inseparable part is the ruling or the reasoning part of it just as the human being at its turn is a whole hierarchical entity governed by reason. However, for the same reason, the human being was assigned a governing role.

Now, the first task of this governor is to enjoy what is already there and not to acquire anything new; Gregory describes this as "the enjoyment (*apolausis*) of the things which were there". This opposition is probably one of the most intriguing discursive structures in the text: the task of enjoyment of the nature implies that there is such a purpose in it; the world as created in order to be enjoyed as a closed act (since there is nothing to be added to it) and therefore, if anything, it should be ruled and enjoyed as such, as a complete system. *Apolausis* also means, according to Mateo-Seco & Maspero (2010, 221), a form of intellectual movement, opposed to desire: it is the form of enjoyment proper to us in relation to God, since God cannot be an object of desire. It is the same kind of act that humanity will manifest at the end of the history, when "there will be a happiness in communion, because all will enjoy the splendor of the other" and "each seeing the beauty of the others, they will be filled with reciprocal joy" (Mateo-Seco et.al. 2010, 278).

This involves deeper employments of the term; Lampe (1961, 199) lists more spiritual meanings like "eucharistic enjoyment", "never giving satiety", with an eschatological aim. So, the current paragraph is consistently illustrating the fact that divine creation is purposefully defined as an act of continuous fulfillment of man by the enjoyment of nature and God. Enjoyment can be sinful or evil (*hybris, amartias* – Lampe 1961, 199) when cut off from the projected purpose of maintaining the active relation to God but otherwise it is the very specific and functional link that human has at disposal for maintaining his living relation with the Creator.

According to Walker (2022, 375), who treats *apolausis* as an emotion, in Christian theology, the term connotes "spiritual pleasure achieved through the satisfaction of desire for union with the divine". Additionally, Walker (2022, 375)notes that *apolausis* indicates "the potential for feelings to burst beyond the bounds of the intellect, to drive the body without moral or rational regulation", pointing towards a contradictory relation between mind and body through this emotion: on one hand, it indicates a strong bondage between mind and body and on the other hand it contrasts to *hedone*, the physical pleasure. It is precisely because of its problematic connection with corporeal satisfaction that *apolausis* was "scrutinized by the early church Fathers" like Gregory of Nyssa who understood the term as "spiritual equivalent of *hedone*" (Walker 2022, 375). The contradictory character of enjoyment is given by the fact that "when it metastasised from enjoyment to pleasure, *apolausis* could cause the body to overtake the soul" (Walker 2022, 377). Therefore, there is a reasonable concern for repressing pleasure or at least for "channeling it toward proper ends and circumscribing its intensity" (Walker 2022, 377).

Gregory designates special faculties for enjoyment so that humans can enjoy both the Divine and the earthly beauty in a differentiated manner, according to specific means:

> "He gives him as foundations the instincts of a twofold organization, blending the Divine with the earthy, that by means of both he may be naturally and properly disposed to each enjoyment, enjoying God by means of his more divine nature, and the good things of earth by the sense that is akin to them" (Schaff et al. 1892, 49; PG 44, 133 b).

These specific faculties, or "instincts", are explicitly referred to as "divine nature" and "senses", respectively. These faculties are *homogeneous* (of the same kind) as the earthly things. On the one hand, this division bears Platonic traces of the division between the intelligible and the sensible but, on the other hand, it has been planned from the very beginning by the Creator according to Gregory's Biblical interpretation. In the section III, he marks the distinction between non-human and human animality by asserting that the previous are "brought into being with a word" whereas man was created "with circumspection ... to liken his form to an archetypal beauty, ... to make for him a nature appropriate and allied to the operations, and suitable for the object in hand" (Schaff et al. 1892, 50; PG 44, 136 a). Both the Platonic division and the Christian Gregory position indicate that the dual constitution of man fits the cognoscible realms of the created environment: the non-human creatures exist by word and accordingly the human is set with circumspection to receive a nature suitable for the object to be grasped.

Whether this cognitive correspondence between human faculties and the realms of the created nature is exactly the meaning of the projected "enjoyment" or not, is difficult to decide. This is especially the case since there is also a sensorial enjoyment involved. It is certain that the intended relationship of man to God is aptly described as enjoyment, encompassing both the sensory, for tangible things, and the intellectual, for the intangible. The goal of enjoyment is to be achieved by the most appropriate kind of activity man can perform, the monarchic.

3. The king of nature and the allegory of God the painter

There is an entire complex of virtues that ornate the human being as a king that bears the image or similitude with the Divine Creator.

"the human nature ... was made to rule the rest, by its likeness to the King of all ... a living image, partaking with the archetype both in rank and in name... but instead of the purple robe, clothed in virtue, which is in truth the most royal of all raiment, and in place of the sceptre, leaning on the bliss of immortality, and instead of the royal diadem, decked with the crown of righteousness; so that it is shown to be perfectly like to the beauty of its archetype in all that belongs to the dignity of royalty" (Schaff et al. 1892, 50; PG 44, 136 d).

This is the first description of the *imago Dei* in the *De opificio: homoiotetos*, *empsychos eikon*, *koinonousa*, similar to the archetype both in importance (*axias*) and name (*onoma*). Human as *imago Dei*, according to this description, is a living image that maintains its status by participating to its archetype. Is this participation another term for enjoyment or not? It shall be clarified later. For the time being it is important to note that the relation of man to Divine is described by three essential terms: enjoyment, participation, and similitude.

The detailing of this similitude is given as a set of advantages over the rest of the creation; thus, humans are superior to nature bywisdom, liberty, and dignities. Wisdom enables human to control both external and internal nature and the body as an instrument, freedom is exercised over will, and the dignities are manifest as virtues (named "purple"), immortality ("sceptre"), righteousness ("royal diadem"). In the fifth section there is the allegory of the painter that Gregory builds to illuminate the status of the human-king. Thus, human as the image of God is presented as a picturesque but realistic copy of the Divine nature, an analogous image painted by God by using colourful transfers of forms such as purity, freedom, blessedness, alienation from evil, love, beauty.

These Platonic concepts such as imitation and participation answer the question regarding the possibility that the corporeal human beings share the beauty of God: it is by an act of self-replication executed by God himself to create the world as God's self-portrait. Within this process, God associates proper colours and tints to imitate the beauty of the original.

"And manifold and varied are the tints, so to say, by which His true form is portrayed: not red, or white, or the blending of these ... nor a touch of black that paints the eyebrow and the eye, and shades, by some combination ... but instead of these, purity, freedom from passion, blessedness, alienation from all evil, and all those attributes of the like kind which help to form in men the likeness of God: with such hues as these did the Maker of His own image mark our nature" (Schaff et al. 1892, 50; PG 44, 137–138 a).

4. The unity of mind

To experience a full participation man enjoys the rest of the creation both by senses and by intellect (horizontal and vertical participation), thus the God-like activity man is meant to experience is unitary: the intellect activates passing through all the organs to understand the nature. In spite of the fact that Thomas Aquinas believed to be using Gregory's *De Natura Hominis* while he was actually quoting from Nemesius of Emessa (Zedler 1968, 35; 54), Aquinas made use of Gregory in his *De Unitate Intellectus Contra Averroistas* and thus made him part of the well-known philosophical debate on the simplicity of the intellect, a problem originated in the Aristotelian *On the Soul*, III, 5. The formulae in the present treaty of Gregory remind of the philosophical position that the intellect is simple and universal:

> "even though the organs formed by nature for purposes of perception may be different, that which operates and moves by means of all, and uses each appropriately for the object before it, is one and the same, not changing its nature by the differences of operations" (Schaff et al. 1892, 51; PG 44, 140a).

Taking position within the traditional debate whether psychological faculties reflect different essences or souls or one soul only (Barnes 2002, 480), Gregory takes the part of the Aristotelian view that there is only one essence, or one soul. Man has a plurality of functions but, still, he is a unity; as the image of God, man's apprehensive faculty imitates the simplicity and the uniqueness of the divine mind: "for there is one faculty, the implanted mind itself, which passes through each of the organs of sense and grasps the things beyond" (Schaff et al. 1892, 51; PG 44, 140a).

As self-portrait image of God, man has its unity given by the unitary *mind* which is *one* and therefore human being has a unique essence and a synthetic functioning. This position can also be traced back to the Aristotelian discussion in the *On the Soul, II, 3*, where the Stagirite makes evident that a single definition must be given to the soul in the same sense as one definition is given to a geometrical figure no matter what its particular form can take.

By their nature, humans are plural and unstable, but it is only by the similitude with God that they can experience the unity. The notion that will successfully explain this conjoint of unity and plurality in Gregory is the *harmonious blend of mind and body:* mind is a copy of Divine, so man is a harmonious blend of Divine and nature or rather of Creator and Creature. Gregory is attempting a description of this blend by narrating the mixture between the reason and the body and the upward position of the human. The vertical position of the body and the use of hands for expressing thinking (as in written language) is part of our logical composition: hands are an instrument of reason; the entire body is organized as a structured compound able to serve reason:

> "*we signify our reasoning by means of the natural employment of our hands in written characters*. It is true that this fact, that we speak by writing, and, in a certain way, converse by the aid of our hands, preserving sounds by the forms of the alphabet, is not unconnected with the endowment of reason" (Schaff et al. 1892, 53; PG 44, 144 b).

5. The unity of mind and body

The multiplicity of human senses forms a harmonious functional structure that is also hierarchical and not antagonistic to the body. The psychology behind this hierarchical division into three parts, which are considered common to the bodily functions and not as separate as in a dualistic view, is again Aristotelian. First, he says that the rational man is a blend of all kinds of soul: vegetative (for nourishment and growth), sensible, and intellectual. The sensible is midway between intellectual and material nature: coarser than intellect, more refined than the material. The three kinds of soul compose a functional mixture. First, the intellectual essence is mixed with the subtle (*lepton*) and enlightened (*photoeides*) part of the sensitive. In the end, by translating into the Pauline vocabulary",man consists of these three: ... the apostle ... says to the Ephesians, ... using, the word 'body' for the nutritive part, and denoting the sensitive by the word 'soul' and the intellectual by 'spirit'" (Schaff et al. 1892, 54; PG 44, 144c).

Thus, the bodily functions or the material nature (*soma*) ensure the nutrition and form the first part of the human, the sensitive function is the *soulper se* (*psyche*), ensuring the perception of the nature, and the intellectual activity (*noerasousias; noeron*) which is finally called *spirit* (*pneuma*) because it perceives the perfection of godly life, are the three functions also named "heart" (*kardia*), "soul" (*psyche*) and "mind" (*dianoia*). A few lines below different names are employed, such as "carnal" (*sarkiken*, responsible with the belly and the connected pleasures), "psychic" (*psychiken*), holding the middle position regarding virtue and vice, respectively "spiritual" (*pneumatiken*), as it perceives the perfection of divine (Schaff et al. 1892, 54; PG 44, 148a).

It appears that Gregory involves a mixed psychology here, unifying Platonism and Aristotelianism into a single synthetic panel of functions. First, he is Aristotelian for at least three reasons: the methodological perspective of avoiding dualism and calling the body a "nutritive part"; the option of attributing to the "psychic" a middle position between virtue and vice (as in the Aristotelian ethical principle of the middle term); then the hierarchical view of the three functions (as in Aristotle, *De an.*, 414a 29–415a 12 – see: Barnes 1984). Despite these, he nevertheless speaks of the power of the "spiritual" to perceive the perfection of the divine, as in the Platonic theory of the knowledge levels in the *Republic*.

The three functions assemble and work together according to a mutual relation that should be guarded or preserved until the *Parousia*. Gregory calls this relation *oikeiosis* (alliance) and *anakrasis*(commixture). Everything regarding the harmonious relation between these functions of the soul is generously and precisely designed and made possible by the Creator, but nevertheless man has the intact possibility to either ensure the good function or to corrupt the design: Parousia will bring the liberation from this task of freely contributing to the preserving God's creation in best possible shape, therefore the Apostle was praying for this preservation to stay intact.

Meanwhile, the man can use the exact necessary organs he has been gifted with to be able to speak (express reason), so reason and body make up a harmonious unity: body is receptive to reason, reason is appropriated by nature through specific organs. This is how the intelligible, *per se* incommunicable and incorporeal, is nonetheless manifested through the instrumental organization of this three-levelled human composition that is capable of actions of translating realities from one level to another: there is a motion in the intelligible that acts like a plectrum over the vocal organs and indicates (*hermeneuse*)the motion behind (Schaff et al.1892, 54; PG 45, 149b).

6. The Allegory of the animated musical instrument

Gregory develops three allegories of the human mind-body relation: the allegory of God as a painter described above, the allegory of the musical instrument, and that of the Governor. One of the most provoking is the allegory of the musical instrument, a powerful depiction of the harmony of the body, soul, and mind. The use of bodily organs compared to the mastering of a musical instrument is far from a simplistic comparison. First, he says that the instrument of the human body is suitable for the use of reason in such a way as the musical instrument is suitable for the use of musicians. Now, the production of music is "according to the form of musical instruments" and "not piping with harps nor harping upon flutes" (Schaff et al., 54; PG 45, 148c), so the organization of the human body is analogically adapted for the creation of a rational behaviour.

> "the human mind being a discoverer of all sorts of conceptions, seeing that it is unable, by the mere soul, to reveal to those who hear by bodily senses the motions of its understanding, touches, like some skillful composer, these animated instruments, and makes known its hidden thoughts by means of the sound produced upon them" (Schaff et al., 55; PG 45, 149b).

According to this analogy, the mind is such a perfect composer because it is the imitation of God: "we cannot strictly say that He gave, but that He imparted them, adding to the image the proper adornment of His own nature" (Schaff et al., 55; PG 45, 149b). The music of the human instrument is a combination of sounds, like in a concerted piece of music. Just like in the final more physiological and medical paragraphs, Gregory enjoys here as well an exaggerated detailed exposition on the musical instruments, showing not only familiarity but also the importance of the analogical argument in use: the analogy is planned to work as a convincing and sophisticated expertise. Teleological thinking is also at its heights when arguing that since it is not by the use of the lips but the hands that we supply food, the lips remain therefore available for the service of reason (Schaff et al. 1892, 55; PG 45, 152b).

On the other part, the body can receive the harmony and perfection of the mind because it is created as a musical instrument and therefore gifted with receptivity, acoustic qualities, so it is not seen as a purely receptive counterpart but as one that supplies the mind with optimal forms of expression or even accompanies the mind in a common activity. Thus, the body as a musical instrument is a sort of dual way activity: ittransmits sounds – *logoi* of the mind *and it receives concepts all the same.* Hearing and speaking are two opposite functions that bring together the logos from the outside and the logos from the inside in a unitary process. Thus, the epistemological grounding for true knowledge lies in the functional unity of human nature. The internal faculties are "a matter of wonder" for their capacity to receive but especially for the special ability to understand the forms received from outside.

> "The operation of the instrument, however, is twofold; one for the production of sound, the other for the reception of concepts from without; and the one faculty does not blend with the other, but abides in the operation for which it was appointed by nature, not interfering with its neighbour either by the sense of hearing undertaking to speak, or by the speech undertaking to hear; for the latter is always uttering something, while the ear, as Solomon somewhere says, is not filled with continual hearing" (Schaff et al. 1892, 55; PG 45, 152b).

Gregory is posing a system of philosophical questions regarding epistemological matters such as: what is the extension of our understanding; what is the substratum of our representations; what is the substratum of memory; how is the mental systematizing possible and at the same time relevant for the knowledge of the things; and how is the visual impression turned into apprehension? It is, nevertheless, for the modern reader a matter of wonder how pro-Cartesian these fragments can sound:

> "That point as to our internal faculties which seems to me to be even in a special degree matter for wonder, is this: – what is the extent of that inner receptacle into which flows everything that is poured in by our hearing? who are the recorders of the sayings that are brought in by it? what sort of storehouses are there for the concepts that are being put in by our hearing? and how is it, that when many of them, of varied kinds, are pressing one upon another, there arises no confusion and error in the relative position of the things that are laid up there?" (Schaff et al. 1892, 55; PG 45, 152b)

All such intricate functions and relations between the different parts are given as harmonious by the divine design which humans are invited to enjoy, use, and understand. A few paragraphs below the epistemological questions multiply by the new problem regarding the nature of mind:

> "What then is, in its own nature, this mind that distributes itself into faculties of sensation, and duly receives, by means of each, the knowledge of things? That it is

something else besides the senses, I suppose no reasonable man doubts; for if it were identical with sense, it would reduce the proper character of the operations carried on by sense to one, on the ground that it is itself simple, and that in what is simple no diversity is to be found" (Schaff et al., 56; PG 45, 153d).

The assembly of the senses and mind looks like a spiritual workshop that is so precise and well organized that it turns itself into a philosophical investigation as such. The new question (what is the nature of mind?) opens a striking theory and presupposition that, behind its harmonious multiplicity, there is a substantial unity of the mind that still "distributes" itself into the functional parts and fulfils several conditions: a) its nature is different from the senses, so that we can recognize the sensations as different from each other, otherwise they would melt into one single perception by a faculty of the same nature as senses unable to perceive their differentiation; b) unitary, since it distributes into different faculties; c) still no different from the faculties due to distribution. Conditions *a)* and *c)* look contradictory but at a closer look they are coherent with the theory of the unitary universal intellect, or the Plotinian interpretation to the Aristotelian problem of the active intellect, as we see for instance in the *Enneads*: "the soul of each individual is one because it is present as a whole at every point of the body, and is really one in this way, not having one part of it here and another there in the body" (Plotinus 1984, IV.9.1).

While the dualist perspective on body and soul contains elements inherited from Origen, the tripartite discussion on the nature of mind seems to come from the competing School of Neoplatonism together with an Aristotelian methodology containing "not only a mingling of the corporeal and incorporeal existences, but a unity" (Bishop 2000, 520; 524; Cross 2002; Zachhuber 2005).

7. The Allegory of the city governor

For the final answer regarding the nature of mind Gregory addresses the Platonic method of analogy a third time. As in Plato's *Republic*, the complexity of mind will be explicit when projected onto a greater object easier to observe, such as a citadel. Since the mind is the governor that sees and organizes everything into human nature, and the city is analogous to the body that has the receptivity to reason and order, a new allegory is at its place. In Gregory, the relation of the city to its governor is again bidirectional: the mind is the governor of the assembly of the senses and their mutual assembly acts like a spiritual workshop. In the analogy of Citadel, Gregory shows that the mind works through senses as the Governor acts through different public instruments, and so the city itself casts signals about its own behaviour.

> "... such city of our mind I seem to discern established in us, which the different entrances through the senses keep filling, while the mind, distinguishing and examining each of the things that enter, ranks them in their proper departments of knowledge" (Schaff et al. 1892, 55; PG 45, 153a).

The sensations that enter through a certain kind of organ are to be received and brought together again in the mind. Some sensations that are foreign to each other enter the same sense ("gate") but they are at the right moment separated again by the thinking. To the same extent, the senses verify each other and bring testimony for reciprocal objectiveness.

> "their community of entrance does not bind them together; ... ; something of the same kind I seem to discern in the spacious territory of our mind; for often the knowledge which we gather from the different organs of sense is one, as the same object is divided into several parts in relation to the senses; and again, on the contrary, we may learn from some one sense many and varied things which have no affinity one with another" (Schaff et al. 1892, 55; PG 45, 153a).

In Plato's comparison of the mind with a citadel and his concept of *oikeiopragia*, the relation is not bidirectional, the contribution from lower faculties to the governor's activity is less desirable and eventually Plato will adopt an isolationist view: "... The ability of everyone to perform his own function is apparently a strong competitor with the city's wisdom, self-discipline and courage" (Plato 2000, 128; 434a-b). In Gregory the same analogy established the existence of an active and dynamic relation between the city and the ruler, where the city and its different components play a functional role that is complimentary and not antagonistic to the ruling part. This is necessarily the particularization of the *Image* that describes the creation but also still compatible with the Platonic theory of imitation.

8. The place of the mind

The mind is beyond our understanding for the same reason: its status as the image of God. Since incomprehensibility of essence is "one of the attributes we contemplate in Divine nature", it is necessary that the image shows its imitation by bearing a similar attribute.

> "But since the nature of our mind, which is the likeness of the Creator evades our knowledge, it has an accurate resemblance to the superior nature, figuring by its own unknowableness the incomprehensible Nature" (Schaff et al. 1892, 56; PG 45, 156b).

The incomprehensibility of the mind is a subject that had travelled a long way through the previous history of philosophy, being perhaps the same old discussion originated in Anaxagoras and entered the psychology of Aristotle and then deeper into late antiquity. For Anaxagoras (B12), the universal intellect is separated from the elements of the *physis* because the *nous* is governing, is supreme and unmixed with nature. Therefore, *nous*, if sensorial, could be identified with just another sense; if separated from the senses but present in each of them, it could not operate distinctions and governance. Aristotle had summarized in his *On the Soul:* "Since everything is a possible object of thought, mind in order, as Anaxagoras says, to dominate, that is, to know, must be pure from all admixtures" (Barnes 1984, 429a18). Gregory rephrased the same argument (see above). On the other hand, like its Divine model, the mind cannot be understood.

One of the most impressive discussions regards the localization of the mind, if there is one, or, in other words, the relation of mind to the space or body. Gregory's questions extend as much as: Where is the mind? – or, what is the corporeal organ that hosts the mind? Does the mind have a place at all? Gregory rejects both the physicist hypotheses like: heart, brain, fire, meninge, liver, but also the literal Biblical common places localizations like heart, reins, even brain. As Bishop points out:

> "Unlike Origen or the Neoplatonists, Gregory acknowledges the necessity of the body, and contrary to Stoicism and Epicureanism, he insists that because mind is a unity, it must permeate the whole: it cannot be housed in a particular organ" (Bishop 2000, 520; 524).

Gregory discusses the question starting with an axiom: "Let there be an end, then, of all the vain and conjectural discussion of those who confine the intelligible energy to certain bodily organs" (Schaff et al. 1892, 56; PG 45, 156c) and then assumes a fully biological terminology criticizing a large array of philosophical, medical, and naturalistic positions. One example is the position that the motion that proceeds from the understanding is akin to the nature of fire (most probably a Greek medical theory traceable as far as Heraclitus); or that the mind is compounded by the heat of the heart, the receptacle of the intelligent nature; that the cerebral membrane must be the site of the mind since it is the substance that gathers different other membranes in the sensorial nature, etc. His main argument, that the mind is equally in contact with all parts of the body, stands on the concept of organized mixture or combination described above (*oikeiosis, anakrasis, koinonia* – PG45, 177b) which is, he says, *indescribable* (Schaff et al. 1892, 57; PG45, 160d). The relation mind-body is not only complex or indescribable but also difficult to characterize as dualistic, deterministic, or instrumentalist, since Gregory concludes that *mind is not placed in one organ but resides in the entire body*, whichis a harmonious unity that receives and expresses reason, therefore judgement functions as harmony of all natural functions.

In conclusion, there is not a single organ responsible for the functioning of the mind but rather the mind is a harmonious functioning of all the organs together. This unity of the compound is not caused by an inner cause but by an external cause, God. The harmony of the beauty of the body comes from the resemblance with the Model, therefore the relation mind-body is the resemblance of the relation of the man with God. To that extent, breaking the relation with God naturally brings upon losing Beauty and Goodness but also losing the similitude or the *imago Dei* status. If mind acts in separation from God the body will lose its connection to the Model, and when body acts in separation from the mind, like in hedonism, it brings about the annihilation of the natural unity with the mind. Therefore, the created mind-body unitywill be lost because of actions either of the mind or of the body. The relation mind-body is both mimetic, since body is at its turn a mirror of the mind just as the mind is a mirror of the Model, and at the same time it is bidirectional (Schaff et al. 1892, 58; PG 45, 161a). It is not only the body but also the mindthat has two directions of acting. Just like thc musical instrument receives harmony from the player but also receives disturbance from outside, the mind is also able to transmit harmony and receive something from the body, therefore the body may corrupt the relation of the mind with God. In Gregory's optical terms,

> "the transmission of the ugliness of matter reaches through the nature to the mind itself, so that the image of God is no longer seen in the figure expressed by that which was moulded according to it; for the mind, setting the idea of good like a

mirror behind the back, turns off the incident rays of the effulgence of the good, and it receives into itself the impress of the shapelessness of matter" (Schaff et al. 1892, 58; PG 45, 164a).

Therefore, the mind is not a part nor a system of the body and there should be no identity of their movements; the multiple functions of the soul are in fact just as many contextual liaisons mind-body. The humans do not act as *bodies* driven by souls, neither do they act as *minds* that govern bodies: the peculiar situations of those *minded bodies* are rather to be described as multiplicity of particular relations mind-body. In other words, the entity that we are in all the particular situations of our lives is a reality defined as a mind-body fasciculate entity. Sometimes the entity focuses on the bodily realities like search for food and instincts, sometimes it is focused on the mind realities like cultural acts. Either way, our mind is bound to the material world in a dynamic way and vice versa.

"The mind is not restricted to any part of the body, but is equally in touch with the whole, producing its motion according to the nature of the part which is under its influence. There are cases, however, in which the mind even follows the bodily impulses, and becomes, as it were, their servant … ; while the mind, receiving such an impulse, furnishes the body by its own intelligence with the proper means towards the desired object" (Schaff et al. 1892, 62; PG 45, 173d).

This may be the main reason why the union of mind-body is unintelligible. We know that soul does not have a place, body is not contained nor contains the soul, and that the soulis operative, working, and alive; the intellect is to be regarded both in the body and around it,

"neither implanted in it nor enfolded with it, but in a way which we cannot speak or think, except so far as this, that while the nature prospers according to its own order, the mind is also operative; but if any misfortune befalls the former, the movement of the intellect halts correspondingly" (Schaff et al. 1892, 63; PG45, 177c).

9. The First Imago Dei

The most important part concerning the concept of *Imago Dei* is chapter XVI where Gregory interprets the idea of man as image of God in Platonic terms: man is themimesis of God, an image or painting made by God as a Self-Portrait. He criticizes the expression "man as microcosm" because human cannot be compared with the created Universe. Man is rather the middle between extremes, both horizontally and vertically. Humanity is not to be magnified by any comparison to the world and not to be minimized by reductionism to naturalist views: they "forget that they are dignifying man with the attributes of the gnat and the mouse: for they too are composed of these four elements" (Schaff et al. 1892, 64; PG45, 180a). No comparison with nature or created world is worth of man, since man as the *image of God* should be the only dignifying comparison.

According to this, humans are not to be considered mortal exactly because they are the image of the eternal creator not of perishable nature. Consequently, human soul is not perishable and not sexuated: the sexual determination belongs to our animal nature, so it appears in a secondary stage of the creation.

The first movement of the creation was the creation "in the image". Gregory splits the Biblical text and says: "then it makes a resumption of the account of creation, and says, 'male and female created He them.' I presume that every one knows that this is a departure from the Prototype" (Schaff et al. 1892, 64; PG 45, 180c). Man was first created neither male nor female, an image of God as a *Perfect form*(God as perfect Creator would not create an imperfect form), "for if the Deity is the fullness of good, and this is His image, then the image finds its resemblance to the Archetype in being filled with all good" (Schaff et al. 1892, 64; PG 45, 180c). According to the first creation, human being is without body but can still multiply in an angelical way, a mystery based on the testimony of the Gospel episode about the woman of many marriages, who had been wife to seven brethren (Luke 20:35–36) and remain to none of them after the Resurrection.

In this first stage of the creation man received "the principle of all excellence, all virtue and wisdom, and every higher thing that we conceive", but above all the absolute freedom and mastery over any bondage to natural powers, along with the power of decision, "for virtue is a voluntary thing" (Schaff et al. 1892, 64; PG 45, 180c). Thus, liberty was received as a primary virtue: to do what we like without limitations from the body. As we can see, Gregory introduces a principle of individuality or multiplication (*diairesis*) directly in the *Imago Dei* creation, saying that the design of God already contains all the multiplicity of individual human development.

Although the first image bears all the similitudes, still, there are differences between Creator and Creation. God is uncreated and man is created, so other incongruences emerge: while God is immutable, man cannot exist without change, its very passage from nonexistence to existence being a certain motion.

Since the notion of *imago Dei* refers to both aspects, first, the humanity as a general name for the common human nature, and second, to every potential individual with its particular limitations and peculiarities, due to the complete knowledge of God, it is reasonable that there are also further consequent differences included in the paradigm of man: the tendency of the motion of man's will, the distinction of male and female (an approximation to the less rational nature), and, on the cognitive level, the fact that man can only imagine the truth, as far as possible, by means of conjectures and similitudes, but does not set forth that which occurs to mind authoritatively but place it in the form of a theoretical speculation:

> "In the Divine foreknowledge and power all humanity is included in the first creation; for it is fitting for God not to regard any of the things made by Him as indeterminate, but that each existing thing should have some limit and measure prescribed by the wisdom of its Maker" (Schaff et al. 1892, 65; PG45, 184–185).

10. The Second Imago Dei

However strange this might appear, sexuality is the addition that God introduced into the nature of man in order to safeguard the race from extinction. This moment of returning and adding something new to the creation is regarded as an act of kindness. Since human nature is the "mean between the Divine and incorporeal nature, and the irrational life of brutes" (Schaff et al. 1892, 64; PG45, 183), and because God foresees the failure of human will to

> "keep a direct course to what is good, … and its consequent declension from the angelic life, in order that the multitude of human souls might not be cut short by its fall from that mode by which the angels were increased and multiplied, … he formed for our nature that contrivance for increase which befits those who had fallen into sin, implanting in mankind, instead of the angelic majesty of nature, that animal and irrational mode by which they now succeed one another" (Schaff et al. 1892, 66; PG45, 188c).

Thus, the second meaning of the *imago Dei* refers to the individual that is prescribed within the general essence, and it is called *the second creation.* It is not departed in time from the first because God's actions are timeless or before time. It is simultaneously with the first Creation when God foresees humans' weakness of will and at the same time decides to add sexuality. The *dual-stage creation* is only performed in case of humans because humanity is an *image of God*. In case of animals, for instance, as they are simple natures, the creation is directly and spontaneously bi-sexuated and *without the council of the Divine persons*. This perspective is advocated within an Origenist framework, as discussed by Zachhuber (2014), which draws upon the dual narratives of creation found in Genesis chapters 1 and 2. This approach interprets these narratives as symbolic of the duality in human constitution, namely soul and body. This combination of attributes is therefore the result of the Divine person's council which resulted in the decision to add a brutal attribute to human nature in order to be able to self-preserve after the fall.

Ianus Biphrons

Man has received, this way, two identities or rather two faces: one directed to God and another to the bestial nature. Each of the two dimensions can be attended to and become stronger. But then, how is it possible to have two identities of man, one paradigmatic and one natural, and still preserve the status of image of God? Gregory compares this dual nature with the *Ianus Biphrons* myth, referring to:

> "Those carved shapes ... tracing out upon a single head two forms of faces; so man seems to me to bear a double likeness to opposite things – being moulded in the Divine element of his mind to the Divine beauty, but bearing, in the passionate impulses that arise in him, a likeness to the brute nature" (Schaff et al. 1892, 67; PG45, 192b).

These two natures can convert each other, for the better or for the worse, and so human nature is a dual *imago Dei* not in the sense of having body and soulbut in the sense that it is at the same time spiritual (Angel-like) and bestial, includes two registers of the creation at the same time. To the extent that nature is itself an image of God (it can be known as creation *per se*; therefore, it offers a path to the knowledge of God as creator), to that very same extent humanity as nature bears the fingerprint of its Creator both as nature and as a rational being.

But these two opposed natures are the extremes of an interval that is proper for natural human action. The conversion of bestial nature into the angel-like, that is, of impulses into virtues, is the aim and complete responsibility of the free man. This is a strong confirmation for the fact that the initial depiction of the creation as composition of opposites (heaven and earth as diametrically opposed, "borderland of the opposition", horizontal participation) that underlie the nature as an interval or realm of motion and change is reiterated in human nature.

In conclusion, humanity is a special kind of creation: not a microcosm, as Gregory protests, not a simple imitation of Divinity. It is an image of God both as Creator, as he contributes to the continuity of Good in the nature by governing the body, and as nature, because he contains all the animal features which humans must assist, understand, and convert into divine, neither fully relying on it, nor completelyallying with it.

References

Aristotle. 1957. *Physics, Volume I*. Translated by Wicksteed, P. H. & F. M. Cornford. Loeb Classical Library. Cambridge, MA: HarvardUniversity Press.

Barnes, J. 1984. *The Complete Works of Aristotle. The Revised Oxford Translation*. Bollingen Series LXXI 2. Princeton: Princeton University Press.

Barnes, M. R. 2002. Divine Unity and The Divided Self: Gregory of Nyssa's Trinitarian Theology In Its Psychological Context. *Modern Theology*, 18(4): 475–496.

Barnes, M. R. 2020. The "Platonic" Character of Gregory of Nyssa's Psychology: The Old Canon. In: A.O. Andrei (ed.), *Jewish Roots of Eastern Christian Mysticism. Studies in Honor of Alexander Golitzin*. Leiden; Boston: Brill, pp. 337–357.

Bell, D. N. 1980. Soul and the Image of God in the Latin Tradition. *Recherches de théologieancienne et mediévale*, 47: 16–52.

Bishop, J. P. 2000. Mind-Body Unity: Gregory of Nyssa and a Surprising Fourth-Century CE Perspective. *Perspectives in Biology and Medicine*, 43: 519–529.

Cross, R. 2002. Gregory of Nyssa on Universals. *VigiliaeChristianae*, 56: 372–410.

Lampe, G.W.H. 1961. *A Patristic Greek Lexicon*. Oxford: Clarendon Press.

Mateo-Seco L.F. &G. Maspero (eds). 2010. *The Brill Dictionary of Gregory of Nyssa*. Leiden;Boston: Brill.

Migne J-P. 1863. *PatrologiaeGraecaecursus completus. [Series Graeca]: ... omnium ss. patrum, doctorum, scriptorum queecclasiasticorumsive Latinorumsive Grœcorum*. XLIV. Parisiis [Paris]

Plato. 2000. *The Republic*. Edited by G.R.F.Ferrari. Translated by T.Griffith. Cambridge: Cambridge University Press.

Plotinus. 1984. *Enneads in seven volumes*. With an English translation by A.H. Armstrong. Cambridge, MA: Harvard University Press.

Schaff, P. & H. Wace. 1892. *Nicene and Post-Nicene Fathers of The Christian Church* (V). New York: Christian Literature Publishing Co.

Walker, A. 2022. Apolausis. Feelings at the Juncture between Body and Mind. In: M. Mullett & H.S. Ashbrook (eds.), *Managing Emotion in Byzantium. Passions, Affects and Imaginings*. London & New York: Routledge.

Zachhuber, J. 2005. Once Again: Gregory of Nyssa on Universals. *Journal of Theological Studies*, 56(1): 75–98.

Zachhuber, J. 2014. *Human nature in Gregory of Nyssa. philosophical background and theological significance*. Boston: Brill.

Zedler, B. H. 1968. *On the Unity of the Intellect against the Averroists*. Milwaukee:Marquette University Press.

The desire to be like God: Addressing temptations coming along with AI

Wolfgang Palaver

1. Introduction

The following article shows in its first part how strongly religion plays a role in debates about technology. Enthusiasts as well as critiques of technology refer to religion in their reflections. The deeper root for this affinity is anthropological. Human beings are characterized by a deep desire that transcends their given existence. This explains our fascination as well as our fear of AI. Before looking into this anthropological challenge coming along with AI this article deals in its second part with dangers connected with weak AI like the threat that social media or certain uses of algorithms mean for democracy. The third part engages with strong AI by addressing the desire to create human robots as well as the human fascination to turn ourselves into machine-like automats. René Girard's mimetic theory helps us to understand that creating robots resembling humans will also create conflictive beings, a danger we most likely will avoid. More dangerous is our desire to become like automats that mimetic theory explains by referring to our longing for self-sufficient autonomy. To seek a godlike independence from all our relations with their mimetic dangers may end up in a complete technological enslavement and in the death of humanity as we know it. The last part addresses with Romano Guardini therefore ways to use technology without being enslaved by it emphasizing an asceticism that allows us to be masters of technology.

2. Technology and Religion

Let me start this section with a short look at my own involvement in the world of technology. Before becoming a theologian, I was trained in electronics and communicational engineering. This was one of the reasons that I accepted the invitation in 2003 to teach ethics for students in computer science at the University of Innsbruck. Since 2004 I teach this challenging course that is quite demanding because I must keep up with the technological developments that transform our world so radically. When I started to work on this course the most astonishing discovery for me was how much religion plays directly or indirectly an important role in philosophical or ethical reflections about technology. Not theologians make primarily such claims but philosophers of technology or leading thinkers in the field of media studies. Media theorist Marshall McLuhan expressed his hope for a more peaceful world by predicting a global Pentecost coming along with the electronic age: "Today computers hold out the promise of a means of instant translation of any code or language into any other code or language. The computer [...] promises by technology a Pentecostal condition of universal understanding and unity". (McLuhan 1994, 80)[1] VilémFlusser, a philosopher in communication studies hoped that the coming telematic society will allow the merging of the Platonic academy with the Jewish sabbath resulting in an "completely unorthodox religiosity" that will allow a "dialogue life" in the sense of Martin Buber and a life of "celebrating God" (Flusser 2002, 165–171): "Only when school and celebration meet, when Academy and Sabbath merge, when space and time negate each other, can one expect the Western tradition to be complete. This is the religious aspect of telematics". (Flusser 2002, 167)

Also, prophets of a coming age dominated by AI like the futurist Ray Kurzweil express the religious aspect of this technological future. His seminal book *The Singularity is Near* plays openly with John the Baptist's announcement in the Gospel of Matthews 3:2 that the "kingdom of heaven has come near" (Kurzweil 2005, cf. Harari 2017, 386). Challenging traditional religions in their task to deal with human mortality advocates of AI like Kurzweil aim to overcome ageing and even death (Noble 1999, 143–171, Harari 2017, 20–29). The historian Yuval Noah Harari ends his book *Homo Deus* with a chapter on the "data religion" describing attempts in our world of today to reduce all live to nothing but algorithms lead-

1 "The computer [...] holds out the promise of a technologically engendered state of universal understanding and unity, a state of absorption in the logos that could knit mankind into one family and create a perpetuity of collective harmony and peace". (McLuhan 1996, 253)

ing to "the creation of a new and even more efficient data-processing system, called the Internet-of-All-Things" that will let *Homo sapiens* vanish (Harari 2017, 386): "By equating the human experience with data patterns, Dataism undermines our primary source of authority and meaning and heralds a tremendous religious revolution, the like of which has not been seen since the eighteenth century". (Harari 2017, 395)

The religious dimension of technology is also addressed by the American computer scientist Jaron Lanier who from a humanist perspective criticizes thc spirituality that characterizes social media of today. According to Lanier, "social media hates your soul" (Lanier 2018, 131–146). In a conversation with the *New York Magazine*, he describes this spirituality as a bad religion: "It's a religion that's completely lacking in empathy or any kind of personal acknowledgment. And it's a bad religion. It's a nerdy, empty, sterile, ugly, useless religion that's based on false ideas. And I think that of all of the things, that's the worst thing about it". (Lanier and Kulwin 2018) Regarding programs like Google's claim to "solve death" he asks why the "religions of the world didn't serve Google with a copyright infringement take-down notice" (Lanier 2018, 139). Lanier calls the business model that currently governs most social media "BUMMER" meaning "Behaviors of Users Modified, and Made into an Empire for Rent" (Lanier 2018, 28) and calls it a dangerous new religion: "The BUMMER business is interwoven with a new religion that grants empathy to computer programs – calling them AI programs – as a way to avoid noticing that it is degrading the dignity, stature, and rights of real humans". (Lanier 2018, 144)

Such critical views of technology that turns itself into a new religion reminds us of religious traditions in which technologies were culturally embedded and religious authorities decided about the use of it. Neil Postman shows that "tool-using cultures" did not see technology as "autonomous" and subjected it to the "jurisdiction of some binding social or religious system" (Postman 1993, 24). Even military technology was controlled by "spiritual ideas and social customs" as, for example, the strong prohibition of the lethal crossbow by Pope Innocent II in the early twelfth century shows (Postman 1993, 23).

A fundamentalist approach may result in a broad rejection of technology. This, however, would result from a very one-sided view of the relation between religion and technology. Both religion and technology stem from the same human root. It is our necessity to transcend nature and ourselves that characterizes our religious nature and explains our technological activities as well. According to the Spanish philosopher José Ortega y Gasset, human beings are not natural beings like a stone or a plant. Close to Jean-Paul Sartre, he understands humans as beings that are an "aspiration to be this or that" (Ortega y Gasset 1962, 113). We need imagination and our life is metaphysically dramatic: "Man [and I think women, too – W.P.] is no thing, but a drama – his [her] life, a pure and universal happening which happens to each one of us and in which each one in his [her] turn is nothing but happening". (Ortega y Gasset 1962, 199–200) This drama of life forces us to become engineers. Technology, however, is according to Ortega y Gasset not the beginning of things. "There exists a first, pretechnical invention par excellence, the original desire" (Ortega y Gasset 1962, 119). With its affinity with Sartre's philosophy, we already come close to Girard's mimetic anthropology. Ortega y Gasset comes even closer to Girard when he remarks that "desiring is by no means easy" and often in need of "a middleman" for orientation (Ortega y Gasset 1962, 119–120). The Spanish philosopher concludes his reflections on desiring in a way that could be part of an introduction into mimetic theory: "Every wish for this or that particular thing is ultimately connected with the person a man wants to be. This person, therefore, is the fundamental wish and the source of all other wishes". (Ortega y Gasset 1962, 120)

Ortega y Gasset's insight into the close relationship between technology and humanity's transcending of nature can also be underlined by Philip Hefner, a contemporary Lutheran theologian who has reflected extensively on technology and its relation to religion. Like Ortega y Gasset, also Hefner underlines the importance of transcendence and imagination for both human nature and technology: "Transcendence is a fundamental element of both human nature and technology – transcendence in the sense of imagining and believing and cocreating what is not actual, and creating the meaning of what is imagined, as well". (Hefner 2003, 83–84)[2] With Augustine

[2] "I said that technology seems to be carried out as a strategy for denying our mortality and death. It is also a means for surpassing finitude and death, in that imagining what is not but might be is a form of transcendence within our mind and spirit. … When we consider how fundamental imagination is to technology and to human life, we also broaden our idea of technology. In his series of 'fantastic events' of which the atom bomb is but the first, Teilhard listed chemistry, genetics, and psychotherapy. He is not

we can understand our restlessness that results from being creatures as a primary cause of mimetic desire. This restlessness seeks union with God but also leads to technology: "Restlessness is as fundamental as meaning, because restlessness is the meaning. Our drive for self-transcendence is an expression of this restlessness. Technology is therefore also an expression of it. We encounter God, share in God, through that restlessness. In my tradition, we could say that technological restlessness is a means of grace". (Hefner 2003, 86)

3. Dangers Coming along with Weak AI

In several meetings Justus Piater, the AI expert at the University of Innsbruck, convinced me that we should not so much focus on utopian or dystopian fantasies that are usually connected with AI of the future but focus on the ethical challenges that are already present with technological systems of today. He follows the distinction between weak or narrow AI on the one hand and strong AI on the other. According to Piater, what is today discussed as strong AI is either impossible or in a rather remote future. Dangers and challenges, however, are already present in applications of weak AI. How are weak and strong AI distinguished from each other? Let's follow the definition given by UNESCO:

> "Weak AI or Artificial Narrow Intelligence [. . .] is the only form of AI that humanity has achieved so far – machines that are capable of performing certain precise tasks autonomously but without consciousness, within a framework defined by humans and following decisions taken by humans alone.

Strong AI [. . .] would be a machine that has consciousness and feelings, and is capable of providing solutions for any kind of problem – that is pure fiction, for now". (UNESCO 2018, 41)

What are possible dangers coming along with weak AI? We could have a full plenary on such dangers, but I will restrict myself to two books that address some of it. The first is Jaron Lanier's book *Ten Arguments for Deleting Your Social Media Accounts Right Now*. Some of you know that

the only one who has interpreted psychotherapy as a kind of technology. It certainly rests on the foundation of human imagination, in its conceptualisation what the self is, as well as in its ideas of what the self can become. We might even speak of religion as a technology". (Hefner 2003, 46)

I have not yet deleted my social media accounts. Nevertheless, the book is a very helpful guide that I use with my students to better understand the impact of social media. It refers also to some problems that are relevant for mimetic theory. I referred to this book already regarding its sound critique of the pseudo-religion that comes along with AI ("social media hates your soul"). Two arguments against social media are especially important in regard to mimetic anthropology: "Social media is making you into an asshole" and "Social media is making politics impossible" (Lanier 2018). Lanier shows how easily social media turns individuals into a pack that strengthens its unity by its enmity against another pack: "The only constant basis of friendship is shared antagonism toward other packs". We know this phenomenon as on offspring of the logic that drives the scapegoat mechanism. Bullying belongs to the pack mode. Lanier recommends leaving platforms that seduce us to become bullies. The business model of many social media needs attention and encourages indirectly those negative news and behaviors that increase attention. "The biggest assholes get the most attention […] and they often end up giving a platform its flavor". Asshole behavior and pack mode undermine our democracies: "Democratic elections are a genuine commingling of ideas, and have historically helped societies find paths forward despite controversy, but only so long as people are switched to Solitary. Democracy fails when the switch is set to Pack. Tribal voting, personality cults, and authoritarianism are the politics of the Pack setting". (Lanier 2018, 48) According to Lanier, "collective processes make the best sense when participants are acting as individuals".

This is definitely true as thinkers like Simone Weil and Hannah Arendt understood, too (Palaver 2014). The emphasis on the responsible individual is also at the center of mimetic theory if we just think of Girard's interpretation of Jesus's treatment of the adulterous woman in the New Testament or his rejection of Nietzsche's view of Christianity: "The Christian individual contradicts the crowd; he or she doesn't join the multitude in the scapegoat resolution of the mimetic crisis, and moreover denounces the very scapegoat mechanism as a murder through the declaration of the innocence of the victim". (Girard 2008, 239–240, cf. Palaver 2020, 58–61)

My second example is a book by the mathematician Cathy O'Neil that refers with its title *Weapons of Math Destruction* to dangers coming along with the careless application of algorithms. Like Lanier, she is also especially concerned with negative impacts on our democracies. She provides many examples how algorithms increase inequality and threaten democracy. Again, religious overtones are addressed when she refers to "mathematical models" that were "opaque [...] like gods" and could only be understood by mathematicians and computer scientists who act like "the highest priests in their domain" (O'Neil 2016, 3). Cathy O'Neil explicitly distances herself from the "evangelists" of Big Data (O'Neil 2016, 12). This is her summary of the impact of these weapons of math destruction: "Promising efficiency and fairness, they distort higher education, drive up debt, spur mass incarceration, pummel the poor at nearly every juncture, and undermine democracy". (O'Neil 2016, 199) According to O'Neil, "mathematical models shoul d be our tools, not our masters" (O'Neil 2016, 207). As we will see soon this is the challenge of today, a task that requires a lot of effort. Fairness, justice are desperately needed but cannot be provided by Big Data processes but rely on "moral imagination" that "only humans can provide" (O'Neil 2016, 204).

The dangers coming along with weak AI demand international regulations and regulations on the state level. They also require responsible data scientist. According to O'Neil, like doctors "data scientists should pledge a Hippocratic Oath, one that focuses on the possible misuses and misinterpretations of their models" (O'Neil 2016, 205). And finally, we should not overlook the users of these systems who also must act responsibly.

4. Becoming Like God: Anthropological Questions Following the Longing for Strong AI

Konrad Zuse, a German engineer who created the world's first programmable computer in 1941 addressed the anthropological challenge of strong AI in a remarkable way: "The danger of computers becoming like humans is not as great as the danger of humans becoming like computers". I concur with his statement and will illustrate every part of this quote with an enlightening example.

I address the first part of Zuse's quote with some episodes from Steven Spielberg's 2001 film *A.I. Artificial Intelligence*. David is a robot child that can experience love. By adding an emotion like love this robot comes closer to what we understand as human beings. We even can observe that suddenly imitation too, influences the relation between the robot child David and Martin, the real child of the couple that bought the robot when

Martin was in a coma and hospitalized. Paul Dumouchel may be right that Spielberg is not up to Girard's insight into mimetic relations nevertheless we can observe conflicts arising between the two boys that roughly stem from mimetic rivalries (Dumouchel 2015; cf. Hefner 2003, 28–33). An especially funny quarrel happens between the boys when they fight for the attention of Teddy, Martin's robotic teddy bear that is an emotionally less developed robot who often behaves therefore much wiser and more rational than David. The conflicts become so intense that the parents finally decide to abandon the robot child David in the woods. To some degree this film illustrates that to develop an almost human robot also means to create the possibility of conflicts. Watching both David and Teddy convince us that it would be better to stay with robots like Teddy not daring to come up with an artificial being that is conflictual like ourselves.

This conclusion matches with an observation called "uncanny valley" according to which a certain uneasiness arises among people as soon as a robot becomes too much like a real human being.[3] Paul Dumouchel and Luisa Damiano are right to connect this observation with the problematic sides of being human: "What we find most unsettling, then, are not the differences between robots and ourselves, but the idea that an artificial agent might begin to act just like a human being, with all that this entails in the way of uncertainty, unpredictability, and danger". (Dumouchel and Damiano 2017, 27) Thinking about mimetic rivalries one can agree with Dumouchel and Damiano that "we do not want robots to reproduce our failings" (Dumouchel and Damiano 2017, ix). From this perspective we understand better why Zuse did not see the main danger in robots becoming humans. We most certainly will avoid this kind of development.

But what about the other side, what about humans becoming robots? I will discuss this part of Zuse's quote by referring to Heinrich von Kleist's story "The Puppet Theatre" from 1810, an essay that became in the 20th

[3] "The uncanny valley is a concept first introduced in the 1970s by Masahiro Mori, then a professor at the Tokyo Institute of Technology. Mori coined the term 'uncanny valley' to describe his observation that as robots appear more humanlike, they become more appealing – but only up to a certain point. Upon reaching the uncanny valley, our affinity descends into a feeling of strangeness, a sense of unease, and a tendency to be scared or freaked out. So the uncanny valley can be defined as people's negative reaction to certain lifelike robots". (https://spectrum.ieee.org/automaton/robotics/humanoids/what-is-the-uncanny-valley)

century a “founding text of all cybernetics” (Rieger 2003, 375).[4] Kleist describes in it the dancing marionettes as more graceful than human dancers, at least with regard to the attractive force they exert on humans. Only the marionettes can emanate self-assurance and inner balance, which is normally reserved only for God, whom Kleist describes as the paradigm of tranquility. Throughout the text, one finds several references to the problems arising from mimetic desire. Grace, the essay’s central issue, is shown to be based on the impression evoked only in others. This is displayed in Kleist’s text through the story of the young man and the “Boy with Thorn” (Dornauszieher), which carries direct parallels to the Narcissus myth. In the story, two young men view the well-known ancient sculpture of the “Boy with Thorn” during a visit to Paris. One of the young men, whose physique bears a striking resemblance to that of the sculpture, points out this resemblance as he and his friend stand in front of a mirror. The young man’s envious friend, however, strongly rejects the resemblance, although, in secret, he shares the observation and admires his friend’s beauty. This rejection causes the graceful young man to doubt his beauty and casts him into ruminations of despair. The conclusion to Kleist’s essay touches on the interconnectedness of human consciousness, the tangible being of marionettes, and God:

> “We see that in the same measure as reflection in the organic world becomes darker and feebler, grace there emerges in ever greater radiance and supremacy. — But just as two lines intersecting at a point after they have passed through infinity will suddenly come together again on the other side, or the image in a concave mirror, after travelling away into infinity, suddenly comes close up to us again, so when consciousness has, as we might say, passed through an infinity, grace will return; so that grace will be most purely present in the human frame that has either no consciousness or an infinite amount of it, which is to say either in a marionette or in a god”. (Kleist 2004, 416)

Mimetic entanglements can lead to a longing for the mechanical world that delivers us from the dramatic struggles that defines human beings who are according to Ortega y Gasset neither natural beings nor things. René Girard described this longing in his first book as the consequence of human attempts to become gods that automatically causes rivalries with others

[4] The following paragraphs are partly taken from (Palaver 2013, 80–81). See also (Palaver 2011).

and results in seeking the tranquility of stones and minerals in a type of a mimetically fueled death-drive:

> "The Other is more fascinating the less accessible he is; and the more despiritualized he is, the more he tends toward an instinctive automatism, the more inaccessible he is. And the absurd project of self-divinization ends up by going beyond the animal to the automatic and even the mechanical. The individual becomes increasingly bewildered and unbalanced by a desire which nothing can satisfy and finally seeks the divine essence in that which radically denies his own existence: the inanimate. [. . .] That end is found in the mineral world, the world of a death which the absence of all movement, of all quivering, has made complete and definitive. The horrible fascination ends in the density of lead, the impenetrable immobility of granite. This is the inevitable termination of that ever more effective negation of life and of spirit, deviated transcendency. The affirmation of the self ends in the negation of self. The will to make oneself God is a will to self-destruction which is gradually realized". (Girard 1966, 286–287)

This danger comes also along with technological attempts to overcome all our anxieties, all our fragilities and all our mimetic dependences and rivalries (Dumouchel 2021). In the modern world we are increasingly obsessed with order and security and do not mind if that means turning human beings into mechanical automata. An early example for this can be found in Jeremy Bentham's *Panopticon Writings*. He applied his idea of a panopticon not only to improve surveillance in prisons but also for institutions like schools. He explicitly recommended to make pupils machine-like to maintain peace. Bentham questioned himself about the outcome of applying the logic of the panopticon to schools: "Whether the liberal spirit and energy of a free citizen would not be exchanged for the mechanical discipline of a soldier, or the austerity of a monk? – and whether the result of this high-wrought contrivance might not be constructing a set of *machines* under the similitude of *men*?" (Bentham 1995, 89) Bentham's answer is clear. He prefers mechanical pupils over conflicts and wars: "Call them soldiers, call them monks, call them machines: so they were but happy ones, I should not care. Wars and storms are best to read of, but peace and calms are better to enjoy".(Bentham 1995, 89)

Today, AI has dramatically increased the possibilities of a universal electronic panopticon. We accept more and more types of surveillance to achieve security. The political philosopher John Gray describes the paradoxical logic of human freedom that accepts self-imprisonment in the following way: "Enclosing the entire population in a virtual Panopticon might seem the ultimate invasion of freedom. But universal confinement need not be experienced as a privation. If thcy know nothing else, most are likely to accept it as normal. If the technology through which surveillance operates also provides continuous entertainment, they may soon find any other way of living intolerable". (Gray 2015, 125, cf. Zuboff 2019)

The danger that we are facing today is what Michel Serres called "death from order", a danger that is not obvious enough for us moderns to avoid it (Serres 1982, 127). The deeper reason for this is, according to John Gray, that Gnosticism has become the dominant religion of today. Kleist's essay is an early example of this tendency. The ending of Kleist's essay refers to the story of the Fall. The frame story of the essay is a dialogue between the narrator and Herr C., the first dancer at the Opera who regularly watches the puppets. The essay concludes with the following exchange between the narrator and Herr C.: "'But,' I said rather distractedly, 'should we have to eat again of the Tree of Knowledge to fall back into the state of innocence?' 'Indeed,' he replied; 'that is the final chapter in the history of the world.'" (Kleist 2004, 416) According to Gray, Herr C. points toward the "religion of Gnosticism" (Gray 2015, 8):

> "In a traditional reading eating the apple was the original sin; but, as Gnostics understood the story, the two primordial humans were right to eat the apple. The God that commanded them not to do so was not the true God but only a demiurge, a tyrannical underling exulting in its power, while the serpent came to free them from slavery. True, when they ate the apple Adam and Eve fell from grace. This was indeed the Fall of Man – a fall into the dim world of everyday consciousness. But the Fall need not be final. Having eaten its fill from the Tree of Knowledge, humankind can then rise into a state of conscious innocence. When this happens, Herr C. declares, it will be 'the final chapter in the history of the world'."

The Gnosticism that we find in Kleist's essay is the forerunner of a spirit that has become much more dominant today, a spirit that characterizes especially current science and technology. Gray mentions Ray Kurzweil as one of the outstanding examples (Gray 2015, 15). Gray connects Kleist's essay with developments in contemporary science: "In the most ambitious versions of scientific materialism, human beings *are* marionettes: puppets on genetic strings, which by an accident of evolution have become self-aware. Unknown to those who most ardently profess it, the boldest secular thinkers are possessed by a version of mystical religion. At present, Gnosticism is the faith of people who believe themselves to be machines". (Gray 2015, 9–10)

Mark O'Connell similarly refers to Kleist's essay where he exposes the pseudo-religiosity if transhumanism: "Transhumanism is interesting less as a set of predictions about our possible technological future than as a religious idea. What transhumanists are after is fundamentally a form of redemption, not through God but through technology. To regain our prelapsarian state of grace, we must become machines". (O'Connell 2023, 42)

We are back to the question about the relation between technology and religion. Whereas the current version of Gnosticism aims at order and security that might result in the demise of humanity. Traditional religion was aware that absolute security is not possible in our world. Medieval Christianity identified the longing for absolute security with the antichrist. Augustine shows in his exposition of Psalm 100 that complete security is not achievable in this world: "Where then is security? Here nowhere; in this life nowhere, except solely in the hope of the promise of God. But there, when we shall reach thereunto, is complete security, when the gates are shut, and the bars of the gates of Jerusalem made fast".[5]

5. How to Use Technology Without becoming Enslaved by It

Technology has been a tool to free ourselves from natural dependences to realize our true being. The anxieties that go along with our dramatic being, however, also causes the temptation to seek in technology the overcoming of all our frailties. We envy machines because they seem to be above our inadequacies, as Paul Dumouchel rightly observes: "Machines escape, to a large extent, the contingency that characterizes human life, or at least that is what we like to believe". (Dumouchel 2021, 102) To seek invulnerability, security, immortality, and a godlike independence from all our relations with their mimetic dangers may end up in a complete technological enslavement and in the death of humanity as we know it.

To avoid this danger, humans must become masters over technology, have to regain power over the power of technology.[6] This, however, can-

5 https://www.newadvent.org/fathers/1801100.htm

6 "Power over the power is required now before the halt is called by catastrophe itself-the power to overcome that impotence over against the self-feeding compulsion of power to its progressive exercise. After the first-degree power, directed at a seemingly inexhaustible nature, has changed into a second-degree power which wrested control of the first from the user's hands, it is now up to a third-degree power to enforce the

not be achieved by desiring to become gods but only by abandoning this desire and by humbly accepting our creatureliness, our insecurity, mortality and fundamental relatedness to others. The German philosopher and theologian Romano Guardini to whom Pope Francis refers in his encyclical *Laudatosi'* to understand the challenges of the "techno-economic paradigm" that we face today reflected again and again on opportunities and dangers related to technology (Francis 2015, # 203, cf. Sedmak 2017, 947–949). In his early *Letters from Lake Como*, he underlined the need that humanity becomes the master of technology: "In appropriate activity we now have to penetrate the new thing so as to gain mastery over it. We have to become lords of the unleashed forces and shape them into a new order that relates to humanity. In the last resort only living people and not the tackling of technological problems themselves can do this". (Guardini 1994) This, however, does not mean less technology but more of it if it is at the same time a more human technology: "What we need is not less technology but more. Or, more accurately, we need stronger, more considered, more human technology". (Guardini 1994) In his later book *The End of the Modern World*, Guardini describes three virtues that are necessary to allow humans to gain power over their technology. He mentions an earnest will to know what is at stake, a courage that exceeds even the courage necessary to face nuclear bombs or bacteriological warfare and finally asceticism. The third virtue is especially interesting because it seems that asceticism is just the opposite of what one thinks one needs to gain power over power. Guardini, however, understands very well that it is humility that allows us to become masters of technology:

> "Man must learn again to become a true master by conquering and by humbling himself. In no other way will he achieve the lordship of his own Power. Only the freedom won through self-mastery can address itself with earnestness and gravity to those decisions which will affect all reality. [...] These deep virtues could breed a spiritual art of government through which man could exercise power over power, through which he could distinguish right from wrong and ends from means. That government would truly measure human dignity and make room even under the strain

---

self-limitation of the rule that carries along the ruler, before it shatters on the barriers of nature. This third degree means power over the second-degree power, which was no longer man's but power's itself to dictate its use to its supposed owner and to make of him the compulsive executor of his capacity, thus enslaving man instead of liberating him". (Jonas 1984, 141–142)

> of labor and battle for man himself to live in dignity and joy. Such a government would be an art, would indeed be *power*". (Guardini 1998, 93–94)

We can understand Guardini's emphasis on ascetism as the rejection of the desire to become God and the humble acceptance to be God's creature that can trust in God's grace. This trust allows us to use technology as a tool and not to become enslaved by our own means.

With Guardini I showed how the Christian tradition can help us to use technology without becoming enslaved by it. I do not claim, however, that only Christianity can help us in this regard. In recent months I was studying the life and work of Mahatma Gandhi who was quite critical about machinery and technology (Gandhi 1997, 107–111). He, however, was not rejecting technology in general. His concern was the danger to become enslaved by machinery: "I am not against machinery as such, but I am totally opposed to it when it masters us" (Gandhi 1997, 166). We can learn from Gandhi – and in this he is close to Guardini – that all mastery requires "self-rule". Controlling our desires will help us to avoid being "attracted by the machine craze" and will allow us to "appropriate what is valuable in modern technologies" (Allen 2019, 130). The more we move forward using artificial intelligence the more we will need this type of self-rule.

References

Allen, D. 2019. *Gandhi after 9/11: Creative Nonviolence and Sustainability*. New Delhi, India: Oxford University Press.

Bentham, J. 1995. *The Panopticon Writings*. London: Verso.

Dumouchel, P. 2015. Mirrors of Nature: Artificial Agents in Real Life and Virtual Worlds. In: S. Cowdell, C. Fleming and J. Hodge (eds.), *Mimesis, Movies, and Media*. New York: Bloomsbury Academic, pp. 51–60.

Dumouchel, P. 2021. Desiring Machines: Machines That Are Desired and Machines That Desire. *Contagion: Journal of Violence, Mimesis, and Culture*, 28(1): 99–110.

Dumouchel, P., and L. Damiano. 2017. *Living With Robots*. Translated by M. B. De Bevoise. Cambridge, Massachusetts: Harvard University Press.

Flusser, V. 2002. *Writings*. Translated by Erik Eisel, *Electronic mediations*. Minneapolis: University of Minnesota Press.

Francis. 2015. Laudato Si': Encyclical Letter of the Holy Father on Care for Our Common Home. Rome: Libreria Editrice Vaticana. https://www.vatican.va/content/francesco/en/encyclicals/documents/papa-francesco_20150524_enciclica-laudato-si.html

Gandhi, M. K. 1997. *Hind Swaraj and other writings*. Cambridge: Cambridge University Press. Original edition, 1909.

Girard, R. 1966. *Deceit, Desire and the Novel: Self and Other in Literary Structure*. Translated by Yvonne Freccero. Baltimore: Johns Hopkins University Press [Original edition, 1961].

Girard, R. 2008. *Evolution and Conversion: Dialogues on the Origin of Culture. With Pierpaolo Antonello and João Cezar de Castro Rocha*. London: Continuum.

Gray, J. 2015. *The Soul of the Marionette: A Short Inquiry Into Human Freedom*. New York: Farrar, Straus, and Giroux.

Guardini, R. 1994. *Letters from Lake Como: Explorations in Technology and the Human Race*. Translated by Geoffrey William Bromiley, *Ressourcement*. Grand Rapids, Mich.: W.B. Eerdmans.

Guardini, R. 1998. *The End of the Modern World*. Wilmington, Del.: ISI Books.

Harari, Y. N. 2017. *Homo Deus: A Brief History of Tomorrow*. New York, NY: Harper.

Hefner, P. 2003. *Technology and Human Becoming*. Minneapolis: Fortress Press.

Jonas, H. 1984. *The Imperative of Responsibility: In Search of an Ethics for the Technological Age*. Translated by Hans Jonas and David Herr. Chicago: University of Chicago Press.

Kleist, H. v. 2004. *Selected Writings*. Translated by David Constantine. Indianapolis: Hackett Publishing.

Kurzweil, R. 2005. *The Singularity is Near: When Humans Transcend Biology*. New York: Viking.

Lanier, J. 2018. *Ten Arguments for Deleting Your Social Media Accounts Right Now*. New York: Henry Holt and Company.

Lanier, J., and N. Kulwin. 2018. 'One Has This Feeling of Having Contributed to Something That's Gone Very Wrong': A conversation with VR pioneer Jaron Lanier on Silicon Valley's politics, being quoted by Mark Zuckerberg, and what went wrong with the internet. *New York Magazine*, 16.4.

McLuhan, M. 1994. *Understanding Media: The Extensions of Man*. Cambridge: The MIT Press. Original edition, 1964.

McLuhan, M. 1996. *Essential McLuhan*. New York: Basic Books. Original edition, 1995.

Noble, D. F. 1999. *The Religion of Technology: The Divinity of Man and the Spirit of Invention*. Harmondsworth: Penguin Books. Original edition, 1997.

O'Connell, M. 2023. Hastening the End. *The New York Review of Books*, 70(7): 40–43.

O'Neil, C. 2016. *Weapons of Math Destruction: How Big Data Increases Inequality and Threatens Democracy*. New York: Crown.

Ortega y Gasset, J. 1962. *History as a System and other Essays toward a Philosophy of History*. New York: W. W. Norton & Company [Original edition, 1941].

Palaver, W. 2011. Gott oder mechanischer Gliedermann? Die religiöse Problematik in Kleists Essay *Über das Marionettentheater*. In: G. Crepaldi, A. Kriwak and T. Pröll (eds.), *Kleist zur Gewalt. TransdisziplinärePerspektiven*. Innsbruck: Innsbruck University Press, pp. 45–62.

Palaver, W. 2013. *René Girard's Mimetic Theory*. Translated by Gabriel Borrud, *Studies in Violence, Mimesis, and Culture*. East Lansing: Michigan State University Press.

Palaver, W. 2014. *Vox populi, vox Dei*: The Pantheistic Temptation of Democracy. In: V. N. Redekop and T. Ryba (eds.), *René Girard and Creative Mimesis*. Lanham, Md.: Lexington Books, pp. 143–159.

Palaver, W. 2020. Transforming the Sacred into Saintliness: Reflecting on Violence and Religion with René Girard. Cambridge: Cambridge University Press.

Postman, N. 1993. *Technopoly: The Surrender of Culture to Technology*. New York: Vintage Books [Original edition, 1992].

Rieger, S. 2003. *Kybernetische Anthropologie. Eine Geschichte der Virtualität*. Frankfurt am Main: Suhrkamp.

Sedmak, C. 2017. Traditional Concerns, New Language? Reflections on *Laudato Si*. *The Heythrop Journal*, 58(6): 942–952.

Serres, M. 1982. *The Parasite*. Translated by Lawrence R. Schehr. Baltimore: Johns Hopkins University Press [Original edition, 1980].

UNESCO. 2018. A Lexicon for Artificial Intelligence. *The UNESCO Courier* (3): 40–41.

Zuboff, S. 2019. *The Age of Surveillance Capitalism: The Fight for a Human Future at the New Frontier of Power*. New York: Public Affairs.

Humanity as Imago Dei in the Theology of Dietrich Bonhoeffer

Noemi Bravená

1. Introduction

Humanity constantly poses questions, as we still ask ourselves: Who is a human being? What are his/her limits? How can we overcome them? If the next stage of human development is found in its connection with technology, then this idea presupposes that every improvement is good for humans. Christian anthropology is also concerned with what is good and perfect for man. In this paper, therefore, we will reflect on the contribution of the theology of the German Lutheran theologian Dietrich Bonhoeffer, who in many ways was ahead of his time in his ideas.[1]

2. Perfection always refers to free choice in human action

Humanity was created by God as His image (*imago Dei*), which is perfect. What does this mean? Bonhoeffer speaks of the fact that the creative work from nothing (*creation ex nihilo*) can also be defined as creation from God's freedom (*creatio ex libertatis Dei*). Bonhoeffer says that "God created man in his own image on earth, that is, in his freedom a person is like his Creator" (DBW 3, 58). The author is not speaking of a physical form, but of the inner likeness of man and the Creator. In the theology of Bonhoeffer, the *imago Dei* is identical to the *imago libertatis*. The likeness between man and God does not imply conformity, because man is not and never will be God. According to Bonhoeffer, this similitude of the Creator to the creature is not even the analogy of being (*in analogia entis*) but is

[1] This paper was created as part of the Cooperatio research project named "THEO: Theology and Religious Studies" of the Charles University in Prague.

a person's ability to relate to the other, that is the analogy of relation (*in analogia relationis*) (DBW 3, 60). Therefore, a person's freedom is always intertwined with the freedom of God, the one who made freedom possible for mankind. This means that man must answer to his Creator for his actions.

The first humans were free. Bonhoeffer defines this in two relational terms. The first is the German concept of "*Freisen für*" ("being free for the other") (DBW 3, 58–59).[2] The content of this concept is that Adam is distinguished from all other creatures by his relationship to another human being. Moreover, Adam acts voluntarily and freely in relation to Eve. At the same time, however, he is dependent on her as his other fellow-human; he needs Eve for his life. The German theologian Sölle drew attention to this idea in her reflection on Bonhoeffer's work (DBW 3, 59–60; Sölle 2006, 81).

The second bond of the free relationship between the first humans is defined by Bonhoeffer as "being free from something" (*Freisein von*), which Bonhoeffer derives from the creational order (Genesis 1: 26–28) in which humans are to have a responsible relationship with God's creation –they may have dominion over it, although of course they are not to abuse it (DBW 3, 60: The self "is not accountable without others", because the self can be characterized as "together-with-others-being-in-the-world". (See also: Michálek 1996, 35).

How do these ideas relate to the idea of transhumanism? Human perfection is always linked to the free choice to act for and against another. In a relationship, we cannot read anyone's mind (yet), so we do not know what the other person's intentions are towards us. To be perfect, according to Christian anthropology, means to be free, that is, not to become anyone's puppet or slave on the one hand, but on the other hand not to cause suffering to other people (nor to take advantage of them). Christian anthropology has a supreme principle – God, to whom one is always accountable for one's own actions. Nonetheless, because pluralism is the prevailing perspective, there is no one principle in the modern world. It is imperative to ask: Who or what will ensure that technology is applied for the good of humanity? Do we know how to stop abuse or misuse in all its forms? Given that we now know that technology is being exploited, how will the freedom of the

---

2 In Bonhoeffer's words, man is "to be-free-for-another" (*frei-sein-für-den-anderen*).

cyborg be defined? The freedom of man, the obligation of the creator of a given technology, the obligation of the user or owner of the technology, and the equipment for safe, purposeful, and environmentally friendly use are all necessary factors to consider if we wish to enhance humanity.

3. Our world is ambiguous and therefore our actions are ambiguous

Every human being, regardless of the particular worldview embraced, perceives that the world contains what seems to us to be good and evil. The problem is that, according to Bonhoeffer, all of reality is as if split, and this makes it difficult for people to orient themselves within the world. Man was created as *imago Dei*, (the image of God), yet man through his free choice has distorted his relationship to his Creator (*corcurvum in se*) (DBW 2, 39).[3]

The story of Adam and Eve in Eden does not merely describe a one-time failure by man, but is, according to Bonhoeffer, the destruction of the original bond between Creator and creation: it affects humans and through humans consequently the whole creation (the world). Everything inside and outside of a person is subject to "inner conflict" (*Zwiespalt*) (DBW 3, 82–86, 105, 127, 130) or "division" (*Entzweiung*) (DBW 3, 82, 84, 95, 115–117, 119, 124–126, 749); see Bonhoeffer 2007, 21, 24, 29, 47, 397),[4] and thus everything in the world becomes as if blurred and unrecognizable to a person. Bonhoeffer says, "It is more than an inner feeling, it not only concerns morality, but it is a complete loss of a person's inner unity with God, with other human beings, and with creation". (Bravená 2010, 72). A person lives in a world that has lost its inner balance, and we see this in people and in global issues. Man is possessive and egoistic, and this determines the nature of all his relationships. This is true even in the case

---

[3] This is the first appearance of this term in Bonhoeffer (cf. pp. 52, 74, 83, 136). Also, in many other places in Bonhoeffer's habilitation it appears that the concept of Adam's sin as *cor curvum in se* is a very significant anthropological category that characterizes man in his natural state, namely without faith and without the acceptance of Christ.

[4] In this concept, Bonhoeffer follows Hans Schmidt and his reflection on the Hebrew words *lustvoll* (Hebrew *tob*) and *leidvoll* (Hebrew *ra*), which we inaccurately translate as good and evil. The influence of Hegel and his idea of the inseparable connection of the two concepts of good and evil as well as their mutual determination on the basis of opposition is also evident in the background. Vik translates the German term *die Entzweiung* with the Czech word *roztržka* ("rupture" or "breach").

of individual, altruistic acts or good deeds for others – even these actions are burdened by the loss of unity with God and with oneself.

Adam and Eve ate the fruit of the tree which the Bible calls "the tree of the knowledge of good and evil" (Genesis 2, 8). According to Bonhoeffer, what has happened is that the concepts of good and evil have lost their unambiguous definition. Bonhoeffer defines this as meaning that the concepts of good and evil (Hebrew *tov* and *ra*) carry a certain opposite in them. Good is not only THAT which is good, but also that which gives pleasure to a particular person (what pleases him and what he himself considers good). Evil is not only THAT which is evil, but also that which causes suffering to a particular person (DBW 3, 115). "Tob and ra are terms for the deepest ambivalence (*Entzweiung*) in every aspect of human life. Their essence lies in the fact that they stand together and in their contradictory nature also belong inseparably together". (DBW 3, 82). And here we see a fundamental problem: that anyone in the world can define that which is good and pleasure-producing (i.e., what pleases a person, is pleasant to him) in different even contradictory ways. Moreover, THAT which is good can be very evil for another person.

Bostrom (2005, 21) writes: "Transhumanists think that if we are generally open and accept new technologies, we have a better chance of turning them to our advantage than if we try to ban them". This statement contains a serious weak point. In a divided world, one person's benefit is always linked to someone else's disadvantage. This cannot be entirely prevented, but it is necessary to converse about its implications. Therefore, every technology should have a defined benefit as well as a defined dis-benefit (e.g., for different target groups). It is also desirable to anticipate situations in which there is a risk of the misuse or abuse of technology.

We know from the fall of man into sin that prohibitions have in them the potential for human error. In my view, the controversy with the author Bostrom is not about the acceptance of technology per se, but about accepting responsibility for the use of technology. Some guidance in this realm of meaning can be found in what is called situation ethics (Fletcher, Bonhoeffer), which points out that there is no one general solution, but that specific situations call for specific solutions. This can be understood to mean that the same-looking situation can bring about different types of good and evil. In this sense, the question of what situational ethics is in relation to specific technologies and their use must also be opened and discussed.

4. Humans and enhanced capabilities

In the perfect pre-fall state, man lacked nothing, yet he disobeyed his Creator's command not to eat the fruit of one specific tree in the Garden of Eden. The question logically arises as to why Adam did this when God said that if he ate of its fruit, he would die (Genesis 3, 3). Man, as the image of God, was free and had a choice because freedom is related to the choice of a particular action according to personal preference.

The text of Genesis does not answer what Adam thought before he tasted the fruit, but states that something happened that permanently disrupted the relationship between the Creator and his creation. Despite the mythological nature of the narrative, we are intrigued by the serpent's speech, which tempts man to believe that "in the day you eat of the tree your eyes will be opened, and you will know good and evil as God" (Genesis 3, 5). The serpent in his promise "*sicut Deus*" (you will be like God) is essentially promising man superpowers (God's very own attributes) (DBW 3, 104). The problem is that man has attained them through disobedience to God, and thus these abilities are undermined. Man apparently did not know what it meant to be equal to God, but what he could have known, according to Bonhoeffer, is that he had an authority over him that limited his possibilities (DBW 3, 79).

The fact that the first humans ate the fruit of the forbidden tree opened a separation in the relationship between man and God. According to Bonhoeffer, the narrative of the sin of the first humans includes the content of the text concerning Cain and Abel. Their story, according to Bonhoeffer, points to the deepest chasm in the relationship between man and God, because the Creator's supreme right is to decide man's being and non-being. In killing his brother Abel, Cain usurped these rights because he decided upon the death of someone to whom he had not given life (Genesis 4, 7–8). This is the new aspect in Cain, the son of Adam, that he himself as *sicut Deus* infringed upon the life of a man (DBW 3, 110).

Based on the narrative of Genesis, man's higher capacities are always connected to man's disunity and his desire to be like God (i.e., to exercise power over the world and over other human beings). Technology is supposed to lead a person toward a more perfect being, that is, also to attain higher abilities. In the Bible, however, perfection apart from the grace of God is always linked to the desire for *sicut Deus*, for God's attributes. We see this also in history, where rulers were often identified with God or had divine attributes.

5. Immortality as a potential possibility

The antediluvian state was related to the immortality of man. Symbolically, man was guaranteed immortality by the fruit of the tree of life. After violating the prohibition, man was denied access to immortality by the Lord. God banished man from paradise (the place of absolute nearness to God) and from the tree of life. Interestingly enough, it was not enough to exile Adam and Eve, God also placed guards by the tree and put a weapon in their hands to protect the tree: "… .and at the east of the garden of Eden he placed the cherubim and a flaming sword that turned every way to guard the way to the tree of life" (Genesis 3, 24). The question is, why didn't God destroy the tree?

The tree of life is part of the biblical text in several places, and it is one of the attributes of the kingdom of God (Revelation 22, 1–3), accompanying the life story of man from his beginning to his eternity. The immortality symbolized in the tree of life still exists as a potential possibility, but it is strictly guarded by certain insurmountable boundaries: angels (Exodus 25, 20), biological death, and the judgment of man (Revelation 7, 2; 8, 3–12; 14, 9; etc.). And this boundary is not directed against man, but against his imperfection before God and his desire to seize the tree for his own benefit. If man were perfect before God, he would have access to immortality, but that is not the perfection that is being sought in connection with technology.

6. Mankind as a new creation

Christian theology speaks primarily of a person's inner change-from a pre-fall state to a post-fall state, that is, from a perfect to an imperfect person. But furthermore, Christian theology recognizes the change from an imperfect to a perfect person. While the first change involved all men, the second change involves only those who come to faith in Jesus Christ as the Son of God and become what is called a new creation (Bravená 2010, 75–78). In non-religious terms, this means that these men have acknowledged a higher principle (God) above them who is perfect, righteous, undivided, and ever-existent (there has never been a time when He has not existed).

Christian anthropology sees the only way out in the post-Fall world, which is affected by the unequal relationship between man and God and between man and the world. Man must become a new creature, undergoing a change that affects his soul, but essentially also his mortal body. The new man is a man pardoned before God, a man who has renounced his egocentrism and has submitted his life to God through Jesus Christ. This means that only the one who has believed that Jesus Christ is the Son of God experiences spiritual union with him (Paul's incarnation into Christ – "*enchristoeinai*") (Souček 1976, 95, 193). And together with him, even as Christ rose from the dead, after his biological death he will rise with a new spiritual body (*soma pneumatikon*) and live with God in the kingdom of God (Souček 1976, 68).

With regard to our topic, this means that partial perfection in Christ will be replaced by complete perfection and immortality after biological death. But there must be a fundamental change that cannot be accomplished by man alone.

According to the Bible, being a new creation has two meanings: one refers to man in his biological body and the other to man after biological death. Man can be a new creation, namely, belonging to Christ already in his biological body. It does not mean perfection of the body, but perfect union with God. The perfect body refers to the spiritual body after a person's death.

7. Conclusion

Christian anthropology acknowledges the perfection of man, which is always connected with the freedom to act according to one's own will. Bonhoeffer pointed out that man's perfection was and is tied to God, who is not only the Creator, but the one who enables a person's better abilities and decides when a person will or will not have access to immortality. Reflecting on the story of Genesis, Bonhoeffer concludes that the whole world, including every human being, is divided and therefore reality is blurred for humans, which manifests itself in the fact that everyone considers something else to be THE good. This also results in a contradiction of views on the topics that surround man. A human being, as the image of God, was created in and for freedom and this means that true freedom manifests itself in a non-egocentric way towards the other. In the fallen state, man is divided, and his main characteristic is a division that can only be overcome in union with God through faith in Jesus Christ.

Christian anthropology's questions on transhumanism are as follows:

- What constitutes human perfection, and what are its possibilities and limits? Does the internally and physically perfect cyborg differ? Experience suggests that these two phenomena often conflict. It is also documented that physical imperfection and suffering can facilitate one's own transcendence (Fromm, Frankl, etc.), and thus, relate to the meaning of life. Might living in a perfect body entail greater suffering? How is biological perfection connected to the experiences of happiness and a meaningful life?
- Having superpowers goes hand in hand with one's responsibility for them. Where are the limits of superpowers and how do they relate to human responsibility?
- How can we ensure individual benefit, but at the same time prevent the misuse of new technologies, especially to control the human mind? Will there be higher and lower order cyborgs, namely can inequalities be predicted already and how will they be addressed?
- If immortality is deemed something to which one is "not entitled" according to Christian anthropology, yet is a component of objective reality (i.e., contingent upon another's decision), this presents a profound Christian thesis that probes why entitlement is denied. This leads to the following question: What consequences might humanity encounter when interfacing with technology?

The desire for power and control of the other, self-interest, the reshaping of one's own truth, the blurring of the boundary between reality in a fictional world (virtual) are all already happening today. Individual self-interest dominates and there is no one system to which one is accountable for one's actions. Religion is the business of those who believe, and there is no general righteous overseer of the good. Who gets to decide on setting boundaries for technology and its use? It is not just a question of rights and responsibilities; it is also a question of what is ethically acceptable and unacceptable. Who will be responsible for the technology implemented – the person who could/could not have influenced the mind or the manufacturer who should have programmed it better?

Christianity warns very strongly against the self-centeredness of man who desires his own benefit and the qualities that would secure him advantages at the expense of other people. The slave in the parable of Plato's cave had the opportunity to leave the shadow realm and know the truth in contact with the sun (Agathon) (Michálek 1996, 66–67). There is a recurring theme in science fiction films suggesting that behind everything lies a concrete, knowable truth that will ultimately prevail. The temptation to manipulate truth for personal gain, to enslave others, and to ensure only the survival of the selected few is profound, and technology facilitates these actions on a broader and more rapid scale.

The only way to resist the misuse of technology is where there is a true understanding of how things work, where there are opportunities for both benefit and misuse. It is therefore necessary to find, ask and seek answers to these questions. Progress cannot be stopped, and technology has served man for many years, and it has also served for good. Nuclear technology has brought man many necessary benefits, but it has also served as a weapon. And it is here that the fragility of existence is revealed. There are situations where we as humans are looking at a potential catastrophe and do not know how to stop it. For example, how do we take nuclear weapons away from those who do not know how to handle them responsibly and thus endanger all of humanity?

The task of the scientific debate is not to be clueless, but to try to define concepts precisely and to anticipate facts. One should be as prepared as possible for the situations that may arise. This is related to the responsibility of which the philosopher Hans Jonas speaks. It is a responsibility for the future that also estimates potential consequences and thinks them through before they occur (Jonas 1997, 143–144). The Apostle Paul said that everything is permissible for man, but that not everything benefits him. Bonhoeffer also wrote of a way of acting that is appropriate to the facts (*Wirhklichkeitgemaesses Handeln*), but which is also responsible for all of humanity (Bravená 2009, 26–28). Human beings possess vast potential for development; however, hand in hand with this potential, they must recognize their capabilities, limitations, and the consequences of disproportionate manipulation of technology and humanity as the image of God. Technology is necessary, but it is not an all-encompassing solution. "It is not technology that endangers man, but man endangers himself with technology where he chooses it as the only means of supporting and benefiting man" (Michálek 1996, 15).

References

Bravená, N. 2010. *Ježíš Kristus, bratr a bližní jednají na mém místě*. Brno: L. Marek.

Bravená, N. 2009. Bonhoefferova Etika a jednání pro druhého. *Evanjelikálny teologický časopis*, 5(1): 24–35.

Bonhoeffer, D. 1998. *Akt und Sein*. In: H.-R. Reuter(ed.). *Dietrich Bonhoeffer Werke 2* (DBW 2). München: Chr. Kaiser Verlag.

Bonhoeffer, D. 1989. *Schöpfung und Fall*. In: M. Rüter and I. Tödt(eds.). *Dietrich Bonhoeffer Werke 3* (DBW 3). München: Chr. Kaiser Verlag.

Bostrom, N. A History of Transhumanists Thoughts. *Journal of Evolution and Technology*, 14 (1): 1–25.

Fletcher, J. 2009. *Situačnietika*. Praha: Kalich.

Jonas, H. 1997. *Principodpovědnosti: Pokus o etiku pro technologickou civilizaci*. Praha: OIKOYMENH.

Michálek, J. 1996. *Topologie výchovy: Místovýchovy v životěčlověka*. Praha: OIKOYMENH.

Sölle, D. 2006. *Stellvertretung*. In: U. Baltz-Otto and F. Steffensky (eds.). *Gesammelte Werke 3*. Stuttgart: Kreuz Verlag.

Souček, B. 1976. *Teologieapoštola Pavla*. Praha: Kalich.

Imago Dei and Transhumanism: Theological Worries

Piotr Orłowski

1. Introduction

The classical doctrine that man is created in the image of God (cf. Gen 1:26–27), which highlights the locus of this imago Dei in man's intellectual nature, appears to align with transhumanist (TH) aspirations for the liberation of the human mind. Transhumanists contend that the mind, which they view as the cornerstone of human identity, should be freed from biological constraints. The transhumanist project thus aims to create a god-like creature through technological progress (Gouw and Green 2022). The concept of a new post-human, enhanced by eliminating factors leading to death, disembodied, and focused on transferring the mind to a non-biological substrate, appears to some transhumanist (TH) groups as a more accurate expression of God-likeness. Does this not then suggest that corporeality itself might not be an image of God, thereby raising questions within Christian theology about the acceptability of transhumanist engineering?

Based on Thomas Aquinas' texts, mainly from the "Summa Theologiae" (q.93), I will draw attention to the reductionism that accompanies such a reading of his teaching on the image of God: for the indication of the role of intellectual nature must be read in a broader context and not in isolation from its anthropological framework. I will then focus on the resolution that Thomas makes in considering whether an angel is more the image of God than a human being, in order to conclude with a reflection on the difference between being the image of God and being like God. The latter option seems to characterize the transhumanist project, and the former the classical version of the theology of the image of God as defined by, among others, Thomas Aquinas

2. The art of differentiation: apparent versus real similarity

Precision in the use of terms is a requirement of any reflection, so it is worth beginning by drawing attention to the actual content of the category of man as 'image of God'. It seems that the argumentation of the proponents of transhumanism as representing the fulfilment of man's vocation and his likeness to God overlooks essential elements of the theology of the image of God, reducing them more profoundly. As it is often pointed out, the proposals of transhumanism have a clear religious context, albeit secularized, and therefore the search for such a justification in classical concepts such as the imago Dei is not surprising, but a significant reinterpretation is made, inscribed in certain historical processes.

The development of the theology of the divine image, marked by a modern departure from perceiving God's reflection in the world and embracing the notion of man's self-constitution, led to a significant shift in perspective from the 19th century onwards. Instead of viewing man as made in God's image, it posited that God is in man's image, thereby becoming a projection of human traits. This trend appears theologically aligned with, or perhaps even a continuation of, transhumanism. Unlike traditional views that see man in relation to God as a creature to the Creator, transhumanism adopts a Hegelian perspective, viewing humanity on an inevitable path toward divinity, embodying the absolute spirit. Thinking formatted against this background in a peculiar way leads the proponents of transhumanism to understand the realization of such postulates as a way of divinizing man (without the help of God!), supposedly leading to the fullness of the imago Dei, since its essence consists in having an intellectual nature. Leaving aside for the moment the way of achieving this goal, which is apparently against God, it is worth reflecting on the actual meaningful scope of the imago Dei as the source of man's dignity in Aquinas' view. For him, what is expressed in this concept is not so much contempt for corporeality (his views are the antipodes of Manichaeism) as it is about participation in the life of God, which is realized in the act of intellectual contemplation, but includes the whole man. Aquinas' anthropological synthesis, which recognizes man not as the 'soul' alone or the body alone, but points to a substantive unity, albeit not without hierarchy (the body lives thanks to the soul, corpus propter animam), perfectly reflects the idea of the imago Dei in classical theology. For this reason, some have seen in

Aquinas – precisely in the concept of the image of God – the key to his entire theological project, which was the *Summa Theologiae*: according to Wilhelm Metz, different kinds of 'images' can be used to distinguish the individual elements of the structure of the three-part Summa: from the *exemplar-exemplata* relationship in creation, through action, including grace, which brings man closer to the divine exemplar, to Christ, the fullness of the divine image, who opens the way to God being the imitation of the Incarnate Word (Nesteruk 2023).

In the rich tradition of reflection on the *imago Dei* in Aquinas, it is worth considering two aspects in particular: the creation of man in the image of God and the essence of this particular likeness, which consists in the possession of an intellectual nature.

Ad imaginem Dei

In the doctrine of the image of God, Thomas notes that while resemblance (*similitudo*) to God is passive, being an image brings in an active element: "Hence it is clear that likeness is essential to an image; and that an image adds something to likeness – namely, that it is copied from something else. For an image is so called because it is produced as an imitation of something else" (ST I, q. 93, a.1c). Creation imitates the goodness of God in many ways, which already led Aristotle to believe that natural forms are even something divine (ScG I, 50), but in the case of the image it is not a matter of sharing only certain common features (*accidens*), but specific differences, species.

Because the Son is the only perfect image of the Father, therefore, Thomas notes that the biblical expression 'in the image' (*ad imaginem*) is entirely appropriate here (ST I, q.93, a.5, ad 4). It expresses a striving, betraying a lack of full adequacy with the image.

This is why St. Thomas, beginning with q.93, states that Christ is the perfect image of God (cf. Col 1:15) and we are imperfect – this, however, is not because of our nature (as if it had lost ontologically through original sin), but because of sin. To be the image of God, then, is to be in the image of Christ, in whom all things were created, combining true deity and humanity. Christ remains always incarnate (the same for ever – cf. Heb 13:8) and thus reveals to us the mystery of the Trinity and what being *imago Trinitatis* is all about.

The Trinitarian aspect further points us to the fact that the true image of God is to be in communion, indicating that Trinity is imaged in creation most clearly in covenantal marriage. The Trinitarian communion of persons, the mystery of which is expressed in the relationship between Christ and the Church, reveals the most important point of reference for Thomas when considering the image of God: not to look for 'structural' elements, but for a profound plan, a Trinitarian reference that sheds light on human personality and action (Long 2016).

Natura intelectualis

Understanding Thomas's anthropology demands a broader metaphysical view, in which man is on the borderline between the material and spiritual worlds, but at the same time constitutes an entity characterized by unity in action. He cannot, therefore, separate one power in him and isolate it from the others: the indication of a certain guiding element or power in human action must be read as a whole. This is the key to understanding Aquinas' statement that the image of God in man is realized in the *natura intelectualis*, but not treated as something static, as a power, but more as an act. And in the act is revealed the integration that takes place; the whole person acts, not just the power; therefore, the person is not the soul – we are not our souls. It is only through action that we come to know power and its habits. The emphasis on the similarity to God in action is due, in Thomas, to the fact that he does not want it to be identified with the potentiality of action, and besides, for him God is not *ens summum*, but *ipsum esse subsistent*. Therefore, the cognition and love of God in the act is the realization of the image of God in man (ST I, 76, 1). And cognition and love are always actions of the whole man, and therefore we are the image as persons and not individual authorities. If Thomas points to them as related to the image, it is in accordance with his way of describing action (e.g. of the authorities), which does not exclude or separate.

It is significant that the identification of the *natura intelectualis* as most similar to God is not exclusive for Aquinas: it is noteworthy that he transfers the reflection on the differences within genus and species, touching on the last difference, to the participation of creatures in the *esse* and the transcendental properties. Recognizing that the creature resembles the Creator by being, secondly, living and thirdly, that creatures reason (*sapiunt vel intelligunt*), Thomas sees that there is no creature closer to God than one possessing intelligence. This is the furthest difference *secundum speciem*, but which builds on the others and is derived from the analogy characteristic of theological adjudication (Reinhardt 2005, 72–73).

The accent placed on depicting God through the prism of intellectual nature, however, does not exclude the body, it includes it, but for the sake of the soul and its intellectuality. At the same time, this emphasises what is common to individuals, male and female, despite bodily differences. Admittedly, in his commentary on the Epistle to the Corinthians, St. Thomas seems to state that man is more the image of God (as *principium* and *finis*), but this must be read in view of the analogies actually between ancient and medieval culture. But these are secondary issues for Thomas, which do not obscure the common dignity flowing from being the image of God.

In this context, it can be seen that contemporary transhumanism accentuates Gnostic reductionism (Marcos and Perez 2019); but it is, after all, 'man' that is in the image, and man is not the soul alone. Therefore, for Thomas, the soul united to the body is more like God than the soul alone (ST, Suppl., q.93, a.1, ad 1.). The body is a vestige (*vestigium*), but just as the soul gives existence to the body, endowing it with a special dignity, so too with participation in the image of God, which, pertaining to the intellectual nature, includes everything in which it expresses itself.

3. Gain or loss? The angelic and human image of God

The tendencies of transhumanism, aimed at eliminating corporeality as a potential source of worry, seem to be a manifestation of the age-old attempts to 'angelise' the human being, by reducing him or her to mere mind. In this key matter, following the presentation of the earlier grammar of Thomistic discourse, it is worth noting that a similar question, albeit in a different context, was posed by Aquinas when reflecting on the image of God. He wondered who was more *imago Dei*: whether an angel, being pure intelligence, or a human being. In the case of the angel, St. Thomas notes, however, the imitation of the intellectual nature does not reach a certain proportionality which man possesses. This refers to the origin of the human being from another human being by begetting, just as God is from God (the Word comes in the manner of the Image, which is a personal name), but also to the presence of the soul in the whole body, analogous to the presence of God in the whole creation (Reinhhardt 2006, 75). He explains this approach in detail in one of the articles of interest in q.93:

> "We may speak of God's image in two ways. First, we may consider in it that in which the image chiefly consists, that is, the intellectual nature. Thus the image of God is more perfect in the angels than in man, because their intellectual nature is more perfect, as is clear from what has been said. Second, we may consider the image of God in man as regards its accidental qualities, so far as to observe in man a certain *imitation of God*, consisting in the fact that man proceeds from man, as God from God; and also in the fact that the *whole human soul is in the whole body*, and again, in every part, as God is in regard to the whole world. In these and the like things the image of God is more perfect in man than it is in the angels. But these do not of themselves belong to the nature of the Divine image in man, unless we presuppose the first likeness, which is in the intellectual nature; otherwise even brute animals would be to God's image. Therefore, as in their intellectual nature, the angels are more to the image of God than man is, we must grant that, absolutely speaking, the angels are more to the image of God than man is, but that in some respects man is more like to God" (ST I, q.93, a.3)

In his commentary on Psalm 8, he notes that man is close to the angels in being God's image bearer, but the difference is that in the angel the imago Dei is by simple intuition of truth, while in man it is *per discursum* (In Ps. 8). It is through cognition and love that man realizes his capacity to know God (capax Dei). But the hallmark of man's being *ad imaginem Dei* is an action that involves a royal government in God's name over creation, a kind of priestly representation of creation before God. The fulfilment of this mission, linked to corporeality, is the purpose of creation: to realize in this way, already eschatologically, the image of God.

Thus, the 'angelisation' of man by depriving him of his corporeality carries with it the detriment of being the image of God. This 'addition,' secondary in the objective order but specific to man and building his identity, expressed in the imitation of God by what is characteristic of man, would be lost as a result of transhumanist transformations.

4. Being in the image of God versus "being like God": Seeking a point of comparison with transhumanism

In Thomas' conception, it can be seen that what matters most is not to draw attention to the 'something' in man (thus reifying the 'image of God' in human being), but the degree of participation in intellectual nature is from the perspective of action: knowing and willing. Having this capacity is the first of three ways of realizing the image of God: at the level of the order of nature, being in the image of God is the capacity to know and love God. At the order of grace, being in the image is the habitual and actual capacity to know and love God, albeit imperfectly, which is accomplished by the power of grace. This image occurs in the just, abiding in grace. The third stage of the realization of God's image is the perfect knowledge of God and his love, which is realized in the saved in heaven. This means that the Christian life becomes a way of perfecting and growing in being in the image of God, which is the goal of grace, and which begins with creation and intellectual nature and, through re-creation, leads to conformity, even participation, in divine nature (Roszak 2018).

It is worth noting that this path of perfecting man as being in the image of God has Trinitarian overtones, because of the emphasis placed on knowing and loving, since these are the constitutive acts of the divine persons in the Trinity (ST I, q.93, a.5). The realization of these acts primarily concerns God himself: "Thus – the image of God existing in man – is found in the word conceived in the mind from the knowledge of God and in the love flowing from this. So, as we can see from this, the image of God in the soul is to be found in the fact that it is directed towards God, or at least has the capacity to be directed towards God". (ST I, q.93, a.8c)

In the last article of q. 93, however, an interesting question arises about the difference between likeness and image, which Thomas considers from a twofold perspective: likeness (*similitudo*) as an expression of what is common when it appears 'before the appearance of the image,' but also after the appearance as an expression of the accuracy and perfection of the image, and this means that the realizationof the image is linked to the virtues (ST I, q.93, a.9c.). It would seem that I would caution this article against an isolationist approach to the 'image,' because although something is an essence, e.g. the essence of the soul belongs to the image because of its intellectual nature, there is a whole series of 'consequences' that affect the whole of existence (Guell et al. 2019).

Will the new man in the sense of the promise of TH still be capax Dei if he is disembodied? The Gnostic character of transhumanism, singling out only the intellectual aspect, seems to forget that faith is not merely an intellectual act, but one in which there is an *affectusboni*, since the intellect is stimulated to knowledge by the will reinforced by grace. The faith of the demons is a faith without this 'goodness,' and this seems to be the aspect that TH is aiming at (Peters 2022). Even the full intellectualization of transhumanism, however, cannot overlook the fact that the lumen fidei for seeing God must be replaced by the gift of *lumen gloriae*.

Crossing the threshold of singularity, and the intention of self-salvation implicit in this, reveals yet another difference, which concerns being 'in the image' and 'being like God,' which has been the temptation of fallen demons. The path of becoming like God is not the same as the path of substituting God and self-soteriology (Gaitan 2019).

For Thomas, functional enhancements of the human being must respect the integrity of his nature: depriving corporeality would lead to replacing the human being with another entity (Asla 2019), and even from the perspective of eternity, the soul aims at reuniting with the glorified body, since the separation of body and soul caused by death is an exceptional and transitory state. The soul holds the memory of identity, but the glorified body is a natural state for the soul.

5. Conclusion

The doctrine that man is created in the image of God, highlighting the natura intelectualis that brings humans closer to God through acts of knowledge and love, should be interpreted within the broader framework of Thomas Aquinas' comprehensive anthropology. The presence of reason in man opens up a series of similarities to the Creator that angels, who are pure intelligences, do not have. This is expressed in the similarities evident in the manner of the soul's presence in the body, man's origin as a human being, but also his rule over others, being the cause of good for others and fulfilling the rule of kingship over creation.

The transhumanist project, akin to Gnostic traditions, reduces humanity to merely an intellectual dimension and obscures not so much the realization of being made in the image of God – of which Christ is the exemplar – but rather the aspiration to be like God, usurping His prerogatives and rendering Him superfluous. A "man" whose soul is not connected to the body but instead resides in an inorganic carrier would not more closely align with "the image of God", since the perspective of grace encompasses the entirety of the human being.

References

Asla, M. 2019. On the limits, imperfections and evils of the human condition. Biological improvement from a Thomistic perspective. *Scientia et Fides*, 7(2): 77–95.

Gouw, A., and Green, B. (eds). 2022. *Religious Transhumanism and Its Critics*. Lanham: Lexington Books.

Guel, F., Echarte, L. E., and Murillo, J. I. 2019. Objectivity and human bioenhancement. The paradox of the natural. *Scientia et Fides*, 7(2): 195–214.

Eberl, J. 2022. Enhancing the Imago Dei: Can a Christian Be a Transhumanist? *Christian bioethics: Non-Ecumenical Studies in Medical Morality*, 28(1): 76–93.

Gaitán, L. 2019. Heaven on Earth: The Mind Uploading Project as Secular Eschatology. *Theology and Science*, 17(3): 403–416.

Marcos A. and Perez, M. 2019. Cave 2.0. The dualistic roots of transhumanism. *Scientia et Fides*, 7(2): 23–40.

Nesteruk, A. 2023. From Deep Incarnation to Deep Anthropology: Hypostatic Union and the Universe in the Image of Imago Dei. *Theology and Science*, 21(1): 81–95.

Peters, T. 2022. Will Superintelligence Lead to Spiritual Enhancement? *Religions*, 13(5): 399.

Woźniak, R. 2014. Materialno-biologiczny wymiar obrazu Bożego w człowieku. *Scientia et Fides*, 2(2): 271–288.

Reinhardt, E. 2005. *La dignidad del hombre en cuanto imagen de Dios. Tomas de Aquino ante sus Fuentes*. Pamplona: Eunsa.

Roszak, P. 2018. La fe y la participación en la naturaleza divina según santo Tomás de Aquino. *Espíritu*,67(155): 153–172.

Long, S. 2016. Creation 'ad imaginem Dei': The Obediential Potency of the Human Person to Grace and Glory. *Nova et Vetera*, 14(4):1175–1192.

COMENIUS'S ANTROPOLOGICAL VISION: INTERPRETING HUMAN NATURE IN HIS KEY WORKS AND THEIR MODERN LERGACY

Martin Kmec

1. Introduction

This paper explores the theological anthropology of Czech theologian, philosopher, and pedagogue John Amos Comenius (1592–1670), whose work transcends his time. The paper has separate but interconnected sections. It starts with Comenius's life and work's historical and philosophical framework, essential for contextual interpretation. Next, Comenius's fundamental theological ideas on human nature, free will, and the divine-human relationship are examined. Each topic is carefully explored using historical and comparative philosophical methodologies. This method helps appreciate Comenius's thoughts in their original context and apply them to modern challenges. The paper then discusses Comenius's present relevance. His religious ideas are compared to modern ethical, educational, and spiritual issues. This section emphasizes Comenius's ageless significance and suggests modern uses.

My main purpose is to show that Comenius's religious anthropology can still inform present discussions of human nature and progress. The study seeks to connect historical religious insights with modern ethical and philosophical issues, providing a unique perspective on past and present human problems. The work is simply a small sample of this large field, and we recognize its limits. However, the paper synthesizes the principles and explores Comenius's legacy for future theological and philosophical research. Each component is meant to inform, challenge, and inspire a deeper understanding of human nature and the pursuit of knowledge and ethics.

2. The Development of Comenius's Anthropological Views

The literary activity of Czech theologian, philosopher, and educator John Amos Comenius (1592 – 1670) was extraordinarily prolific, both in the volume of writings and their thematic focus. This study presents his view of man through selected works, primarily from his output up to the age of 50, before 1645, i.e., before writing his grand utopian work on the reform of all things based on the principle of pansophy, *De rerum humanarum emendatione consultatio catholica* (A General Consultation on the Improvement of Human Affairs). *Consultation* offers a more elaborated and philosophically profound conception of man (cf. Čížek 2016). He began its composition during his stay in Elblag, now Poland, but most of the work falls into the last, Amsterdam period of his life and work (1656–1670).

Comenius's anthropological views contain selected thoughts in his didactic work, in Latin *Opera didactica omnia* (Amsterdam, 1657). In the English edition, we refer to the system of didactics written in Leszno, *DidacticaMagna* (Great Didactic). This writing is an extension of the *Didactics* previously written in the Czech language, also in Polish Leszno, and is contained in the first volume of *Opera didactica omnia* (hereafter ODO). Volume I of ODO contains writings from his first period of exile in Leszno, 1628–1641, where he worked as a teacher at a higher brethren school, later as a rector of a gymnasium, and, among other tasks, wrote educational works. Comenius's anthropology is also found in his Czech philosophical-religious writings, especially *Centrum securitatis* (The Center of Safety), written in 1625, published in 1633 in Leszno, and in other pre-pansophic (preparatory) and pansophic writings.

3. The Place of Man in Creation and imago Dei

Man, as a being placed among other living creatures, is a creation of the Creator. Comenius's fundamental Christian starting point is that man and everything on Earth has its origin in God. In Comenius's conceptual hierarchy of existence, ranging from elements (earth, water, fire, air) and minerals (stones and metals), through plants and animals, up to angels, humanity holds the highest position. This elevation underscores humanity's central role in God's design. The first chapter of *Didactica Magna* (Great

Didactic) is aptly titled: “Man is the most perfect, the strangest, and the most remarkable creature”. Humanity is deemed the most perfect creation due to its reason or alternatively, its soul. It is also considered the strangest, for in humans, the temporal and the eternal, the visible and the invisible, converge. Finally, humans are deemed the most glorious among all creatures, being the rulers of creation, crafted in the image of God, imago Dei (Great Didactic, ch. 1).

From this understanding flows the notion that humans should conduct themselves with gravity and virtue, recognizing only one Creator, preserving their dignity, and not succumbing to slavery – either to other humans or to their own bodies. They are to use all things for service, for the needs of others, and properly govern their actions and movements, both external and internal (Great Didactic, ch. 4). These implications highlight the dignity and freedom of humanity, emphasizing independence from earthly matters that could divert attention and energies from higher goals – service for the common good. Comenius perceived all humans as created in God’s image, tasked with emulating Christ and fully utilizing God’s gifts (Atwood 2009, 389). The glory of humanity does not lie in dominion itself but in being a good ruler, created in God’s image. Secondly, humans are imbued with a desire for knowledge and the capacity to understand themselves and all things. Thirdly, an innate desire for God marks humanity as remarkable (Great Didactic, ch. 5).

This stewardship over creation is also derived from the fact that humans are not merely rulers within creation, but part of its greater unity (Atwood 2009, 384). Comenius poignantly captures this sentiment in a quote from his later works: “We all sit together in the great theater of the world. Whatever happens here affects all. The sun provides light for all” (Unum necessarium, p. 80). This statement reflects the interconnectedness of the world and its origin in God, emphasizing that human actions should aim for the greater good of others.

An enlightening illustration can also be found in Comenius’s early pre-pansophic work, *Labyrinth of the World and Paradise of the Heart* (1623), where he draws from the German mystic Jacob Boehme: “The world is a simple organism, not dead matter; it is a tree with roots and branches, and God is the root of that tree . . . ” (Vliet &Vanderjagt 1994,86). This imagery conveys a worldview in which the world is interconnected, with its origin in God, signifying that everything that transpires affects everyone, thereby directing human activity towards the good of others.

In another of Comenius's early works, which delves more seriously into philosophical questions than his preceding so-called consolatory writings, *Centrum Securitatis* outlines a dichotomy between the Creator God and the created image. Divine wisdom ensures that each creation maintains its essence, its natural center. However, humanity is composed of two parts, spiritual and physical, hence possessing dual natures (centers). The body is subject to decay, but the spiritual part is rooted in the immortal soul, which originates directly from God. The soul is to cling to God, serving as a mediator between the Creator and creation (Centrum Securitatis, ch. 2).

As the world is created by God, God is its stable center – the hub of the wheel. Similarly, humans (in their spiritual aspect) have their center in God, as the spokes of a wheel have their stable point (center) in the hub. This is the center of essence or existence. The second place where the spoke is fixed, on the wheel's circumference, is called the center of place. For the soul, this mediating role is the center of place, meaning to stand in submission to the Creator and to rule over one's own body and other beings (Centrum Securitatis, ch. 2).

Compared to the rest of creation, humans possess specific abilities, attributed to their embodiment of the imago Dei (image of God). This includes a profound desire for knowledge and an admiration for encompassing all that can be known. Human knowledge constantly deepens; the mind is a depth capable of absorbing everything that can be known on Earth (Great Didactic, ch. 5, 76). Mirroring the divine archetype, humans are creative and social beings, inherently driven towards work and knowledge, and the engagement with others. Comenius observed a natural inclination towards work and even strenuous effort, coupled with a curious desire to know and learn something new, evident even in early childhood (Great Didactic, ch. 5, 43).

Moreover, humans possess innate senses (communes notitiae). Criegern (1881) finds throughout Comenius's didactic works, among these, the concept of language – regardless of how different individual languages may be, for Comenius, they share something fundamental, hinting at an original, superior state of humanity. This includes a sense for truth and goodness, intellect (illuminated by Holy Scripture), and free will (various places in ODO, II. 29, 36, 148, 245). Comenius speaks of "common notions" as some innate notions, in alignment with English deists of the 17th century, such as Herbert of Cherbury, and later, John Locke (Criegern 1881, 113–114).

The composition of the human being, or rather the aspects of the soul, vary according to the period in Comenius's work. In his early period, Comenius addressed the question of human composition solely in terms of the body and soul. However, in his later period, he proposed a model of unity comprising the body, spirit, and soul (or mind) (Čížek 2016, 180). Comenius identifies three higher parts of human beings, three aspects of the spiritual life that we possess thanks to the imago Dei: 1. thought (mens), 2. will (voluntas), and 3. action (facultatesoperatione) (ODO IV, 68). Occasionally, he adds language, speech (sermo), as a fourth fundamental mental ability (ODO III, 731). The elements of this tripartite division are not constant, and at times interchange, for example, memory, reason, will (Centrum Securitatis, ch. 3). From this, we infer that Comenius did not have a fixed or harmonized terminology for the fundamental mental capabilities.

4. The Consequences of Fall into Sin for the Human Capabilities

From a theological perspective, the human condition underwent a significant transformation following the fall into sin. This change consequently altered anthropology, the understanding of human capabilities, and even the imago Dei, which was in some ways influenced by the corrupted nature of humanity. For Comenius, the fall into sin primarily signified a substantial diminution of mental strength. He spoke less about the traditional theme of the sinfulness into which humanity fell after the original fall. Instead, he emphasized that our perception of reality is inadequate and flawed, characterized by a lack of understanding of the world, a deficiency in wisdom, and moral judgment (Criegern 1881, 119). Post-fall, the state of human existence is such that J.A. Comenius, in *Centrum Securitatis*, created two unique Czech terms to describe it:

1. "Jinudost" (German: Anderswo) signifies a displacement from one's rightful center, being in the wrong place. This implies that humans are not fulfilling their intended purpose and mission for which they were created. Humans are somewhere other than where they should be, their path leading away from God and self-improvement according to God's will (Centrum Securitatis, ch. 6).

2. "Samosvojnost" (German: Selbstsucht) represents a closure in self-absorption, devoid of regard for God or the world, essentially self-love. This results from the loss of the essential center, the essence, which should have been in God. Now, humans are independent, detached from God, and focused inward, encompassing selfishness, envy, and other vices, essentially aspiring to be their own gods (Centrum Securitatis, ch. 5).

Human will and its freedom, while belonging to mental dispositions, gain theological significance in the aftermath of the Fall. Comenius rejected the Calvinist doctrine of total depravity from the Synod of Dort (1618–1619), arguing scripturally that piety can be learned. In the matter of free will, he leaned towards the views of Philip Melanchthon and Erasmus of Rotterdam (Atwood, 2009, p. 389). Comenius's emphasis on free will grew with his increasing optimism about humanity and its potential for self-improvement. His thought overall considers the impact of original sin on all humanity while emphasizing the necessity of actively participating in one's salvation. His reformative efforts imply lofty expectations that could not be propagated without a robust activity of human will. For orthodox confessional theology, Comenius's stance might appear as a deviation from a clear course. However, his hopes are seen by J.M. Lochman and A. Molnár as an eschatological hope in the reconciling power of Christ, anticipating Christ's victory (Hábl 2010, 3–4). The significance of human will is first recognized by Comenius in *Centrum Securitatis*, a period before his exile (Čížek 2016, 179). Reason, according to Comenius, elevates humanity above other creatures (p. 180). In his later writings, there is a noticeable shift in the view of human possibilities, where free and limitless will is considered the primary disposition of the soul (Čížek2018).

There exists a natural inclination in humans towards God, as mentioned earlier in the context of *Great Didactic*. However, in the world and within ourselves, there are many causes for deviation and displacement from this center, such as other creatures, the devil, and our own desires (Centrum Securitatis, ch. 3–4). The resolution, proposed by Comenius in *Centrum Securitatis*, consists in reorientation towards God as the center. The closer we are to the center, the better it is for us. Liberation from this post-fall state or the state of having fallen from the center is possible only with God's help. The solution is akin to the narrative in the *Labyrinth*. For a person to find God's mercy and reap all benefits from Christ, one must leave the world, turn away from it, ascend, or abandon all things, even to step out of oneself and find peace in the immovable center, in God (Centrum Securitatis, ch. 9–10).

> "[...] and having abandoned everything, including his self, he sets out towards the depths of God's mercy in Christ and disappears from his will and reason; surrenders himself fully to God's will and His providence in order to do with Him what He wants to do, the way He wants to do it, when He wants to do it, where He wants to do it, if He wants to do it. [...] That is what we call resignatio: the surrender of one's will to God". (Centrum Securitatis, ch. 9.; quoted in Čížek 2016, 169).

Comenius's fundamental view remained unchanged even in his later period: free will is the crown of human mental capabilities, but for our salvation and eternal life, it must be subordinated to God's will. In this development, the focus is on the central theme of Comenius's theology: the human inclination towards God and the necessity of aligning the human will with divine will for true liberation and salvation. This theme resonates with the broader Christian theological tradition, highlighting the tension between human freedom and divine providence.

5. Conclusion: The Legacy of Comenius Theological Anthropology

When we consider the contemporary relevance of Comenius' theological anthropology, it is clear that his findings may be reduced into three essential themes. At least two of these categories can be used effectively in public discourse to promote humanity, mutual respect, and appreciation of an individual's dignity and uniqueness. The fact that Comenius' ideas can inspire people from all times and worldviews, even those who do not share a biblical viewpoint on the world, demonstrates their ongoing cultural value.

Comenius' teachings provide a perspective through which to view and confront current personal, familial, and national difficulties. Comenius' understanding of human nature, particularly in the aftermath of sin and its consequences, necessitates a serious and honest assessment of individual and communal inadequacies. This perspective can be especially revealing in an era marked by unrestrained optimism about human progress and technical achievements. Recognizing the gravity of sin and the inherent defects in human nature, as Comenius advises, allows us to take a more balanced view of humanity's potential and limitations. This awareness can lead to greater resilience in the face of personal misfortune and a more empathetic attitude to societal concerns. In a world increasingly divided by ideological and cultural differences, Comenius' emphasis on human imperfection may foster a more compassionate and tolerant society, one that accepts fallibility and is committed to mutual support and understanding.

The second part of Comenius' legacy is his strong trust in the human capacity for knowledge and self-improvement. This notion resonates well in today's environment, when lifelong learning and personal development are widely regarded as necessary components of a meaningful existence. Comenius's belief that humans are born with an insatiable need for knowledge and understanding provides a solid foundation for advocating educational and personal development programs in today's world.

This viewpoint is consistent with the present emphasis on lifelong learning and flexibility in an ever-changing global landscape. The idea that people are not only capable but also predisposed to learning and self-improvement can motivate educational policies and practices that accommodate varied learning styles and lifelong educational journeys. It also emphasizes the notion that education should not be limited to intellectual pursuits, but should also include moral and ethical learning, preparing students to manage the challenges of modern life with insight and integrity.

The third and possibly most important part of Comenius' legacy is his notion of free will, specifically its subordination to divine will. This concept is important in current spiritual discourse because it provides a worldview that balances personal autonomy with a greater, transcendental purpose. Comenius's advocate for aligning human will with God's will is consistent with the current search for meaning and purpose beyond monetary accomplishments and cultural recognition. In a culture dominated by individualistic ambitions and self-centered goals, Comenius' theology calls for a reorientation toward a greater purpose, aligning personal desires with divine designs. This approach does not diminish personal agency; rather, it elevates it by connecting it to a greater, more fundamental sense of life's purpose.

This notion can be seen in contemporary Christian theology and spiritual practice as the pursuit of a life that is not only self-serving but also contributes to the larger good, led by spiritual principles and values. It pushes believers to think about not only their goals, but also their obligations as part of a greater, divinely organized plan. Furthermore, Comenius' concept of "resignatio", or surrendering one's will to God, provides a counter-narrative to today's emphasis on self-actualization. It implies that true fulfillment and tranquility are found not in constant self-assertion, but in modest acceptance of one's place within God's plan.

References

Atwood, C. D. 2009. *The Theology of the Czech Brethren from Hus to Comenius*. University Park, PA: The Pennsylvania State University Press.

Cizek, J. 2018. John Amos Comenius and his Philosophy of Man. *Bruniana and Campanelliana*, 1(24):155–163.

Cizek, J. 2016. *The Conception of Man in the Works of John Amos Comenius*. Frankfurt am Main: Peter Lang.

Comenius, J. A. 1978. *Centrum securitatisto jest, Světlévymalování, jak v samém-jediném Bohu, a pokorném se jemunavšeckujehovůlioddání a poddánívšeck-adokonalápřítomnéhoživota Bezpečnost, Pokoj, a Blahoslavenstvízáleží [The Center of Safety]*. Leszno, 1632 [1625]. In: Johannis Amos Comenii Opera Omnia / Dílo Johna Amose Komenského. Sv. 3. Prague: Academia, 1978, pp. 473–564.

Comenius, J. A. 2021. *The Labyrinth of the World and The Paradise of the Heart*. London: Ekklesia Press.

Comenius, J. A. 1957. *Opera didactica omnia*. Prague: Nakladatelství Československé akademievěd.

Comenius, J. A. 1967. *The Great Didactic*. Trans. M.W. Keatinge. New York: Russell & Russell.

Comenius, J. A.1958. *Unum necessarium*. Translated by Vernon H. Nelson. Bethlehem, Pennsylvania: Moravian Theological Seminary.

Criegern von, H. F. *Comenius als Theologe*. Heidelberg, 1881.

Hábl, J. 2010. Komenskýčasový a nadčasový: problémtakzvanéaktuálnosti Komenskéhoodkazu. *Komenský*, (135(2): 47–53.

Patočka, J. 1966. Komenskéhonázory a pansofickéliterárníplányod-spisůítešnýchkeVšeobecnéporadě. In: *Komeniologickéstudie II*. Praha: Oikúmené, 223–270.

van Vliet, P.; & Vanderjagt, A. J.(eds.). 1994. *Johannes Amos Comenius (1592–1670): Exponent of European Culture?*. Amsterdam: North-Holland Publishing Company.

‘TRANSHUMANISM’, A CATEGORY MISTAKE: INSIGHTS FROM BRUNO LATOUR

Mendo Castro Henriques

1. How did ‘Transhumanism’ emerge?

How can we talk about transhumanism if we still do not know completely, nor we will ever know, who the human being is? It is with this question in mind that we must approach transhumanism that, for decades, has trumpeted its increasingly ambitious proposals. Transhumanists advocate the enhancement of the human condition by promoting sophisticated technologies that increase all kinds of human capabilities, longevity and cognition. They strongly enhance the benefits of emerging technologies that would overcome what they call “human limitations”; some of them believe that humans may be able to transform into beings with abilities so greatly expanded from the current condition as to merit the label of “posthuman”. The pinnacle of the transhumanist dream is, apparently, the downloading of “human consciousness” into a computer RAM (Hayles 1999) a variant of the “ghost in the machine” argument, a category mistake.

A categorical mistake is a semantic or/and ontological error in which things belonging to a particular category are presented as belonging to a different one; alternatively, it occurs when a property is attributed to a thing that could not support it. The term was introduced by Gilbert Ryle in *The Concept of Mind* (Ryle, 1949) against Cartesian metaphysics. Gilbert Ryle failed to understand that Descartes was a methodical dualist, able to overcome mind-body dualism through the enigmatic unity of man in *The Passions of the Soul* (1649). Nevertheless, Ryle’s argument is formally correct; the mind is usually misrepresented as an object made of an immaterial substance. Such argument is useful to deconstruct the transhumanism discourse that speaks about humanity as if we already knew it as a ‘nature’, ‘substance’, or ‘value’, which is not the case.

In 1924, the British biochemist J.B.S. Haldane published *Daedalus; or science and the Future* where he states that great benefits would result from the control of human genetics and science in general. He predicted a society with abundant energy, where genetics would make people more perfect in body and mind, and where fetuses would be gestated in artificial wombs. As militant Stalinist he stated: "The chemical or physical inventor is always a Prometheus. There is no great invention, from fire to flight, that has not been hailed as an insult to some god". (Haldane 1924, 6)

Haldane's essay was a bestseller and started a chain of forward-looking debates, including J.D. Bernal's *The World, the Flesh, and the Devil* (1929). Apparently, the word 'transhumanism' was coined by Julian Huxley, biologist and first Director General of UNESCO and founder of the WWF a member of the famous Huxley family and grandson of Thomas Henry Huxley, commonly referred to as 'Darwin's bulldog'. In *Religion Without Revelation* (1927) he wrote: "Perhaps transhumanism will solve the problem: man remaining man, but transcending himself by realizing new possibilities *of* and *for* his human nature". Along with the launch of the transhumanist project, the first critics appeared. Aldous Huxley (Julian's brother) criticized the social impact of technological transformation in *Brave New World*, (1932). He presented a dystopian caste-based and conformist society in which psychological conditioning, promiscuous sexuality, biotechnology, and drugs, keep the population "serene" through the agency of world controllers.

Keeping these predecessors in mind, I will try to submit contemporary transhumanist goals to the analytical framework of the philosopher and anthropologist Bruno Latour (1947–2022). He never wrote explicitly about *transhumanism*, but his mighty work helps to clarify it as a category mistake. He envisaged the uncertain boundaries between the human and the non-human, freeing us from the modernist and dualistic image of man. In *An Inquiry into Modes of Existence* he wrote about his previous book *We have never been moderns*: "It didn't take a genius twenty years ago to feel that modernization was going to end, as it became more and more difficult by the day – indeed, by the minute – to distinguish facts due to increased mixing between humans and non-humans". (Latour 2013a, 9)

2. Latour's work and why it matters about transhumanism

Bruno Latour's work is multifaceted, a cabinet of curiosities according to his best interpreter (De Vries (2016). For a long time, he was relatively unknown, and even the target of some academic hostility, in his native France; but he kept his maverick identity. He received the 2013 Holberg Prize, the social sciences equivalent of the Nobel Prize and then the Kyoto Prize in 2021, just before his death in 2023. His research is wide: laboratory life at theSalk Institute; the shared history of microbes, microbiologists, and society in Pasteur's France; the tragic fate of ARAMIS, an innovative public transport system; law enacting in the French Supreme Court, *Conseil d' État*; geopolitics in the epoch of the Anthropocene; Christian and catholic profession of faith; economical organization and morality; ethnopsychiatry; modernity questioned; the city of Paris; politics of nature and environment; philosophy of science. He uses different methods to capture the intricacies of the human and non-human factors: "The smallest AIDS virus takes you from sex to the unconscious, then to Africa, tissue cultures, DNA and San Francisco, but the analysts, thinkers, journalists, and decision-makers will slice the delicate network traced by the virus, for you, into tidy compartments where you will find only science, only economy, only social phenomena, only local news, only feeling, only sex". (Latour 1999, 2)The surprising connections of everyday reality are proof that no abstraction, no essence – transhumanist or humanist – will substitute for what we are looking for.

Latour is one of the stars of a galaxy of 20th philosophers – Bergson, Whitehead, Adorno, Teilhard de Chardin, James, Rosenzweig, Péguy, and others – who rejected the tradition of essentialism. They did it on different grounds but they all shared an enhanced sense of experience. Bergson's philosophy of life; William James' philosophy of experience; Wittgenstein's late philosophy of language, Rosenzweig's philosophy of religion; Whitehead's philosophy of organisms; Adorno's negative dialcctics; Kuhn's debates on rationality; Péguy's meaning of repetition; Teilhard's evolution to Christogenesis. After Darwin, it became plausible to view present-day humanity not as the endpoint of evolution, but as a transitional phase. Darwin shifted biological thinking from essentialism to population thinking. From the beginning of the twentieth century, great philosophers explicitly recognized his work and applied his evolution theory to epistemology and anthropology. As Latour says: "We have finally understood that there was no Idea of a Horse to guide the proliferation of horses. Here ends, on this point at least, the quarrel of the Universals". (Latour 2013a, 102)

When Latour says that "a mode of existence is instituted by being experienced", he does not mean quite "empirical evidence". He incorporates William James' and Alfred Whitehead's critique of "matters of fact" and speak s about "matters of concern". In *Essays in Radical Empiricism*, James (1996 [1912]) argued that Locke, Berkeley, Hume, and Mill, the classical empiricists, defended an amputated concept of experience. They conceived experience in terms of discrete objects and atomic units, losing sight of its flow, the parts of which have no boundaries, each leading and interpenetrating the next. Rationalists tried in vain to correct the inconsistencies of empiricism with the addition of unifying agents, substances, categories, and intellectual powers, or "selves" (James 1996 [1912], 43). The result was a long history of mistakes. We must keep in mind how contemporary transhumanists are limited by such "bad empiricism".

Conceiving experience as a flow, James (1996 [1912], 42) argues that "the relations that connect experiences must themselves be experienced relations, and [that] any kind of experienced relation must be considered 'real'". Similarly, in *Science and the Modern World* (1925), Whitehead outlined "the foundations of an objectivist philosophy adapted to the requirements of science and the concrete context of human experience" (Whitehead 1967 [1925], 89). He argued that since the 17th century, the beginning of modernity, the dominant cosmology presupposed the ultimate fact of irreducible brute matter, meaningless, valueless, purposeless; such prejudice is inadequate to the status of science which [in 1925] through quantum mechanics and relativity theory requires a new theory of nature. Modern metaphysics suffered from the 'fallacy of the displaced concrete', that is, the expression of concrete facts under the guise of abstract logical constructions (Whitehead 1967 [1925], 50–51). He argued that matter is reality plus a specific way of formatting and locating events and entities: "the whole concept of materialism only applies to very abstract entities, the products of logical insight". (Whitehead 1967 [1925], 79)

Latour needed a philosophy to articulate his own scientific insights. He is not looking for a theory of nature (like Whitehead), neither a philosophy of religion (like James). He seeks for an anthropology and a conceptual apparatus in tune with human experience articulated by sciences and humanities. In such anthropology, there is no place for subject and object, neither primary and secondary qualities, and the stuff of modernempiricism and rationalism.[1] Along thirty years of Science Studies, he provided alternative descriptions of science, technology, politics, law, and other key institutions of modernity. He evaluated his own accomplishments arguing that the dominant descriptions of modernity are faulty. Science does not allow us direct access to reality – as a "double click" thought; chains of procedures are necessary to establish facts. Philosophical Anthropology requires a new starting point.

The history of science shows us that modernity defines and justifies its activities at odds with its practices. Latour proposes irreductivism as a new starting point. He wrote *An Inquiry into the Modes of Existence*, a book of nearly 500 pages, on which he worked for some 25 yearsas an "interim report" (Latour 2013a, xix, 476). In a website www.modesofexistence.org with data and a glossary, the readers are invited to contribute "to extend the work [. . .] with new documents, new sources, new testimonies and most importantly [. . .] [to modify the questions correcting or modulating the project in relation to the results obtained" (Latour 2013a, xx). He worked in science studies and actor-network theory and offered the conclusion that the usual epistemological dualities – fact and value, nature and society, mind and matter, word and world – are always completed through the use of "translations", or mediations.

Classified as a treatise on "empirical philosophy", *An Inquiry into the Modes of Existence*, is written by an anthropologist who questions the enigmas and embarrassments of modernity as he tries to explain values in science, technology, religion, politics, law, literature, emotions, morality, and economics. He does not worry much about specificities and technical details. Whereas most of his earlier work has focused on describing how actor networks are set, now Latour attempts to record what goes on in actor networks. The anthropologist has a toolbox to experiment what means to be human; he needs no labels, humanist or transhumanist; instead of talking

---

1 "It is thus crucial that students of science learn how to achieve greater proximity to their object of study and circumvent the pitfalls of critical or subjective discourse. Then, we might be able to use Powers's resources for giving our own descriptions the kind of grasp on reality that we can understand conceptually through the work of William James and Alfred North Whitehead".(Latour 2008, 94)

about different "interpretations" and conflicting "cultures", he researches different modes of existence.

A 'mode of existence' is defined by five characteristics: (1) Gaps that need to be overcome; (2) A trajectory, i.e., continuity through associations; (3) Felicity conditions of these translations; (4) Beings that are instituted as events; (5) Alteration as being-as-other.

The anthropologist deals with each of these five issues in each specific mode of existence. (Latour 2013a, 488–489) The following applies to science: (1) As regards *gaps*, science must take account of dissimilarities, using samples and data (2) *Trajectory*: Science must create inscriptions that make a bridge between gaps, allowing information about samples to go down the translation chain until the scientist can communicate. (3) *Happy/Unfortunate Conditions*: Bring Back/Lost Information. Scientific translations must allow full access to previous steps, to bring back lost information. (4) *Beings to be instituted*: 'Reference' is the mode of science (5) *Alteration*: Science uses reference to reach remote entities, accessible through instruments and calculus, not through "double-click" thought, of subject vs object type.

Transforming epistemology into ontology is a hallmark of Latour's work. In earlier work, he defended this turn by pointing to ethnography; Now, to create an ontology on empirical grounds the anthropologist checks whether his redescriptions of reality do clarify conflicts between values, institutions and cultures.

3. Focusing on construction and instauration

Let us focus on one achievement that enables us to dismiss the transhumanist discourse as a category mistake. I am speaking of Latour's "deconstruction" of the concepts of construction and constructivism. He was for a long time considered a member of the so-called constructivist studies of Social Science. His first big book was *Laboratory Life*; *The Social Construction of Scientific Facts* (1979) co-authored with Steve Woolgar. It is an anthropological approach to scientific culture and how the social world of the laboratory produces papers and other "texts". It was based on field work done by himin Roger Guillemin's laboratory at the Salk Institute.[2] A second edition (1986) with an extended postscript scraps the term "social"from the subtitle, as Latour breaks with the "sociology of modern science", not without some academical scandal.

This shift into a "new empiricism" has strong consequences for the "construction of facts". It is easy to answer that reality exists': that something is constructed does not exclude its being real; but why is it so difficult to construct a fact? Why does it take so much effort, and why do scientists fail so often?

Latour's answer is that 'construction' tries to say too many things at once, namely three different things. (Latour 2013a, 158–9). First, *to 'build' means to make it happen, to make someone or something, do something.* Engineers build machines and make them do what they need to do. "When someone acts, others move, take action" (Latour 2013a, 158). Secondly, "to say of something that it is constructed is *to make the direction of the vector uncertain*". Balzac tells us that creating a novel is like is to be "dragged along by characters", who force the author to write about them. (Latour 2013a, 158) Thirdly, "to say of a thing that is constructed is *to introduce a value judgment*, not only about the origin of action but [also] about the quality of the construction" (Latour 2013a, 159). To build well is what keeps creative and caring people awake: is the literary character properly constructed? What was built in the lab is a fact or an artifact? Is the medication properly administered? Is the person being taken under care?

To overcome the equivoques of construction, Latour elects the term "instauration" taken from Étienne Souriau. It encompasses better what 'construction' is supposed to mean. An artist, says Souriau, is not a Prometheus, but the creator of a work that requires something from him. A sculptor knows that he is the author of a statue; *to build is to make* [1st sense above]. He also knows that the statue *requires an orientation* [2nd sense above]. Moreover [3rd sense above], *there is appreciation*, for the excellence of the work produced: the sculptor wakes up in the middle of the night because he must do what needs to be done, to finish the work or fail. (Latour 2013a, 160) Having presented this concept of 'instauration' Latour draws an important conclusion: "[The] act of instauring must provide the opportunity to encounter beings capable of worrying us. Beings whose ontological sta-

2 Roger Guillemin (born January 11, 1924) received the Nobel Prize in Medicine in 1977 for his work on neurohormones.

tus are still open, but who are nevertheless capable of forcing us to do something, to worry us, to insist, to force us to speak well [...]. Articulable beings to which the establishment can add something essential for their autonomous existence. Beings that have their own resources". (Latour 2013a, 161)

Why do a scientist and a novelist or a nurse or a caretaker wake up at night? What worries them? Are they afraid of becoming the stock laughter of colleagues if they are faulty? Or is it because the responsibility of their work weighs on them, because they feel different kinds of normative forces, according to the mode of existence and the relationship in which they are involved?

The human being is "a being with its own resources" and articulated through another being. What makes a novelist, a scientist, a nurse, or a judge, do something? How do their modes of existence require a grip, a normative force upon what they do? Writing a novel implies a commitment to characters waiting to be properly committed to paper. Scientific research implies that data must be handled, and calculations done in a way to preserve reference. Making a promise supposes that someone is expecting the promise to be fulfilled. When the novel is not yet written and the fact not yet established, the defendant not yet judged, those *who must do things with words* worry about how to speak and act; the ontological status of beings-with-other is open, "articulable beings to whom [its] establishment can add something essential to their existence". They have normative force. Now, "what is good for the goose is good for the gander". What is adequate for a being in relation is adequate for the human being. If human beings are able *of forcing us to do something, to worry us, to insist, to force us to speak well*, they are being-as-other.

Here we come across the main reason why transhumanism is either a redundant concept or a category mistake: it takes humanity as being-as-the-same and not as being-as-other. Transhumanism does not care about the simultaneous characteristics of instauration: making things happen; focusing on the goal that attracts; and pursuit of excellence without a prior model. It does not overcome the bridge between facticity and normativity, between facts and values as it remain stuck in thetypical modernist contrast, summed up by Lotze's phrase: 'Seiendesist, Wertegelten' – 'what exists is, values hold.'

4. Humanism or transhumanism; the same narrative?

As Latour established a new kind of relationship between facts and values, he expanded the notion of 'experience' as being-as-other, incorporating normativity. There *is responsibility for a character in a novel*, *there is responsibility for facts in science*, and there is *responsibility for "beings whose ontological status is open*". He followed a path opened by Kant, to whom knowledge was a normative concept, thus opening the way for researching other forms of normativity, other concepts, and actions where responsibility is at stake. Concepts and actions do not dominate us; other beings call us. They keep us awake, force us to speak to them, and care about them.

This framework is crucial to evaluate the usual narratives of transhumanism such as, "the enterprise of transcending our natural limits". (Bostrom 2006) Bostrom'shistory goes back to... prehistory! His narrative can also be presented as a history of humanism because it is nowhere written what our (human) "natural limits" are. Again: transhumanism is redundant, indeed, or a category mistake.

Since at least 30.000 BC there are ceremonial burials and from the invention of writing onwards, there are documents showing how humans suffered the death of those whom they loved. The belief in an afterlife went along with efforts to prolong earthly life. In the Gilgamesh epic (circa 1700 BC), the hero sets out in search of immortality; as he takes a miraculous herb that grows at the bottom of the sea, a snake steals it before he can eat it. This well-known tale reappears in the search for the 'fountain of eternal youth'; in the alchemic 'elixir of life'; the esoteric Taoists strive to control the forces of nature. Be it myth or pseudo-science, one thing seems certain; there are no "natural limits" to human beings. To be human is to be in thc open as showed by the variants of the Prometheus myth. What happened to the Titan who stole the fire from Zeus and gave it to man? In Sophocles' version, Prometheus is persecuted. In thc carlier Hesiod version, Prometheus is freed by Heracles.

Middle Age Christians had conflicting opinions about the alchemists who tried to transmute substances, to create *homunculi* in tubes and invent *panaceas*. Pope John XXII and the Avignon school promoted these endeavors of which the work of Opicinus de Canistris around 1330, rediscovered in the 20th century, stands out as an outstanding example. Scholastics such as Albertus Magnus,Thomas Aquinas and Roger Bacon somehow defended the practice of alchemy claiming continuity with Aristotleand against the anti-experimentalist teachings of Augustine.

Renaissance humanism developed the ideal of the integral human being. Giovanni Pico della Mirandola's *Oration Concerning Human Dignity* (1486), thus proclaimed:

> "22. We have made you neither of heaven nor of earth, neither mortal norimmortal, so that you may, as the free and extraordinary shaper ofyourself, fashion yourself in whatever form you prefer.23. It will be in your power to degenerate into the lower forms of life, which are brutish. Alternatively, you shall have the power, in accordancewith the judgment of your soul, to be reborn into the higher orders, thosethat are divine". (Mirandola 2012, 148)

The aspirations of this manifesto of Humanism began to be consolidated in modernity by René Descartes' *Discourse on Method* (1637) as he envisioned a medicine that would grant humans both a better health, a stronger mind and a way to god. Science and morality and religion were joined in this 17th century early Enlightenment, which combined critical reason with religious revelation, as confirmed by Isaac Newton.

We could carry on Bostrom's description of humanity's dream to transcend humanity, but it would miss the major point argued by him and transhumanists in general. They argue that contemporary science – and its twin sister, contemporary technology – changed everything about the human future. They argue that the exponential acceleration of computer science and nanotechnology in the 21st century transformed humans and non-humans. They argue that we are about to reach singularity, the moment in history when artificial intelligence will overcome human intelligence (AA. VV. 2017 and AA. VV. 2012).

The conversation about singularity began almost 70 years ago. The mathematician Stanislaw Ulam wrote in 1958 about John von Neumann: "Our conversation centered on the ever-accelerating progress of technology and in the changes in the human way of life, which seems to be approaching an essential singularity in the history of the race beyond which the human affairs, as we know them, could not continue". (Ulam 1958, 5)Gordon E. Moore stated in 1965 that the number of transistors on a chip grows exponentially over the years. The so-called "Moore's Law" states that computing power doubles roughly every two years. Ray Kurzweil claims that he documented similar rates of exponential growth in other technologies. Transhumanists such as Marvin Minsky, Hans Moravec, Ray Kurzweil, and Nick Bostrom indicated that singularity would be attained sometime in the first half of our 21st century.

The singularity hypothesis states that technological changes will lead to some sort of discontinuity in human history through self-improving artificial intelligence. In 1965 I.J. Good formulated its usual "mantra": continued progress in artificial intelligence could lead to the creation of machines that think in the same general way as humans. "Define an ultra-intelligent machine as a machine that can overcome by far all the intellectual activities of any man, no matter how smart he is. Since machine design is one of these intellectual pursuits, an ultra-intelligent machine could design even better machines; Unquestionably, then there would be an "intelligence explosion", and man's intelligence would be much behind. Therefore, the first ultra-intelligent machine will be man's last invention".[3] Vernor Vinge discussed this idea in more detail in a 1993 article: "Within thirty years we will have the technological means to create intelligence superhuman. Soon after, the human age will end".[4]

Another big driver of transhumanist ambitions is nanotechnology. In its mature form, it could help us abolish most diseases and aging, makingit possible to "revivify" patients maintained in cryogenics, allowing colonization of space, and leading to the creation of arsenals of lethal weapons. In 1986, Eric Drexler published *Engines of Creation*, an exposition of molecular engineering. His subsequent book, *Nanosystems* (Drexler 1992), provides a more technical analysis. In recent years, helped by big business, nanotechnology is providing spectacular advances in Medicine. (Moriarty 2022)

"Transevangelists" (Vidigal 2012) are interested in the augmentation of the self, the enhancement of socicty and better governance. Transhumanist missionaries are of another kind. In 1962, Robert Ettinger published *The Perspective of Immortality*, launching the idea of cryogenic suspension. However, the technology did not become popular. Another transhumanist,

---

3 Good 1965, https://www.historyofinformation.com/detail.php?id=2142. Stanley Kubrick consulted Good regarding aspects of computing and artificial intelligence when filming 2001: A Space Odyssey (1968), one of whose principal characters was the paranoid HAL 9000 supercomputer.

4 Vinge 1993, https://historyofinformation.com/detail.php?id=2141.

FM Esfandiary, who later changed his name to FM-2030, formed a group of optimists known as *Up Wingers. Are you a transhuman?* (1989) described the signs of the emergence of the "transhuman"; the "transitional human", through technology, cultural values, andlife-styles, constitutes an evolutionary link to the approaching "f-human era". Signs of this transhuman status included prosthetics, plastic surgery, heavy use of telecommunications, cosmopolitan and androgynous lifestyles, mediated reproduction (such as in vitro fertilization), and irreligious, and non-traditional family values. As Nick Bostrom, himself a transhumanist, drily commented: Why someone who, for example, rejects family values, gets rhinoplasty, and spends a lot of time on airplanes is closer to post-humanity than the rest of us?

The pet project of transhumanism is the "upload of the human mind into a computer" whatever this means for the many personalities, institutes, and big money interested in such fantasy. Most science fiction movies and books move around such "mantra": 2001: A Space Odyssey (1968) The Matrix (1999) V for Vendetta (2005), Oblivion (2013), The Giver (2014), Ex-Machina (2014) Multiverse (2021). Posthumanism and Transhumanism Studies, are also driven by the persistent need to develop, update, upgrade and relentlessly move forward such conceptual fantasy.[5] On one side, the gap between sci-fiction and sci-fact, between literary imagination and technoscientific realities, is being bridged and literature can stimulate scientific development, as in the case of Primo Levi's 1966 novel *The Sixth Day and Other Tales* that preceded the actual invention of the 3D printer in the 1980s. On the other side, when aligned with utopianism, Sci-Fi becomes a powerful mass entertainment. The question is how close the huge powers of technology that feed transhumanism are to dystopian nightmares revealed by the tale of the, the sorcerer's apprentice, and Frankenstein.

[5] Bostrom (2011) offers a "description" which is a typical category mistake of the steps for uploading: a) create a rigorous image of a specific human brain, perhaps deconstructing it with nanorobots or inserting thin slices of brain tissue into scanning tube microscopes for automated image analysis; b) from this image, reconstruct the neural network that the brain developed by combining it with computational models of different types of neurons; c) emulate the entire computational structure in a powerful supercomputer. If successful, the original mind, memory, and personality, intact, would be transferred to the computer, where they would exist. Individual transhumanists have different views on these philosophical questions.

What is redundant about Transhumanism? Artificial intelligence and molecular nanotechnology are certainly transforming the human condition as they enable a long menu of achievements: virtual reality; preimplantation genetics; genetic engineering; medicaments for memory, concentration, alertness, and mood; drug performance enhancers; cosmetic surgery; prostheses; anti-aging medicine; closer human-computer interfaces. (Moriarty 2022) Transhumanists want to make these technologies safe and available to anyone, and more relevant in the future. Such agenda is a fancy fueled by a category mistake.

5. Back to Latour and the Turing machine

After this "orgy" of transhumanist projects let us go back to see how Bruno Latour offers a framework to think about singularity and its consequences. As expected, he has an indirect approach to deflate the balloon of transhumanist expectations. He did not elaborate anti-transhumanist arguments; he reminded us that the frontier between humans and no humans is much more complex and richer than we usually imagine. He has no use for the myth of *uploading consciousness into a computer* exactly because this kind of dualistic and double click thought ignores the uncertain boundaries between human and non-human. He brings no less than Alan Turing and Jesus Christ to ground his arguments, or to speak in a more sober way: he analyses the internal limitations of artificial intelligence through a reading of Turing's 1950 famous article about the "imitation game" (Latour 2008); and he deals with the external limitations of singularity through his appropriation of Judeo-Christian religion, notably in his book *Rejoicing*. (Latour 2013b)

The main point of Latour's 2008 article is that science and engineering as well as literature and art have much in common to say about the boundaries of "being human". "Great scientists and great artists bring us closer to a common problem of what it means for entities to exchange properties through the artificial construction of language". (Latour 2008,21) Most readers of Turing's 1950 article, yet ignored its deliberate ambiguity, only retaining the *imitation game* and the first formulation of the human mind as computational and whether machines can think. Now in this article and subsequent lectures, Alan Turing himself considered such question "too meaningless to deserve attention", an amazing indictment of all upload/download approaches of human intelligence and the usual "transhumanist discourse". Put in another way: Turing was not a transhumanist.

Turing's much debated test is still fairly controversial. He apparently chose learning from experience as best approach to achieve machine intelligence and he spent several years with chess-playing to illustrate his conversational question-answering 1950 paper. Some of the epistemological roots of the so-called Turing test – scarcely observed in the secondary literature – came out of a controversy of Turing over the cognitive capabilities of digital computers, with the computer pioneer Douglas Hartree, the philosopher Michael Polanyi, and neurosurgeon Geoffrey Jefferson. Seen from its historical context, Turing's 1950 paper is a reply to a series of challenges posed to him by these thinkers against his view that machines can think. (Gonçalves, 2022)

Now, in the first half of his paper, Latour analyses the American novelist Richard Powers, namely three of his novels: *Galatea 2.2* (1995), *Gain* (1998), and *Plowing the Dark* (2000), a rewarding source of philosophical inspiration. Powers perceives science as James and Whitehead, circumventing the pitfalls of critical discourse. He is not a science-fiction novelist presenting *cyborgs*. As Latour says "typically, cyborgs establish a connection between the average definition of a brain, the average definition of a computer, and the average definition of psychology, and fuse the three together in a classic – sometimes strident – character/background/story amalgamation". (Latour 2008, 3) Powers' characters, on the contrary, are not silhouetted out of a background and inserted into a story; they are hybrids, or beings-as-other. His novels connect and fuse domains of reality:the uncertain deployment of what a computer is; the controversial multiplicity of what a brain is, and the wavering achievements of psychology theyare related in a narrative. Latour appreciates Powers for instauring plausible, fleshy characters, things, and stories, as Balzac had suggested.

Engaging the "imitation game", Latour notes that automata have fascinated human imagination since Antiquity because they *complicate all our ideas about freedom, about the obligatory choice between autonomy and construction*. Anthropomorphic automata were fabricated, since Alexandria to modernity. Descartes observed the automata in the Paris gardens as raising the question of mankind's limits. Richard Powers asks what it means for a character to be realistic; Turing asks the crucial question of what an *automaton* is. The problem is the same since it is never clear what sort of *autonomy* an automaton possesses. We should not be forced by the fundamentalists' dilemma: either it is constructed *or* it is autonomous; we should not forget about mediations or translations.

Latour envisages Turing not just as a mathematician, engineer, and scientist, but also as a *creative thinker*; following his discourse and not only his conclusions, he stresses that Turing was more influenced by the reality of unproved conjecture rather than designating reality through deductive proof. Alongside his mastery of electronical computation and logical calculus, Turing presented persuasively what he was doing.[6]

Turing elaborated his most famous paper – *On Computable Numbers* (1936) – to conceive the computer as an abstract mathematical concept or algorithm. There he gives a negative solution to *Hilbert's decision problem*, thus, showing the intrinsic paradox of automation: it is impossible to systematically predict what a certain function will do before you execute it. Turing's 1950 article, brings the same point in non-mathematical language:

> "The popular view that scientists proceed inexorably from well-established fact to well-established fact, never being influenced by any unproved conjecture, is quite mistaken. Provided it is made clear which are proven facts and which are conjectures, no harm can result. Conjectures are of great importance since they suggest useful lines of research". (Turing 1950, 49)

According to Turing himself, the thought experiment of the "imitation game" creates novelties that no formal description would have predicted and that force us to change our definition of what an automaton is. One of those surprises is that "input" is not a good term to describe what you put "into the machine". Turing heavily criticizes how Ann Lovelace sums up *Babbage's Analytical Engine* in a memoir that is a description of that 19th-century contraption they both created. Ann Lovelace states that 'The Analytical Engine has no pretensions to *originate anything*. It can do "*whatever we know how to order it* to perform (her italics)" (Latour 2008, 17). This is the usual mantra of AI experts "that since all the robot's outputs include nothing but our inputs, it can originate nothing. Such is the normal, usual, reasonable, logical conception of what a computer is and what an input is". (Latour 2008, 17)According to Turing, such silly approach supposes that, from first principles you can "work out the consequences" without

6 While 'the Turing test' is widely known Gonçalves filled the gap of scholarly studies on its genesis (Gonçalves 2022)

surprises. *Turing is saying, in effect, that all formal descriptions of the computer as an input/output logical entity are a category mistake.*

Thus, Latour detects a complex metaphysics of agency in Turing: a computer is not only a calculus machine: it is also an artifact, a thing. Machines and facts – everything and each thing – are born as *things*, not as *objects*. Heidegger, of all people, would have considered a computer as a typical *Gegenstand*(object); he would have reserved his enthusiasm for a "thing" such as Van Gogh's painting of the peasant's boots, or a jug made by hand which mobilizes heaven and earth.

After stating that Turing's 1950 text allows for "*metaphors, tropes, anecdotes, asides and self-description*", Latour creates a new type of Turing test. Can one distinguish between a novel of realist literature and the scientific realism of Turing? If one is sufficiently fooled, then Latour "will have at least indicated that matters of concern might be best accessed through the joint inventions of literature and science". (Latour 2008,20). In his vocabulary "matters of concern" not matters of fact, are the proper object of scientific research. As he says, "It's not true that we live in a world of senseless matters of fact to which the human mind alone would be able to add, through imagination, morality, and sensibility, a little bit of superficial meaning". (Latour 2008,21)

Latour's test terminates any significant difference between "an important scientific text and an important novel" precisely insofar as one cannot distinguish "dealing with demonstrations while the other deals with rhetoric, one dealing with proofs while the other deals with stories[. . .]" (Latour 2008,21). Latour even jokes that Alan Sokal would no doubt have interpreted it as a hoax. It is no wonder that Turing's friend and logician Robin Gandy said of the 1950 essay that, "it was intended not so much as a penetrating contribution to philosophy but as propaganda. Turing thought the time had come for philosophers and mathematicians and scientists to take seriously the fact that computers were not merely calculating engines but were capable of behaviour which must be accounted as intelligent; he sought to persuade people that this was so". (Turing 2004, 433). According to Latour, Humanities should claim Turing as a kindred spirit as, again, he does not support the transhumanist's claims.

6. "Love's labor lost"

Another Latour's approach to the human/non-human complex and convolutive boundaries is through his very personal "variety of religious experience", to borrow William James' formula. His approach strikes a contrast with the usual transhumanist outright rejection of religion: "The modernist tragedy consists of having been mistaken at the same moment, by means of a ricochet, so to speak, about Science and about Religion" (Latour 2013a, 321). Epistemologists get it wrong when they try to define objective knowledge as 'Double Click communication' forgetting that galaxies, microbes, and electrons are only detectable with instruments. "Theology falls in a similar trap [. . .] *forcing theologians to escape faith through a misconception of knowledge*" (Latour 2013a, 305).

When Latour says that "to be religious" is outside the scope of conventional anthropology; he asserts that a 'religious being' is empirically recordable. As an anthropologist, he describes the religious experience through protocols. Its condition of happiness is 'to save, to bring into presence'; its trajectory is to 'engender people'; the instaured beings are 'carriers of presence'; its hiatuses or gaps are 'intervals in time'. Religion is a mode of existence that directs us in a direction opposite of science. Religious discourse does not refer to a remote entity; it makes present 'God', as a person, through love.

In his original French book *Réjubiler*, Latour helps us understand why religion is not about reference but about presentation, as he learned with Charles Péguy. The language of human love is the best way to understand Judeo-Christianity, as attested by *The Song of Songs*. Latour does not speak about other religious traditions because Christianity is the one where he feels at home. He suggests one can find in human love "a kind of prefiguration, a scale model of the conditions of happiness of religious discourse" (Latour 2013b, 118). If a woman asks his partner [or the other way round]:

> "Do you love me?' and the partner replies (without irony) 'Yes, but I told you that last year', it would be difficult to find more decisive evidence that she [or he] has stopped really loving. He took the request for love as a request for information [. . .]. By the quality of the answer, any impartial observer would understand that the lover did not understand anything. The fact is that his girlfriend did not ask if he had loved her, but if he loves her now. That is the request, the supplication, the challenge" (Latour 2013b, 25).

The worn-out cliché "I love you" does not transmit news; the one who says it and the one who hears it, both feel transported, transformed, shaken, altered, and reorganized; if there are no words of love, they feel alienated, flattened, forgotten, mothballed, humiliated. Many sentences uttered every dayare likewise not intended to give reference, but to produce either proximity or distance. (Latour 2013b,26) "Caring is not saving" (Latour 2013a, 304). Latour distinguishes love talk from other forms of producing subjectivity and interiority because it addresses a person, not a self; Then he uses the discourse of love as a model to describe the religious experience, of 'person', 'soul', and 'self'. The religious discourse "has no reference – just like love exchanges" (Latour 2013b,28). Religious speech does not refer to "God, up there in heaven; it does not refer at all; what it does, we can learn by going back to the lovers' dialogue".

The love language is often reduced to words that lost their meaning to a large part of the Moderns, both a) the secularized who defend radical humanism; a) the spiritually minded who do not accept revelation; and atheists and transhumanists against religion.

Latour is sending two distinct messages: to the Moderns who consider themselves religious – as he himself does – and to fully secularized Moderns that reject religion. He warns secularized Moderns, among them transhumanists, that religion is about "making present"; he warns modern religious people that there are better and alternative ways of explaining their experience. In the vocabulary of secularized moderns, there is no place for words like 'God', 'salvation', 'souls', and 'angels'; *'to save' is associated with saving files, not with love.* Latour asks them to think about the discourse of love and then, observe that the affectionate conversation does not ask for anything in return, it does not refer to a substance, to a thing. If someone says, 'I believe in God', he is not referring to a remote entity to which adequate objectivity would give access. 'God' is not an extraterrestrial life form. Religion and science are two totally different modes of existence that should be contrasted.

Latour's message for religious people is "change the current accounts of your experience because they are not convincing". Religious discourse does not refer to the past; there is no "God" to refer to. Religion is not a 'belief' in something. "The word 'God' cannot designate an assumption; it designates, rather, the renewal of a subsistence, constantly at risk [. . .]" (Latour 2013a, 309). God is also a being-as-other. "This [religion] is enlightenment itself: start again, start again, go back to starting point again and again, it repeats itself, improvises, innovates: moreover, it never stops describing itself, self-reflexively, as the Word" (Latour 2013a, 306). It is all about speech, incessant renewal of speech by speech itself, *reprise par excellence*. Péguy had already grasped it, in content and style. "The religious mode should be at home in natural language" (Latour 2013a, 306). "Words that correct must be comprehensible, this is the first condition [of the happiness of religious discourse]; they must be said in the language of the person addressed" (Latour 2013b, 54) – a conclusion that the Roman Catholic Church was slow to adapt; only in 1965 did the Vatican allow the use of the vernacular language *en masse*.

7. What about modernity?

The "modes of existence" enabled Latour to explain the ambivalence of modernity. We must free ourselves from the *fallacy of misplaced concreteness* – denounced by Whitehead – that the so called 'primary qualities' – nuclear particles, chemical elements, etc. – describe nature, matter, the world; and the so-called 'secondary qualities' – are subjective. There are multiple valid forms of human experience, in art, religion, science, law, engineering, literature, and technology. The modernist approach that privileges science as the unique way to the world is only a perpetuation of the gap between humanistic and scientific cultures. All varieties of human experience must be treated in a particular context; they must be redescribed by protocols, to be articulated as different "modes of existence". Latour does not relativize those modes. Their value and form of eloquence must be recorded in their own terms. He does not relativize science, and even less intends it to be "a social construction", "a culture". He is not a postmodernist, nor is he a skeptic or a relativist. He is not downgrading the value of science; he upgrades what moderns cherish – human rights, health, scientific progress.

Latour's whole endeavor leads to a reappraisal of modernity. In accounting for their values and institutions, Moderns become confused when they talk about different "cultures" allowing for conflicting views about the same "substance". Moderns become totally confused when they consider science as just another 'culture', one that by its 'half rationality' cannot account for all the other values they hold dear.

Moderns are at a loss to describe their own values. Appraising Ulrich Beck's social theory as one of the most relevant forms of sociology developed in recent years, Latour thinks that Beck misunderstood the problems we are confronted with. Beck thinks that contemporary problems have emerged because society has changed; according to Latour the crisis of modernity is much more profound: we can no longer live with our self-image as Moderns.

What is this self-image? Until the middle of the 20th century, the answer seemed clear. "We" – meaning the people of Europe and the Westernized world – self-consciously declared ourselves to be Modern, that is, no longer bound by traditional social practices and values. To be enlightened, in Kant's words, was *to be released from man's self-incurred tutelage*. Science enabled us to control nature, we thought; democracy and the rule of law guaranteed political freedoms, we thought; economic growth would allow prosperity for the greater number, we thought. These keystones defined societies as 'modern'; but they hide an ambivalence. Latour proposes a new picture of modernity, an alternative account of its values and institutions. He registers constraints, and complaints and he detects category mistakes through rough key concepts of hiatus, trajectory, conditions of happiness, beingwith-other and instauration. Once the values of modernity are identified, Moderns will be less confused and in a better position to present themselves before others – pre-moderns and post-moderns; transhumanists will be confronted with their category mistake and the error of maintaining dualities without mediations. However loud and clear the transhumanist diagnoses may sound, they repeat the non-mediated dualities characteristic of Émile Durkheim and Max Weber, exposing the profiles of industrial societies. Latour managed to answer in his 2013 book the questions about modernity he left unanswered in the 1993 book. "If we were never modern, what happened to us? What should we inherit? Who have we been? Who are we going to become? Who should we connect with? Where will we be from now on?" (Latour 2013a, 11).

He raises these questions in the context of what he perceives as an existential crisis, of humanity and of the planet. At the beginning of the 21st century, we face ourselves and our planet, with 'Gaia' (no New Age undertones) "a stranger figure doubly composed of science and mythology used by certain specialists to designate the Earth that surrounds us and that we surround" (Latour 2013a, 9). We need a better diagnosis of our situation, a more realistic description of Modern values, a "comparative analysis" of the anthropology of the Moderns instead of contrasting "Us, Moderns" with "Them", other peoples".

What comes out of Latour's new reading of modernity? What should we keep from the pre-moderns who esteemed religion? And of the moderns who gave us human rights and scientific progress? And what about the deconstruction and constructivism in post-moderns? Latour (1993, 135 [fig. 5.1]) summarizes his conclusions:

	What is retained	What is rejected
From the moderns	- Long networks - Size - Experimentation - Relative universals - Final separation between objective nature and free society	- Separation between nature and society - Clandestineness of the practices of mediation - External Great Divide - Critical denunciation - Universality - Rationality
From the pre-moderns	- non-separability of thing and signs - transcendence without a contrary - multiplication of non-humans - temporality by intensity	- obligation always to link the social and natural orders - scapegoating mechanism - ethnocentrism - territory - limits on scale
From the post moderns	- Multiple times - Constructivism - Reflexivity - Denaturalization	- Belief in modernism - Critical deconstruction - Ironic reflexivity - Anachronism

We are distant from the Ancients, or pre-moderns, due to our Great Division between nature and society, an extension of the inner Great Division between mind and matter. Yet, as contemporary science imploded this inner division, the outer division also disappeared, replaced by timescale differences. Anthropology and Comparative History allow us to understand the pre-moderns in a better way. Pre-modern collectivities were accused by Moderns of mixing things, creating scapegoats, and ethnocentrism. We no longer feel constrained by their totems and taboos, although we do not adopt them anymore, as we understand their intentions: non-separability of things and signs; transcendence without a contrary; multiplication of collectivities; and an intense feeling of temporality.

What should we keep from the Moderns, asks Latour? A lot, but not trust in modernity itself. The legacy of modernity is the proliferation of hybrids, expanded networks, and multiple vestiges, produced through successive approximations. Modernity may have been mechanistic, but it created human rights, giving dignity to each individual, and increasingly freed mankind from servile labor through technical wonders. The audacity, innovation, bricolage, and wide scale of action of the Moderns enabled the creation of a world of useful tools that enhance human life. On the other hand, we cannot keep the illusions of generality, the illusion of pure objectivity, pure critique, or historicism, i.e, modernism triumphant. Such illusions of modernism separate society from nature and keep the subject at war with himself.

Post-moderns – as expressed by the Frankfurt School, French Postmodernism, and Transhumanism – deserve scrutiny because they know how to express the crisis of Modernity. Latour writes that *if we take from post-moderns what they think about the moderns, their vices become virtues, non-modern virtues*. What to Latour seems inadequate is the post-modern despair, discouragement, nihilism, and self-criticism; all these characteristics are dependent upon a misplaced conception of Modernity, never taken seriously or practiced; the overall optimism and triumphalism of transhumanists is a mirror attitude of the depressed post-modernists and inadequate, too. It is important to stick with deconstruction; if it becomes constructivism, it is no longer linked to self-destruction; the refusal of naturalism is good – nature being recognized as complex. This refusal does not distance us from science but brings us closer to it. We can retain a strong taste for reflexivity if it is shared by everyone, and it loses its parody deficiencies. The post-modern refusal of a coherent and homogeneous time is good – if we do fall into anachronism.

8. Some conclusive hints

It is easy to agree with transhumanists that the increasing pace of technology is radically transforming the human condition in the 21st century. This reality imposes the duty to think about future scenarios and to work out ethical implications. It is easy to agree with transhumanists that new technologies bring huge medical possibilities for the enhancement of human life, provided the side effects are controlled. Transhumanists emphasize the enormous potential for genuine improvements in human well-being that can be achieved through technological transformation. We should appreciate more the fact that we can derive great value from venturing beyond our limitations and certainly consider it a crime against humanity to proceed without a thorough risk analysis and the instauration of adequate ethical and legal guarantees.

What transhumanism should not do is distract us from the way every and each thing enters our world, including nanotechnology and computers, as well as literature and religion. The boundaries between humans and non-humans are constantly being redesigned in a convolutive way, as Bruno Latour's anthropology shows. The debate about human values eroded by technological advances is a misplaced formulation of the evolution of humanity, a consequence of the category mistake that Bruno Latour identifies in modernity. Latour's philosophy clearly offers a "changed attitude because he asks us to change the common sense of the Moderns, on nature, science, politics, religion, and society. He is not the only 20th philosopher who has realized that an alternative is required. What makes Latour stand out is that he has formulated not only the philosophical groundwork of an alternative worldview but also has offered the means to empirically explore it.

References

AA. VV. 2017. *Futuros No limiar da autodeterminação da inteligência artificial.* Lisboa: APDSI.

AA. VV. 2012. *Beyond Artificial Intelligence: The Disappearing Human-Machine Divide.* Eds. Romportl, J., Zackova, E., and Kelemen, J. Springer International Publishing.

Beck, U., A. Giddens & S. Lash. 1994. *Reflexive Modernization – Politics, Tradition and Aesthetics in the Modern Social Order*. Cambridge: Polity.

Bernal, J. D. 1969. *The world, the flesh & the devil; an enquiry into the future of the three enemies of the rational soul*. Bloomington: Indiana University Press.

Bostrom, N. 1998. How long before superint *elligence*? *International Journal of Futures Studies*, 2(1): 1–9.

Bostrom, N. 2003. Are you living in a computer simulation? *Philosophical Quarterly*, 53(211): 243–255.

Bostrom, N. 2011. Una historia del pensamiento transhumanista. *Argumentos de Razón Técnica*, 14(1): 157–191.

Bostrom, N. 2014. *Superintelligence: Paths, Dangers, Strategies*. Oxford: Oxford University Press.

Capek, K. 2004. *R.U.R. (Rossum's universal robots). Penguin classics*. London: Penguin Books.

Darwin, C. 2003. *The origin of the species. Barnes & noble classics*. New York: Fine Creative Media.

De Vries, G. 2016. *Bruno Latour*. Cambridge, UK: Polity Press.

Drexler, K. E. 1985. *Engines of creation: the coming era of nanotechnology*. London: Forth Estate.

Drexler, K. E. 1992. *Nanosystems: molecular machinery, manufacturing, and computation*. New York: John Wiley & Sons, Inc.

Esfandiary, F. M. 1970. *Optimism one; the emerging radicalism*. New York: Norton.

Ettinger, R. C. W. 1972. *Man into Superman; the startling potential of human evolution – and how to be part of it*. New York: St. Martin's Press.

Floridi, L. 2010. *The Cambridge Handbook of Information and Computer Ethics*. Cambridge: CUP.

FM-2030. 1989. *Are you a transhuman?: monitoring and stimulating your personal rate of growth in a rapidly changing world*. New York, NY: Warner Books.

Gonçalves, B. 2022. Can machines think? The controversy that led to the Turing test, 1946–1950. *AI & SOCIETY*,38(6): 2499–2509.

Good, I. J. 1965. Speculations concerning the first ultraintelligent machine. *Advances in Computers*, 6(1): 31–88.

Haldane, J. B. S. 1924. *Daedalus; or, science and the future*. London: K. Paul.

Hayles, N. Katherine N. 1999. *How We Became Posthuman: Virtual Bodies in Cybernetics, Literature, and Informatics*, Chicago, Chicago U. Press.

Henriques, M. 2022. O futuro da democracia na era digital. In: *APDSI. Sociedade da Informação. 20 anos de promoção e desenvolvimento*, pp. 72–80. Lisboa: Sílabo.

James, W. 1996 [1912]. *Essays in Radical Empiricism*. Lincoln and London: the University of Nebraska Press.

Huxley, A. 1932. *Brave new world*. London: Chatto & Windus.

Huxley, J. 1927. *Religion without revelation*. London: E. Benn.

Kurzweil, R. 1999. *The age of spiritual machines: when computers exceed human intelligence*. New York: Viking.

Latour, B. 1977 (French); 1984 (English). *Les microbes – guerre et paix suivi de Irréductions*. Paris: Éditions A. M. Métailié.

Latour, B. 1993. *We Have Never Been Modern*. Cambridge (Mass.): Harvard University Press.

Latour, B. 2008. The Powers of Fac Similes : a Turing Test on Science and Literature application. In:S. J. Burn & P. Demsey (eds.), *Intersections Essays on Richard Powers*, p. 263–292. Dalkey Archive Press.

Latour, B. 2013a. *An Inquiry into Modes of Existence – An Anthropology of the Moderns*. Cambridge (Mass.): Harvard University Press.

Latour, B. 2013b. *Rejoicing – Or the Torments of Religious Speech*. Cambridge: Polity.

Latour, B. & S. Woolgar. 1979. *Laboratory Life – The Social Construction of Scientific Facts*. Beverly Hills and London: Sage Publications.

Latour, B. & S. Woolgar. 1986. *Laboratory Life – The Construction of Scientific Facts*. 2nd ed. Beverly Hills and London: Sage Publications.

Moriarty P. 2022. *Nanotechnology A Very Short Introduction*. Oxford: Oxford University Press.

Moore, G. E. 1965. Cramming more components onto integrated circuits. *Electronics*, 38(8): 114–118.

More, M. 2003. *Principles of extropy, Version 3.11* 2003. [online]. http://www.extropy.org/principles.htm.

Oliveira, A. 2019. *Inteligência Artificial*. Lisboa: Fundação FMS.

Orwell, G. 1949. *Nineteen eighty-four, a novel*. New York: Harcourt.

Pico della Mirandola, G. 2012. *Oration on the dignity of man*. Cambridge, Cambridge U.P.

Russell, B. 1924. *Icarus; or the future of science*. London: K. Paul, Trench, Trubner& Co., ltd.

Ryle, Gilbert 1949*The Concept of Mind*, Chicago, Chicago U. Press

Shelley, M. W. 1818. *Frankenstein; or, the modern Prometheus*. London: Lackington, Hughes, Harding, Mavor, & Jones.

Tegmark, M. 2019. *Life 3.0, Ser-se Humano Na Era da Inteligência Artificial*. Lisboa: D. Quixote

Turing, A. 1950. Computing machinery and intelligence. *Mind*, 59: 433–460.

Turing, A. 2004. *The Essential Turing*. Edited by B. Jack Copeland, Oxford, Clarendon Press

Ulam, S. M. 1986. John von Neumann 1903–1957. In: *Ulam, S. M., Reynolds, M. C., & Rota, G. C., Science, computers, and people: from the tree of mathematics*. Boston: Birkhäuser, 169–214.

Vidigal, L. 2012. *Questões epistemológicas e ontológicas para o estudo do e-government. Do ato ao pensamento*, ISCSP / CAPP. Lisboa: Universidade de Lisboa.

Vinge, V. 1993. The coming technological singularity. *Whole Earth Review*, Winter issue. https://www.aleph.se/Trans/Global/Singularity/sing.html

CULTURAL AND IDEOLOGICAL PERSPECTIVES

Intersections of Transhumanism with Cultural Ideologies and Ethical Systems

THE OPPORTUNITIES AND CHALLENGES OF TRANSHUMANISM: INSIGHTS FROM CONFUCIAN PHILOSOPHY AND ANTROPOLOGY

Dong Tai Nguyen

1. Introduction

Transhumanism changes our view of human potential and limits. Transhumanism advocates the enhancement of human capacities through biotechnology and artificial intelligence, which goes against traditional humanistic beliefs. This study examines the dynamic relationship between transhumanism's lofty goals and Confucian anthropology's profound discoveries. Transhumanism's use of technology to overcome biological limitations poses important ethical and philosophical problems. These problems challenge the very nature of humanity, a question central to modern and ancient philosophy.

With millennia of thinking and practice, Confucian anthropology presents a complex tapestry of ideas on human nature, society roles, and ethics. This school of thinking offers a distinct perspective on transhumanism. Confucianism emphasizes morality, collective harmony, and balancing individual demands with societal requirements, in contrast to transhumanism's individualism and technology. This study juxtaposes these two realms to understand the difficulties of this modern technological revolution and find a balance between technology and tradition.

This paper argues that transhumanism offers unparalleled chances for human advancement and the ability to cure some of humanity's most pressing problems, but it also raises serious ethical and philosophical issues. This study proposes that Confucian anthropology, which emphasizes moral development and societal harmony, might give ethical standards and a framework for comprehending transhumanism's human effects. By combining Confucian and transhumanist values, we can navigate this new frontier's ethical environment while respecting human dignity and scientific development.

This paper compares transhumanism and Confucian anthropology using comparative analysis. Philosophical literature, historical studies, and current scholarly discussions must be critically examined. The paper uses mixed techniques to examine the similarities and differences between these two perspectives using qualitative analysis and philosophical argumentation. Comparative analysis helps explain how Confucian ideas may influence transhumanism's ethics. By using Postmodernism, Utilitarianism, Systems Theory, and Social Constructivism, this paper's analysis becomes more complex. Postmodernism may challenge large narratives and ideologies like transhumanism's techno-utopian vision and illuminate Confucian philosophy's cultural and historical contexts. Utilitarianism helps analyze the ethical implications of transhumanism, notably the pros and cons of human enhancement technologies. Systems Theory is used to examine these philosophical ideologies' intricate relationships and their effects on persons and civilizations. Finally, Social Constructivism highlights how transhumanist and Confucian philosophy is impacted by societal structures and beliefs.

This approach allows a full examination of transhumanism's prospects and difficulties through Confucian anthropology's wide and varied lens. It analyzes transhumanism's philosophical, ethical, and societal aspects and critically evaluates its consistency with and departure from Confucian values. Creating a balanced discourse that appreciates technology's revolutionary potential while rooting it in ethical and human-centered principles is the goal.

This study argues that while transhumanism provides revolutionary ways to enhance and evolve humans, it also faces enormous ethical and philosophical issues that Confucian anthropology might help solve. Transhumanism's technocentric focus is balanced by Confucianism's emphasis on morality, societal harmony, and human goodness. This study proposes that transhumanist ideals and Confucian ethics can lead to a more ethical and humanistic approach to technological growth. The overall idea is that such a synthesis enhances human enhancement discourse and encourages a more comprehensive and balanced view of human progress in the age of advanced technology.

2. Transhumanism: Definition and Historical Overview

Transhumanism emerges as a revolutionary movement aspiring to transcend human biological limitations through technological means (Manzocco 2019, 1–2). This ideology envisions a future where humans, augmented by technologies such as nanotechnology and gene therapy, could surpass their current capabilities, potentially achieving what has long been perceived as the ultimate human aspiration: immortality (Huxley 1957, 17).

At the existential core of transhumanism lies the quest to overcome human vulnerabilities, notably the inevitability of death. This timeless human desire for prolonged life, enhanced health, and superior intellectual capabilities, while not new, finds a unique expression in the current era where science and technology promise tangible paths to these once-elusive aspirations.

The philosophical roots of transhumanism can be traced back to the Renaissance, particularly to Giovanni Pico della Mirandola's influential work, "Oration on the Dignity of Man" (1486). Mirandola portrayed humans as beings capable of transcending their earthly bounds and reaching towards divine-like existence, a concept echoed in Dante's notion of 'transumanar' in his "Divina Commedia – Paradiso", symbolizing the transcendence of the human condition (Mirandola 2012; Manzocco 2019, 2).

Julian Huxley, an evolutionary biologist, officially coined the term 'transhumanism' in 1957. Huxley's perspective encapsulates the essence of the movement: humanity not only evolving but transcending itself by realizing new possibilities of human nature (Huxley 1957, 17).

Nick Bostrom, a pivotal figure in contemporary transhumanist thought, presents the ideology as an extension of secular humanism and Enlightenment values. In his work, Bostrom advocates that human nature is improvable through rational methods, foreseeing a future where human health-span, intellectual and physical capacities, and control over mental states are significantly enhanced through scientific and technological means (Bostrom 2013, 28–53).

The evolution of transhumanism is also marked by the establishment of several organizations and groups dedicated to its promotion and development:

a) **Humanity+**: Originally the World Transhumanist Association, it focuses on promoting transhumanism within political and academic spheres. Their manifesto envisions broadening human potential by overcoming aging, cognitive shortcomings, and our confinement to planet Earth (Humanity+ 2012).
b) **The Extropy Institute**: Founded in the early 1990s, it played a crucial role in shaping transhumanist thought before dissolving in 2006 due to unmet objectives.
c) **The Terasem Movement**: Aims to create a 'trans-religion' centered around the concept of self-replicating machines, exploring the intersection of technology and spirituality.
d) **Institute for Ethics and Emerging Technologies**: Affiliated with Humanity+, this institute publishes the Journal of Evolution and Technology, contributing to the academic discourse on transhumanism.
e) **Future of Humanity Institute**: Aligned with the University of Oxford, this institute delves into the broader implications of technological advancements for humanity's future.
f) **Methuselah and SENS Research Foundations**: Both founded by Aubrey De Grey, these organizations focus on research and initiatives aimed at prolonging human life.
g) **Foresight Institute**: Advocates for research in nanotechnology, biotechnology, and longevity, exploring the frontiers of technological advancement.
h) **Center for Responsible Nanotechnology**: Concentrates on the socio-ethical dimensions of nanotechnology, highlighting the need for responsible innovation.
i) **Machine Intelligence Research Institute**: Dedicated to the development of benign artificial intelligence, ensuring AI advancements are safe and beneficial for humanity.
j) **Singularity University**: Despite its name, this institution is not a university in the traditional sense but offers specialized courses and programs that align with transhumanist objectives.

These organizations, along with others such as the Acceleration Studies Foundation, Alcor and Her Sisters, Ascender Alliance, and Biocurious& Co, form a vibrant ecosystem that shapes and influences the transhumanist landscape, each contributing in its unique way to the advancement of this transformative ideology.

3. Ethical and Philosophical Dimensions of Transhumanism

Transhumanism, at its core, grapples with profound ethical dilemmas that strike at the heart of our understanding of life, identity, and the human condition. Julian Huxley's vision of humanity transcending its biological and cognitive limitations through technology outlines a future where the boundaries of human existence are radically redefined (Huxley 1957, 17). This transcendence, as envisioned by Huxley, is not merely physical but also intellectual and spiritual, suggesting a fundamental transformation of the human experience.

Nick Bostrom, a leading thinker in the field, extends this vision by advocating for the possibilities of a posthuman future. In his view, transhumanism represents a natural extension of human progress, a step towards realizing our full potential through the enhancement of our physical and cognitive abilities (Bostrom 2013, 28–53). Bostrom's perspective is rooted in a profound optimism about the role of technology in overcoming our innate limitations, including aging, disease, and even death.

However, this optimistic view of transhumanism is not without its detractors. Francis Fukuyama, among others, raises critical concerns about the impact of such radical transformations on human dignity and the fabric of society (Fukuyama 2003, 42–43). Fukuyama's critique centers on the notion that transhumanism, in its quest to enhance and extend human capabilities, might inadvertently erode the very essence of what it means to be human. The pursuit of immortality, the alteration of cognitive functions, and the potential creation of disparate classes of beings – enhanced versus unenhanced – pose significant risks to the equality and dignity inherent in the human experience.

Moreover, the transhumanist movement raises fundamental questions about the nature of evolution itself. The idea of directing our evolutionary trajectory through technological means represents a paradigm shift from natural selection to a more deliberate, design-oriented approach. This shift brings with it a host of ethical considerations, including the responsibility of making decisions that could irrevocably alter the human species.

The central tension in transhumanism thus lies in the delicate balance between the pursuit of advanced capabilities and the preservation of inherent human qualities. As we stand at the precipice of potentially revolutionary technological advancements, this balance becomes increasingly crucial. The lure of transcending human limitations – achieving enhanced intelligence, physical prowess, and even immortality – presents a seductive vision of the future. However, it also raises profound questions about the essence of human identity and the ethical boundaries of such enhancements.

4. Confucian Anthropology: Insights into Human Nature

Confucian anthropology, with its roots steeped in moral philosophy, presents a compelling contrast to transhumanism. Central to Confucian thought is the belief that while human nature is innately similar, it diverges substantially through practice and cultivation (Confucius, The Analects, Yang Hua). This divergence is not merely a consequence of biological predispositions but is significantly influenced by moral and ethical choices.

4.1. Confucius and His Conceptualization of Human Nature

Confucius, a seminal figure in Eastern philosophy, posited a nuanced view of human nature. One poignant illustration comes from 'Nan Hua Jing' by Chuang Tzu, where Confucius' disciple, Zi Gong, encounters a gardener resistant to mechanical innovation. The gardener's response highlights a fundamental Confucian principle: the importance of maintaining a natural, unadulterated connection with the Dao, or the ultimate truth. This story underscores the Confucian preference for simplicity and harmonious existence with nature, diverging markedly from transhumanism's reliance on technological augmentation (Nguyen 1994, 280).

Confucius himself stated, "By nature, men are nearly alike; by practice, they get to be wide apart". This aphorism encapsulates the Confucian view that while humans share a common nature at birth, their paths diverge due to their choices and actions. This inherent similarity lays the foundation for universal equality, untethered by societal status or intellectual capability, with moral rectitude being the distinguishing factor (Confucius, The Analects, Yang Hua).

4.2. Mencius and the Intrinsic Goodness of Human Nature

Mencius, another pivotal figure in Confucianism, advanced the idea of intrinsic human goodness. He argued that human nature, imbued with qualities like benevolence, righteousness, propriety, and wisdom, is fundamentally good. These virtues are not external additions but are integral to the human psyche. Mencius' philosophy emphasizes the potential for moral development inherent in every individual, a stark contrast to transhumanism's focus on external enhancements (Mencius, Mencius: Gao Zi I).

He also distinguished humans from animals based on moral awareness rather than instinctual drives, suggesting that the essence of humanity lies in its moral and ethical dimensions. Mencius postulated that the difference between humans and animals, although subtle, is crucial and resides in the capacity for moral judgment and ethical conduct. He believed that moral sensibilities such as compassion, shame, and respect are innate to humans and form the basis of a virtuous life. This perspective posits that the true nature of humanity is not defined by physical or intellectual capabilities, but rather by the ability to cultivate virtue and wisdom (Mencius, Mencius: Li Lou II).

Mencius' assertion that "benevolence, righteousness, propriety, and wisdom are not infused into us from without" aligns with the Confucian belief in the inherent potential of humans to achieve moral excellence. His teachings emphasize self-cultivation, suggesting that humans can realize their innate goodness through introspection, learning, and ethical behavior. This intrinsic approach to human development, focusing on internal moral and ethical growth, forms a stark contrast to the transhumanist emphasis on enhancing human capabilities through external technological means. Moreover, Mencius' philosophy underscores the importance of preserving one's inherent human qualities in the face of external influences and temptations. In the modern context, this can be seen as a call to maintain our core human values and ethics in an era increasingly dominated by technological advancements and artificial enhancements. Mencius' teachings thus provide a foundational ethical framework within which the implications of transhumanism can be critically examined and assessed.

This gives us good reasons to claim that Mencius' insights into human nature present a compelling argument for the intrinsic goodness and moral potential of humanity, emphasizing the importance of ethical cultivation over physical or technological enhancement. This perspective offers a vital counterpoint to transhumanist ideals, highlighting the enduring relevance of Confucian thought in contemporary ethical debates surrounding human enhancement and technological progress.

5. Intersecting Visions: Transhumanism and Confucianism

The juxtaposition of transhumanism and Confucianism initiates a multifaceted dialogue, juxtaposing the former's pursuit of technological transcendence against the latter's commitment to moral integrity and societal cohesion. Transhumanism, with its visionary aspirations for human evolution through biotechnological means, inherently challenges the Confucian ethos, which places paramount importance on ethical conduct, social harmony, and the cultivation of virtues.

Transhumanism's emphasis on extending human capabilities, potentially to the point of achieving immortality, directly confronts Confucian ideals. This ambition to transcend human biological limits not only raises fundamental ethical questions but also poses a threat to the intrinsic human values championed by Confucian thought. The pursuit of immortality and superhuman abilities, as espoused by transhumanist philosophy, risks diminishing the significance of core human qualities such as compassion, humility, and righteousness. Francis Fukuyama, in his critique of transhumanism, underscores this potential erosion of human dignity and the destabilization of societal norms, cautioning against the unbridled advancement of human capabilities without ethical constraints (Fukuyama 2003, 42–43).

Confucianism, with its focus on the cultivation of personal virtue and social responsibility, offers a critical lens through which to view and potentially temper transhumanist ambitions. It advocates for a holistic approach to human development, one that balances technological progress with moral and ethical considerations. This Confucian perspective emphasizes the importance of maintaining a harmonious relationship between humanity and the natural order, suggesting that true human advancement lies not solely in physical or cognitive enhancement, but in the nurturing of moral wisdom and ethical conduct.

The intersection of these two philosophical realms calls for a nuanced approach that respects the transformative potential of technology while ensuring that it serves the greater good of society. This balanced approach would integrate the innovative aspirations of transhumanism with the ethical and humanistic principles of Confucianism. It invites a dialogue that does not merely accept technological advancements as an end in themselves but rather views them as a means to further human flourishing within the bounds of moral and societal norms. So we can see that the interplay between transhumanism and Confucianism presents an opportunity to reexamine the goals of human enhancement. It prompts a thoughtful consideration of how emerging technologies can be harnessed not just for physical or intellectual augmentation, but also for the enhancement of moral and ethical understanding. In this dialogue between transhumanism and Confucianism, there is an opportunity to explore how technological advancements can be aligned with the Confucian values of harmony, balance, and the betterment of society as a whole.

This intersection challenges us to reconsider the goals and implications of human enhancement. While transhumanism advocates for overcoming human limitations and expanding capabilities, Confucianism invites a reflection on the nature of these enhancements and their impact on human virtues and societal ethics. The pursuit of immortality and superhuman abilities, as envisaged by transhumanists, raises critical questions about the essence of human life and the moral boundaries of our existence. Confucianism, with its focus on the cultivation of personal virtues and social ethics, offers a framework to assess these developments, ensuring that technological progress does not come at the cost of losing sight of what it means to be human. Moreover, this juxtaposition encourages an examination of how technology can be employed to foster ethical growth and societal well-being, in line with Confucian ideals. Instead of viewing technological advancement and moral development as mutually exclusive, this perspective suggests a synergistic approach where technology is used as a tool to enhance human virtues, promote social harmony, and contribute to the common good.

6. Addressing Transhumanism Challenges through Confucian Ethics

Confucianism can provide a framework to address the ethical challenges posed by transhumanism. It advocates for prioritizing ethical considerations over biological enhancements and accepting the change in human nature while preserving core human values (Chavalier and Gheerbrant 1997, 957). Confucianism's emphasis on societal harmony and individual moral development offers insights into creating a society where transhuman advancements coexist with traditional human values, ensuring that technological progress does not compromise ethical standards and social responsibilities.

6.1 Prioritizing Ethics over Biology

The rise of transhumanism, with its radical emphasis on surpassing human limitations through technology, collides with core Confucian tenets, posing significant ethical and societal challenges. Confucianism stresses moral consciousness over biological attributes, countering transhumanism's prioritization of biological enhancement. Confucianism's foundational belief in 'learning to be human' through education and self-cultivation contrasts with transhumanism's reliance on genetic modification and technological augmentations, which could marginalize those without enhancements. Furthermore, the potential disruption of family structures in a transhumanist society challenges the bedrock of Confucian morality, emphasizing the need to maintain societal and familial harmony in the face of technological progress.

6.2 The Notion of Static Human Nature Redefined as a Dynamic Concept

The dynamic nature of human nature, as discussed in Marxist philosophy and Buddhism, offers a flexible framework to understand the transformative potentials of transhumanist technologies. These perspectives suggest that human nature is not a fixed, unchangeable essence, but rather a mutable construct shaped by societal interactions and spiritual relations. This fluidity of human nature is crucial to accommodate the ethical and societal implications of transhumanism.

6.3 Bridging Transhumanism and Traditional Ethos

Transhumanism's ambition to advance the human condition through technology presents a challenge to Confucianism's emphasis on cosmic harmony. Confucianism advocates for a holistic connection between humans and the universe, suggesting that true liberation and transcendence lie in aligning with the cosmological order. This perspective is vital in navigating the ethical dilemmas posed by transhumanism, emphasizing the importance of compassion, empathy, and moral integrity. In this context, Confucian teachings offer a counterbalance to the transhumanist pursuit of technologically driven evolution. They remind us that progress should not only be measured in terms of physical or intellectual enhancement, but also in the cultivation of virtues that define our humanity. This includes maintaining respect for the natural order and recognizing the interconnectedness of all things.

Ly Tu Tan's poetic reflections on human and cosmic harmony illustrate this beautifully, suggesting that our technological advancements should not sever our intrinsic ties to the cosmos. Instead, they should enhance our understanding of our place within it, enriching our lives with a deeper sense of purpose and connection. As human individuals and societies grapple with the rapid advancements in technology, Confucianism's emphasis on moral integrity and social responsibility provides a framework for ensuring that these innovations are used ethically and for the greater good. The challenge lies in creating a symbiotic relationship between transhumanism and traditional ethos, where technological progress is harmonized with our moral and ethical responsibilities.

7. Conclusion

By examining transhumanism through the lens of Confucian anthropology, this study has investigated both the opportunities and the challenges that it presents. Despite the fact that transhumanism ushers in new frontiers in human growth and capabilities, Confucianism functions as an essential ethical framework that enables individuals to manage these advancements. The combination of these philosophies hints at a future in which the advancement of technology maintains a healthy equilibrium with a profound reverence for human nature, the growth of morality, and the maintenance of social harmony. As we move forward into an era of technological capabilities that have never been seen before, the incorporation of Confucian ethical principles has the potential to lead us to a future that is more harmonious and ethically grounded. This is provided that we pay attention to both the opportunities and the challenges that the new age of technology is bringing to us.

References

Bostrom, N. 2003. Human Genetic Enhancements: A Transhumanist Perspective. *The Journal of Value Inquiry*, 37(1): 493–506.

Bostrom, N. 2004. Transhumanism: The World's Most Dangerous Idea? [online]. https://nickbostrom.com/papers/dangerous (accessed June 27, 2023).

Bostrom, N. 2013. Why I want to be a posthuman when I grow up. In: M. More & N. Vita-More (eds.), *The transhumanist reader: Classical and contemporary essays on the science, technology, and philosophy of the human future*. Oxford: John Wiley.

Chavalier, J. & Gheerbrant, A. 1997. *The Penguin Dictionary of Symbols* (Tudienbieutuongvanhoathegioi). Translated by Phạm Vĩnh Cý. Da Nang: Da Nang Publishing House.

Confucius. [n.a.]. *The Analects of Confucius* (Lun Yu 論語). [online]. https://ctext.org/analects/zh (accessed June 27, 2023).

Fukuyama, F. 2003. *Our posthuman future: Consequences of the biotechnology revolution*. New York: Farrar, Straus and Giroux.

Hansell, G. R. & Grassie, W. (ed.). 2011. *H±Transhumanism and Its Critics*. Philadelphia, USA: Metanexus Institute.

Hauskeller, M. 2016. *Mythologies of Transhumanism*: London: Palgrave Macmillan.

Ho Chi Minh. 2005. *Ho Chi Minh's poems* Nghe An: Nghe An Publishing House.

Humanity+. 2012. The Transhumanist Declaration. [online]. https://www.humanityplus.org/the-transhumanist-declaration (accessed June 27, 2023).

Huxley, J. 1957. New Bottles For New Wine, London: Chatto & Windus Ltd.

Huy Bich, T.A.B. 1958. *Imperial Selection of Vietnamese Poetry and Literature, Vol. 2*. Hanoi: Culture Publishing House.

Manzocco, R. 2019. *Transhumanism – Engineering the Human Condition: History, Philosophy and Current Status*. Chichester, UK: Springer International Publishing.

Mencius, M. [n.a.]. (Mengzi 孟子) [online]. https://ctext.org/mengzi/zhs (accessed June 27, 2023).

Mirandola, P.D. 2012. *Oration on the dignity of man: a new translation and commentary*. Cambridge: Cambridge University Press.

Nguyen, D.C. 1992. *The Quintessence of I Ching*. Ho Chi Minh City: Ho Chi Minh city Publishing House.

Nguyen, H.L. 1994. *Chuang Tzu and Nan Hua Jing (Trang Tuvà Nam Hoa Kinh)*. Hanoi: Culture and Information Publishing House.

Nguyen, T. 1971. *Uc Trai Collection (Uc Trai tập), Volume I*. Translated by Hoang Khoi. Sai Gon: Secretary of State for Culture.

The Book of Change. 2023. (I Ching 周易) [online]. https://ctext.org/book-of-changes/zhs (accessed June 27, 2023).

Confucian Concept of Man in the Context of the Fourth Industrial Revolution: Vietnam's Experience

Hung Quang Nguyen

1. Introduction

Confucianism, along with Buddhism and indigenous religions, forms one of the spiritual foundations of Vietnamese people and traditional Vietnamese culture. Confucianism originated 2500 years ago in East Asian agricultural culture and has had a significant influence on Vietnamese society. The fourth industrial revolution, on the other hand, represents the transition into a post-industrial era driven by technological advancements. It is a global phenomenon that presents challenges for all nations, including Vietnam. Given this context, it is pertinent to explore how the concept of human nature and human existence in Confucianism will adapt to the new challenges brought by the fourth industrial revolution. This paper aims to provide initial and suggestive remarks on the topic, highlighting the need for further in-depth studies to gain a more comprehensive understanding. By investigating this issue, we can gain insights into the potential transformations and adaptations that Confucianism may undergo in the face of contemporary changes and developments.

2. The concept of *the Human* in Confucius's *Analects*

There have been numerous books written on the concept of humanness within Confucianism, as it is one of the fundamental categories found in Confucius's texts and teachings. However, this article specifically focuses on the *Analects*. But what exactly is meant by "humanness"? In simple terms, humanness refers to the qualities and characteristics that make a person truly human. According to the Confucian viewpoint, humans are an integral part of the world. While they may hold a significant position within the natural order, they cannot transcend it, and therefore must abide by the laws of nature. The metaphysical question of the origins of the world is not discussed extensively, but it is believed that everything is governed by Heaven. This includes human beings. Even individuals with exceptional talents and intelligence have their limits and cannot surpass the will of Heaven. Every aspect of daily life, from the most basic elements such as life and death, is believed to be subject to the dictates of Heaven (Confucius 1950, 107). In Confucianism, going against human morality is considered to be contrary to nature and is believed to go against the reason of Heaven. Such actions are believed to invite punishment from Heaven. The punishment can be administered at different levels: human punisher, demon punisher and the highest is Heaven punisher because people or demon/ghost can make mistakes, but Heaven will never fail. "The Heaven's net is high and majestic, although it is sparse, but it is difficult to penetrate"(Lao Tzu, chapter 73) is a maxim in the *Tao Te Ching*.

The *Analects* begins as follows:

> "Confucius said, "Is not it amusing for those who study morality and practice daily to become proficient and skillful? If you have friends who are passionate about morality, listen to your voice, and are people of great virtue, and don't mind coming to visit you from afar, wouldn't you be happy? Even though I am an educated and virtuous person, not many people know me. I am not sad or angry because of that, am I not a gentleman?" (Confucius 1950, 5).

Indeed, it is important to distinguish between the word "human" (人) in the sense of a human being and the word "human" (核) in the sense of personality, morality, and virtue. Understanding the concept of humanness in terms of virtue requires clarification. Firstly, humanness is seen as a virtue, an essential quality of a gentleman. Secondly, humanness is understood as the love for fellow human beings. Lastly, humanness involves the cultivation of morality through adherence to rituals. Confucius primarily focused on the socio-ethical aspects of morality rather than other areas of human activity. Humanness is considered a deeply rooted value within the heart of a person. It surpasses worldly temptations, and the contrast between the body and the soul represents the distinction between the mundane and the noble.

However, the expression of humanness is reliant on rituals. Humanness and ritual are not separate; they are interconnected. The relationship between humanness and ritual can be understood as the relationship between the inner and outer aspects of a person. While humanness forms the root, if it is not expressed through ritual, there is no means for people to understand one another. If rituals fail to accurately represent the essence of being human, they become mere formalities, no longer true to their intended purpose, thus diminishing virtue.

Mr. Nhan Uyen asked about humanness. Confucius replied:

> "Being humane is self-restrain, obedience to ritual, that is, overcoming one's lusts and delusions, and following etiquette. On the day that we are stoic, worshiping, on that day people in the world will naturally empathize and follow humane. So humanness is due to me (…) If the beauty is not ritual, we should not look, if the voice is not respectful, we should not listen, if the word is not respectful, we should not speak, if it is not appropriate, we should not do it. Those four things are the items of that humane (…) when leaving the house, they must keep their dignity and respect as if they are about to meet a distinguished guest; when I send people to do public work, I fervently and cautiously (…) No one resent me in the country; At home, no one hates me. That is the happiness of a man who has humanness". (Confucius 1950, 181).

What is humanness? Confucius did not have really a clear definition of this category, but used many expressions to describe different aspects of humanness. "Mr. Phan Tri asked about humanness. Confucius replied, 'Humanness is compassion for people.' Ask about wisdom. He replied: 'Wisdom is knowing, understand people.'" (Confucius 1950, 193). Elsewhere, Confucius explains his understanding of humanness somewhat more clearly. Humanness is not something completely stranger, but close to people, in the conscience and feelings of each person. Love others as you love yourself. Whatever you don't want, don't force others to do it. "Mr. Phan Chi asked about humanness. 'When I'm at home, I keep my face humble; when I go to work, I do it respectfully; When dealing with people, I stay loyal. Even if I go to the Eastern and Northern bands, I still do not give up the three virtues of friendship, respecting, and loyalty; such is man had humanness.'" (Confucius 1950, 207).

Indeed, humanness is closely associated with the qualities and character of a gentleman. A gentleman is considered to be a virtuous and morally upright human being. On the contrary, a petty person is seen as lacking in humanness and moral virtue. A virtuous person acknowledges their errors and feels remorse or repentance for their actions. In contrast, an unrighteous person may show indifference towards their transgressions and continue to engage in immoral behavior. Attaining humanness and becoming a gentleman is considered to be a challenging and rare achievement. "A gentleman never forsakes humanness, even for about a meal! A gentleman is never forgetting humanness, even in a rush, while leaning forward, people are also in accordance with the benevolent (. . .) when observing each person's faults, we can know whether that person has humanness or not". (Confucius 1950, 53)

In the *Analects*, Confucius discusses the concept of humanness (ren) extensively, and its interpretation varies depending on the context. Confucius describes humanness as a stable core or foundation, comparing it to the solidity of a mountain. This suggests that humanness is an inherent quality within individuals that serves as a moral compass. Mr. Hien asked: "If a person has the qualities of being such as eager to win, boasting, resentful, and lustful, but he knows how to hold back, not letting those qualities reveal themselves, can such a person be called humane?" Confucius replied, "To overcome these desires can be called doing difficult things. Whether it is humanness, I am not sure". (Confucius 1950, 215)

Humanness does not stop at an act, nor does it even within a virtue or character of human behavior. Humanness is a noble and invaluable human quality and virtue. "A humane person must have a talent for language; People who have language skills are not necessarily humane. People with humanness have courage; a brave person is not necessarily humane (. . .) A gentleman sometimes fails to act humanely; But I have never seen a petty person who can do humane things". (Confucius 1950, 217)

Confucius emphasized formality, but at the same time criticized the ostentatious, overly formalism that was common among later Confucians. "Whosoever speaks with beautiful words; the face is elaborate, the shape is stylish, the clothes are flashy; He must be a man of low humanness". (Confucius 1950, 5) In order to gain respect from others, it is essential for an individual to conduct themselves in a dignified manner rather than exhibiting a careless attitude towards appearances. The foundation for earning respect lies in self-respect. However, it is crucial to strike a balance and avoid excessive focus on formalities that may overshadow the true essence of one's character. It is important to recognize that individuals should not be solely judged based on their external appearance. This distinction can be observed between Confucius and later generations of Confucians who emphasized the significance of adhering to formalities, prioritizing rituals over human respect, and relying on etiquette instead of humane governance.

The humane aspect of an individual is not external, requiring a search for its acquisition. Rather, it is an inherent virtue that resides within a person. However, this virtue is not automatically present from birth; it must be developed through the process of self-cultivation and cultivation of others. At times, it may necessitate undertaking rigorous practices to attain this virtue. "Humanness is more essential to the people than water and fire. However, I have seen people step on water and fire and die. I have never seen anyone who has ever stepped on virtue and died (. . .) A person who specializes in humanness, whenever he encounters a human thing, he is happy to do it immediately, not yielding to his teacher". (Confucius 1950, 253)

Humanness represents the utmost value within individuals. Without humanness, qualities such as courage or wisdom lose their significance. Furthermore, a person who possesses humanness is characterized by loyalty to their ruler, nobility, and incorruptibility. Virtues such as courage, wisdom, moderation, and integrity are indeed noble manifestations, but they do not necessarily encompass humanness in its entirety. Merely possessing loyalty, honesty, or courage does not automatically denote true virtue. Not everyone who exhibits loyalty adheres to principles of honor and loyalty, nor does every honest official abstain from exploiting the people. Likewise, not all individuals who possess courage demonstrate benevolence or advanced intelligence. These qualities are undoubtedly noble and rare to find in the world. However, individuals who possess these qualities alone may not embody humanness. Those who possess humanness occupy a much higher position than individuals of high virtue. (Confucius 1950, 75)

A humane person can be defined as someone who embodies certain qualities, with honesty and sincerity being essential attributes that align with the inherent nature of human beings. Confucius, in his teachings, does not appear to make a clear distinction between humanness and a humane person. Individuals who possess humanness are not solely focused on their own lives but prioritize setting an example for others as a primary objective. He explained:

> "A humane person is someone who can do the five virtues that are universal in the world. It is from being dignified, having a generous heart, having true faith, being quick to be diligent, being kind and generous. If I am dignified, no one will dare to despise me. If I have a generous heart, I win people's hearts. If I have true faith, people will trust me. If we are quick and diligent, we can do useful work. If I do good deeds, I can command people". (Confucius 1950, 273)

Humanness serves as the foundational and overarching value that encompasses all other virtues. Without humanness, there is a lack of intrinsic worth in this world. It is important to note that individuals who possess knowledge and can comprehend the workings of the heavens do not automatically possess humanness. Similarly, wisdom and courage do not guarantee the presence of humanness either. Humanness is also a vital requirement for rulers to govern their people in a sustainable manner. Ultimately, human life is multifaceted, involving various responsibilities, worries, and challenges. However, it is important to acknowledge that alongside these difficulties, there are also numerous joys and positive experiences to be enjoyed. "A gentleman has three things to fear: fear of the Mandate of Heaven; fear of great people, people of great position, high virtue; fear the teachings of the Saints. Ignorant petty people do not understand the Mandate of Heaven, so they have no fear: they despise great people, they despise the teachings of saints". (Confucius 1950, 263)

A humane person is one who must keep his word, know how to choose friends to keep his dignity, loyalty, and faithfulness:

> "If a gentleman has no self-respect, that means he does not respect his words, gestures and deeds, is not majestic, people do not respect (. . .) Must take loyalty, faithfulness as the goal. You should not be friends with people who are not like you, that is, you must choose friends among those who are educated, moral, and like you. If I make a mistake, I must have the courage to repent". (Confucius 1950, 7).

Confucius frequently mentions and criticizes the opposite of a humane person and a gentleman, which he refers to as petty individuals. These two classes of people possess contrasting moral qualities, akin to water and fire or goodness and badness. Confucius openly expresses disdain for petty individuals, equating them to thieves who scale walls and break through barriers. Their focus lies solely on pursuing fame and personal gain, without consideration for the rights of others. Confucius highlights the stark contrast between gentlemen and petty individuals by employing various dichotomies, such as good and bad, righteousness and self-interest, honor and cunning, glory and infamy, nobility and lowliness, humility and conceit, and more. The world contains numerous noble expressions of human kindness, just as it harbors many forms of evil exhibited by petty individuals. The relationship between virtue and inhumanity is not one of dialectical balance, like yin and yang, but rather an antagonistic and mutually exclusive dynamic. The humane person cannot find any compromise with the petty person. Confucius consistently includes criticism of petty individuals whenever he discusses humane persons. By emphasizing these contrasts and distinctions, Confucius underscores the immense value he places on virtues and those who embody them, while simultaneously expressing disdain for petty and inhumane individuals. This feature of Confucian ethics is evident in the way it presents a strong dichotomy between good and evil, good and bad. In comparison, Western moral conceptions often attribute evil actions to a lack of understanding or knowledge of goodness, as seen in Socrates' perspective, or view evil as an incomplete form of goodness, as argued by Augustine. These differences highlight the distinct nature of Confucian ethical thought.

Confucius identifies the petty person through various manifestations. Externally, they may appear dignified in their attire, but internally they possess a volatile temper. They tend to be talkative and boastful, lacking the ability to uphold what is right. They are also prone to flattery. Initially, their outward appearance can deceive others. The petty person can also be someone who possesses talent, bravery, wisdom, and education, but unfortunately lacks humanness. Becoming a humane person and a gentleman requires constant cultivation in daily actions, gestures, and thoughts, which is a challenging endeavor. On the other hand, it is relatively easy to become a petty person due to the numerous temptations and societal pressures that lead individuals to adopt negative habits. A gentleman governs through principles of kingship, whereas a petty person exercises rule through dominance. A country governed by a gentleman experiences peace and prosperity for its people. In contrast, a country ruled by petty individuals resembles a hellish existence. The nobility of humanity is indescribable, just as there are no words to fully capture the vulgarity exhibited by petty individuals.

Every moral system emphasizes the virtue of filial piety towards one's parents, and Confucius is no exception. He places great importance on filial piety, considering it to be the foremost quality that distinguishes an individual as virtuous. Confucius famously stated, "find a loyal servant in the home of a filial son" (Confucius 1950, 59). Being a filial person is closely intertwined with possessing humanness, as filial piety is considered a fundamental aspect of humanness itself. In the Confucian hierarchy of social and moral values, while humanness is seen as a lofty aspiration attainable only by the truly noble, filial piety holds the utmost significance for all individuals. It serves as a defining characteristic that sets humans apart from animals. Filial piety extends beyond merely serving and caring for one's parents while they are alive; it also involves making sacrifices and demonstrating respect even after their passing.

> "As long as you are children, while your parents are still alive, you must serve them respectfully; when the parents are finished, they must be buried with ceremony; then, when making sacrifices, you must also keep enough politeness to be dignified (. . .) Nowadays, whenever someone sees someone who can take care of his or her parents, someone praises him as a filial person. But animals like dogs and horses, people can keep them too. So, if you don't respect your parents, what's the difference between that and raising animals?" (Confucius 1950, 17–19)

The central focus of Confucius has been a subject of debate among researchers, with differing opinions on whether it lies in humanness, rituals, or another category. The content of the Analects suggests that the primary emphasis is on the human aspect, although rituals and other categories are also reiterated throughout. Humanness is regarded as the foundational principle from which all other virtues emanate. While rituals hold significance, the absence of rituals alone does not negate the presence of humanness. Confucius does place importance on upholding rituals, including the promotion of the legitimacy of hierarchical relationships such as "emperor to emperor, servant to servant". However, he leans more towards the governance of humans based on humane rule rather than strict adherence to etiquette alone.

3. Confucianism in Vietnam: Tradition and at Present

Confucianism was introduced to Vietnam in the first centuries AD, but its profound influence on the spiritual life of the Vietnamese people was not fully realized until later. This occurred during a period of independence, particularly after the establishment of the Le Dynasty (1428–1778), which designated Confucianism as the state religion. The Le Dynasty emerged after a ten-year resistance war against Ming invaders, and upon gaining independence, Vietnam aligned itself culturally and politically with Chinese Confucian traditions. During the 15th century, the influence of Confucianism was primarily concentrated in the capital city of Thang Long (now Hanoi) and its surrounding areas. (Tran 2003, 487–501). The influence of Confucianism continued to expand during the Nguyen Dynasty (1802–1945) in Vietnam. The Nguyen rulers established political institutions that were built upon Confucian moral and political principles. As the dynasty expanded its control southward, the sphere of Confucian influence also extended throughout the Vietnamese territories.

> "In the fifteenth century as well as today, religion, to be precise, ancestor worship, plays an important role in marriage, in building a family (. . .) Indeed, in marriage of Vietnamese people, religion does not come to add another element of pure humanity (. . .) It must be said that marriage, the contract between two men and women, is a part of religion; this is one of the main acts of worship in the family (. . .) The second remark, that is the preeminent role of ancestors in the wedding rituals (. . .) the third point about the nature, about constitutive factors of marriage in Vietnamese. I think that factor is consensus". (Cadiere 2010, 73–74)

Traditional Vietnamese society is undoubtedly a Confucian society. As Tran (1994, 206) correctly observes,

> "Confucianism is a theory based on the family to visualize the world, following the model of a peaceful family to build an ideal society. Humans are therefore generally family people. From the Son of Heaven to the peasants, businessmen, everyone takes cultivation as the root. Everyone's moral cultivation is basically to cultivate the qualities of that family person. The family has received special attention from Confucianism not only because it pays much attention to building the family, upholding the role of the family in social life, but also because it advocates organizing the state and society according to the model family".

Confucianism created the traditional Vietnamese social institution according to the family model. The family was considered the fundamental unit of society, with the broader society seen as one large family. The legacy of Confucianism in Vietnam can be summarized in three main aspects. Firstly, Confucianism contributed to the establishment of a Confucian absolute monarchy in Vietnam, which endured during the Le and Nguyen dynasties from the 15th century until the first half of the 20th century. The principles of Confucianism shaped the political system and governance, emphasizing the importance of hierarchical relationships and the ruler's responsibility to govern with benevolence and virtue. Secondly, Confucianism fostered the development of a scholarly class and a tradition of Confucian education. This led to the creation of a well-educated intellectual elite that perpetuated a long cultural tradition in Vietnam. The values of "respecting teachers and respecting religion" (ton sutrongdao) were deeply ingrained, emphasizing deference to teachers and the cultivation of moral virtues. Thirdly, Confucianism influenced the formation of family institutions centered around ancestor worship. Ancestor veneration, along with the worship of village lords and communal deities, became foundational elements of Vietnamese culture and spirituality. The reverence for ancestors and the preservation of family lineage were integral to maintaining harmony and continuity within society.

Confucianism in Vietnam exhibits distinct characteristics that differentiate it from Confucianism in China. While Confucianism was introduced and took root in Vietnamese society during the Chinese occupation period, its profound influence was primarily felt during the Le dynasty in the 15th century. In terms of doctrine, Confucianism in Vietnam leans towards Song Confucianism but does not adhere strictly to either Song or Han Confucianism in an extreme manner. Vietnamese Confucians incorporated Confucian teachings at different stages, adapting them through a process of "accidental entry" to make them compatible with Mahayana Buddhism and indigenous religions and beliefs. The patriarchal nature of Confucianism was adapted to the matriarchal environment of Vietnam's indigenous culture. This adaptation allowed for greater flexibility and a blending of different cultural influences within the framework of Confucianism. Overall, Confucianism in Vietnam demonstrates a degree of flexibility and adaptation to local cultural and religious contexts.

One of the unique aspects of Confucianism is that it functions as a secular religion, often coexisting and integrating with other religious traditions. In both China and Vietnam, Confucianism is often complemented by Mahayana Buddhism, Taoism, and indigenous religions. In the context of filial piety, which is a central concept in Confucianism, having a successor to carry on the family lineage is considered important. It holds the second position on the hierarchy of values, just after loyalty. Among the three forms of unfilial behavior (not taking care of parents while they are alive, not making sacrifices to them after their passing, and having no successors in the family line), suicide is regarded as the most severe form of unfilial conduct. However, in order to have children and ensure the continuation of the family line, infertile couples may seek help from the Bodhisattva or rely on the assistance of Taoist midwives for a safe childbirth. This illustrates that Confucianism alone cannot fulfill all the religious and spiritual needs, thus necessitating the integration and tolerance of multiple-religious practices. Throughout history, there has never been a period in China or Vietnam where a single religion could exist in isolation. The interplay and integration of Confucianism with other religious traditions have been essential for the religious and cultural landscape of both countries.

Vietnam, being a country situated in both East Asia and Southeast Asia, possesses a cultural identity that encompasses elements of both regions. While it is widely acknowledged that the spiritual foundation of the Tonkinese people draws upon the Chinese "three teachings", credited to Rhodes as the first to document this connection, it is important to recognize that Vietnam also possesses indigenous elements that distinguish it from Chinese culture. These indigenous elements cannot be disregarded when considering the unique characteristics of the Vietnamese culture. (Rhodes 1994, 44) As one moves deeper into the Central and Southern regions, the influences of Champa and Khmer cultures, closely tied to Indian heritage, become more pronounced. However, it's crucial not to overlook the significance of indigenous Southeast Asian beliefs. These local beliefs mold and adapt external cultural influences entering the region. In Vietnam, Catholics integrate ancestor worship, while Islam adheres to the principle of 'customary entry' for establishment in Southeast Asian society. Hinduism in Champa (Vietnam) or Bali (Indonesia) notably differs from its Indian roots. Cham Ba Ni represents a localized form of Islam in Southeast Asia, reflecting the unique variations both Hinduism and Islam undergo upon arrival here. This localization is why Southeast Asia, despite its significant Muslim population, isn't a hub for Islamic terrorism. These instances highlight the rich diversity inherent in Vietnamese culture.

However, there is no doubt, besides Buddhism and indigenous religion and beliefs, Confucianism is one of the spiritual foundations of traditional Vietnamese. Generalizing the spiritual foundation of Vietnamese culture, Tran Quoc Vuong said:

> "The infrastructure of farmers-agriculture – villages of Great Viet – traditional Vietnam (…) in terms of religion-religion – a structural component and product of culture in general – the Vietnamese people's mind is openness, pluralism, diversity (…) there is the 'rationalism' of Confucianism (rationalism in the style of western agricultural technology. East, not the old Western commercial rationality, and the new Western industrial rationality from the eighteenth century to the present); there is the 'spirit' of the Buddha, there is the 'transcendence' of Taoism and there is the superstition of the 'ghosts' of the small farmer's identity. This is 'traditional heritage,' before Vietnam contacts with the West". (Tran 2003, 495–496)

Within the historically tolerant Southeast Asian milieu, it appears that conflicts among the "three teachings" have been notably subdued, primarily evident in literary works. Vietnam's history has been devoid of religious conflicts and notably unfamiliar with religious wars, a departure from the frequent occurrences in various other civilizations.

In the cultural landscape of East Asia, a distinctive challenge emerges in the relationship between the secular state and religion. Contrary to perceiving the "three teachings" as entirely harmonious, history reveals numerous clashes between the Confucian state and religions. Max Weber (1988) noted a significant disparity in lifestyles between Confucians and Buddhist monks and shamans in China, leading to mutual mockery and attacks. Temples were often subjected to state interference to extract coins and forge weapons for wartime purposes. Chinese officials harbored a disdain for Buddhist monks, categorizing them as "parasitic" due to their perceived lack of direct material wealth production, rendering them exempt from taxation in the eyes of authorities. (Weber 1988, 285)

Traditional Vietnamese society exhibits a notable divide: while the upper class predominantly aligns with Confucianism, employing Chinese grammar and deeply embracing Confucian principles and Chinese culture, the lower classes are more inclined toward Buddhism and Southeast Asian indigenous culture. This dichotomy sparks conflict between the patriarchal Confucian ideals of "respecting men and despising women" and the indigenous Southeast Asian culture that emphasizes the status of women. As described by A. Woodside (1971), Vietnamese Confucians mirror the attire and mindset of Chinese culture, adorned in tunics, turbans, wooden clogs, steadfastly valuing loyalty and filial piety, all within their Southeast Asian context. (Woodside 1971, 199–200) This elucidates the recurrent occurrence of peasant uprisings in Vietnamese history. These uprisings arise not solely during periods of natural calamities, enemy interventions, crop failures, or famines, but also during times of abundance, as observed during the reigns of Kings Thai To and Thai Tong, "rice were all over the fields but buffaloes didn't want to eat". Notably, these uprisings were predominantly led by individuals influenced by Buddhism and indigenous religions. The chronic nature of peasant revolts in the country extends beyond mere material poverty, encompassing a significant aspect of spiritual oppression. Instances where temple bells were confiscated by the state for coining currency and especially for crafting weaponry and military apparatus, even amidst civil conflicts, underscore the multifaccted nature of these uprisings.

During the Tay Son dynasty in Vietnam, the state's appropriation of bronze bells emerged as a significant issue. This dynasty, born amidst a civil war involving the Trinh lords in the North and Nguyen lords in the South, played a pivotal role in initiating the country's reunification after more than two centuries of division. However, the persistent warfare led to economic stagnation and burdened the populace with exorbitant taxes, perpetuating impoverishment.

Upon the ascent of the communists to power, there were initial movements against Confucianism in various forms, albeit not as extreme as China's Cultural Revolution. Anti-Confucian sentiments were primarily channeled through slogans targeting remnants of feudalism, followed by campaigns against superstition in rural areas. The waning influence of Confucianism had ramifications not only on socio-ethical grounds but also on socio-cultural aspects, weakening the traditional family and societal structures rooted in Confucian institutions. The decline of Confucianism has led to significant consequences, wherein the introduction of Western cultural elements, though crucial in advancing Vietnamese society amid globalization, remains insufficient to fill the void left by Confucianism.

4. The Confucian *humane* in the context of fourth industrial revolution

In contemporary context, the concept of humane and the essence of being human, fundamental to Confucianism, undergoes an evolution. Initially, within Confucian thought, "humanness" pertains to a person but doesn't encapsulate the entirety of human essence. It signifies a developed individual in terms of character and personality. Primarily, the term "humane" in this context revolves around moral and intellectual values, akin to the soul in Western philosophies, typically dissociated from the physical body. Confucius emphasized courage as a critical trait of a noble person. While traditional Eastern philosophies acknowledge the importance of the human body and temperament, with regard for the elderly and physical attributes, the connection between virtue or inhumanity and physical condition or age is indirect.

Secondly, in considering the human soul, Confucianism places significant emphasis on human dignity through the lens of morality and ethics, prioritizing these aspects over other values such as intelligence, skills, creativity, and various human qualities. The essence of being humane in the modern context within Confucian thought thus continues to prioritize moral and ethical principles over other human attributes.

There is no doubt that the Confucian concept of the human being is still valid in today's society. The use of artificial intelligence will become extremely dangerous if it falls into the hands of some people who are irresponsible to their fellow human beings, into the hands of inhumane humans, or 'inhumans.'

> "The inhuman cannot endure poverty, cannot rest for long in pleasure. The benefactor is at peace with his humane, in every scene is still peaceful and relaxed; Wise people know how to take advantage of humane, depending on the occasion to increase their humane (. . .) Only a humane person knows how to love and hate people in a righteous way (. . .) If you really focus on being humane, you won't commit evil". (Confucius 1950, 51)

Fundamental aspects of humanity encompass the dual nature of individuals, embodying benevolence and forgiveness towards those sincerely striving to rectify their mistakes while maintaining a stern attitude towards those adhering to trends, upholding their beliefs, and voicing their opinions. The Vietnamese adage "hit those who run away, no one will hit those who run back" signifies the endorsement of strictness towards obstinate individuals and simultaneous tolerance and altruism towards those seeking guidance. Emphasizing form without becoming a slave to it, the dichotomy between good and evil, between the virtuous and the trivial, persist as enduring values. Across societies, there exists a universal reverence for goodness and a collective condemnation of wrongdoing. The notion of "Being a general when alive, being god after death" underscores the eternal relevance of contributing positively to the world, leaving an indelible mark on humanity. Despite embracing Western influences in the landscape of international cooperation and integration, Vietnamese society and culture remain rooted in numerous traditional values, which remain indispensable.

The concept of human dignity encompasses not only fundamental moral and ethical values, which are intrinsic and essential facets of an individual, but extends beyond these foundations. Within the spectrum lie two distinct categories: the strong and the virtuous, recognizing the challenge of achieving virtuousness for those with weakened or ailing bodies. However, this forms just one facet of a larger issue. Delving into human value systems entails not solely moral and ethical principles, but a diverse array of other value systems. Ho Chi Minh once acknowledged parallels between the philosophies of Confucius and Christ, aspiring to learn from both. Over half a century ago, he underscored the correlation between talent and virtue. Presently, the maxim "With virtue but without talent, it is difficult to do anything. Having talent without virtue makes a person useless" remains pertinent. The essence of an individual, particularly a leader, lies in possessing a lucid mind, a sense of justice, discernment between right and wrong, and a comprehensive perspective. Human talent manifests in myriad domains, encompassing not only comprehension and adherence to ethical norms but also spanning intellectual prowess, experiential wisdom, scientific and artistic ingenuity, adeptness in acquiring and applying skills, and the cultivation of soft skills essential to meet the demands of specific professions, among others.

Confucius' concept of humanness extends beyond affection solely for fellow humans, encompassing a profound regard for numerous animals beneficial to humanity. Implicit in Confucius's virtue is the cultivation of love not just for fellow beings but also for animals, emphasizing harmony with the natural world – a crucial aspect often overlooked in many nations' approaches to environmental concerns. Confucius' interpretation of humanness is both grand and lofty, presenting a virtue that appears immense and challenging for individuals to embody. Yet, conversely, it also manifests in simple, everyday acts, emphasizing kindness not only toward people but also toward animals closely intertwined with human existence. This dual essence underscores the significance of being compassionate in both human and animal interactions, promoting harmony within the living environment. "The Master fished, but did not use a net. He shot, but not at birds perching (...) Confucius said, 'Is kindness far from me? If we want to be benevolent, then that benevolence will come to us right away.'" (Confucius 1950, 113)

In our contemporary era, there's a pronounced demand for a high level of specialization. Modern individuals are required to possess a spectrum of skills that weren't necessarily requisite for individuals in agrarian civilizations of centuries past. We're well acquainted with metrics such as IQ (intelligence quotient), EQ (emotional quotient, or emotional intelligence), and various other parameters that serve as benchmarks for assessing individuals worldwide. These metrics encapsulate numerous facets of psychology and logical reasoning, spanning intelligence, emotional acumen, problem-solving capabilities, and adaptability in addressing challenges. While the cultivation of moral philosophy and ethical values remains an enduring priority in education, human development now necessitates a focus on a multitude of intellectual and creative capacities to engender a well-rounded individual. Within the traditional Confucian ethos, an individual embodied nearly all the essential values of humanity. However, in the contemporary landscape, there exists an imperative for an array of vital value systems beyond the traditional ones, constituting an essential and indispensable framework, yet not exhaustive in defining an individual's entirety.

Confucianism predominantly examines individuals within the context of society, emphasizing their roles and relationships within both family and broader societal structures. Central to Confucian ethics is the notion of responsibility – a constant consideration of one's duties and obligations to family based on hierarchical order and to society in accordance with one's social standing. In this framework, an individual's happiness aligns with the well-being of their family, where blessings upon the individual signify blessings upon the household. The prevailing mantra is "Everybody for everyone", prioritizing collective welfare over personal concerns. Personal or private aspects of individuals remain understated within Confucian discourse, often regarded as sensitive and intimate to each person. The concept of freedom and equality, prominent in Western ideologies since modern times, remained largely foreign to Confucian societies. However, since the colonial era, the influx of Western ideologies and cultures has propelled attention toward the personal and private realms of individuals, as well as the recognition of fundamental human rights. To complement the prevailing ethos, there's a necessity to incorporate "Everyone for each person" into the paradigm, thereby forming an ideal model for the relationship between the individual and the community. The trajectory of Vietnamese society from the colonial period to the present reflects a merging of traditional Confucian values of duties and responsibilities with Western notions of individual rights. Notably, Ho Chi Minh, in the Declaration of Independence, referenced both the United States' Declaration of Independence and France's Declaration of Civil Rights, signifying the infusion of Western philosophical and cultural values into Vietnamese society during the twilight of the colonial era. (Ho Chi Minh 1998, 434–440).

Indeed, certain traditional Confucian notions have lost relevance over time. Similar to ancient and medieval Western philosophy, Confucianism historically placed less emphasis on material values and the human body, somewhat downplaying worldly emotions and desires. Confucius doesn't explicitly engage with discussions about the body, yet doesn't necessarily dismiss its significance. While the Confucian framework acknowledges the "face" of a person, encompassing appearance, physique, and demeanor, as part of a woman's four qualities alongside work, speech, and virtue, the emphasis typically sways away from material dignity and the mundane, often deeming them as secondary or even disregarding them due to their association with potential moral pitfalls. In contrast, Western thought from the Middle Ages has adopted a more comprehensive approach, prioritizing both intelligence and virtue while acknowledging and respecting the role of the body. This divergence in perspective becomes apparent when comparing traditional Asian thinking to modern Asian thought emerging from the colonial era. In essence, it's conceivable that if Confucius were to return, he might also concur that an individual possessing virtue wouldn't be someone physically weak or ailing. This viewpoint would likely align with the recognition that an individual's physical condition holds significance in complementing their virtuous character.

The preceding analysis highlights an error when viewing the Confucian understanding of the human condition solely through the lens of historical narrative. Contrary to such a limited perspective, its significance transcends the confines of Asian cultural boundaries and holds universal relevance for humanity. This observation stands as a primary indication supporting discussions on the relevance of Confucianism amidst the challenges of modernization and its pertinence within the context of the ongoing fourth industrial revolution.

5. Vietnamese Confucian society in the context of fourth industrial revolution: opportunities and challenges

Confucian society operates on the institutional framework of the family, wherein each family unit mirrors a cell within the broader societal structure, portraying society as a larger familial entity. This essence is distinctly evident in the everyday communication patterns of Vietnamese people, wherein personal names and modes of address are determined by the familial hierarchy and age. Over fifty years ago, L. Cadiere cautioned about the ramifications of familial deterioration, asserting that if the family unit were to weaken, it would inevitably precipitate numerous crises within Vietnamese society.

> "There are indeed too many reasons to explain the present moral decline; but one of the most powerful causes is the loosening of family bonds; it is the individual's escape from the influence of family education formed as a mechanism where the living follow the example of the dead, where each member is responsible for the common honor of all (...) Well, I would like to make a wish that please do not use any method that threatens to weaken the family in this country of Vietnam, on the contrary, strengthen it by all means. Alas! Is it possible! Will it be able to resist changes with so much force!" (Cadiere 2010, 115)

Vietnamese society has grappled with challenges stemming from the absence of Confucian principles over the past century. However, it's crucial to acknowledge Vietnam's current status as a developing nation undergoing a transition from an agrarian society to an industrialized one by the projected year 2030. In the era of the fourth industrial revolution, what trajectory will Vietnamese society take? To be direct, Confucianism, akin to many major religions, originates from ancient times, emerging within an agricultural civilization. In stark contrast, the fourth industrial revolution stands as a pinnacle of modern scientific and technological advancements, largely attributed to the Western world's dominance. This dichotomy prompts an essential query: what hurdles will Confucianism and traditional Vietnamese culture encounter within the realm of the fourth industrial revolution?

First of all, the assumption that the fourth industrial revolution brings only challenges to Vietnamese culture should be reconsidered; within these challenges lie opportunities. Nearly two millennia of Vietnamese history vividly demonstrates the remarkable adaptability of Confucianism. As previously discussed, despite fluctuations, contemporary Vietnamese society remains reliant on Confucian values. The advent of the colonial period in East Asia during the latter half of the nineteenth century marked the onset of Confucianism's decline across the region. Consequently, the Korean peninsula, China, and Vietnam shifted away from Confucian-based authoritarian monarchies, embracing secular republican state models imported from the West. Despite this shift, the Confucian educational system persisted alongside the secular education systems implemented by colonial governments. In Vietnam, the last administration of the Confucian examination occurred in 1919, after which the public education system fully embraced the Western model.

Yet, this historical context did not prompt Vietnamese society and culture to entirely abandon fundamental Confucian values. A century ago, during colonial rule, Vietnamese nationalists engaged in debates concerning national rejuvenation. Figures like Phan Boi Chau (1867–1940) and Tran Trong Kim (1883–1953) highlighted the era as one of "European rain, American wind", acknowledging Vietnam's grasp of Western scientific achievements. However, they advocated for maintaining a firm foothold in Confucian principles, encapsulated in the mantra of "Western science, Vietnamese Confucian spirit". Conversely, other Western-educated Vietnamese scholars, such as Phan Chu Trinh (1872–1926), Nguyen Van Vinh (1882–1936), and Pham Quynh (1892–1945), chose a path of modernization inspired by Western models, particularly drawing from France as their prototype.

Despite the presence of two primary ideological currents concerning the path towards national independence and self-sufficiency, both generally concur on the enduring relevance of Confucianism in contemporary Vietnamese society. Their critique typically doesn't target Confucianism as a whole, much less in an overtly negative light. Rather, the focus lies on specific antiquated notions or drawbacks within Confucianism that impede the nation's progress, recognizing their incompatibility with the present circumstances.

Vietnam, viewed from both a cultural and regional standpoint, embodies not solely a Confucian East Asian identity but also holds the essence of a Southeast Asian nation. Particularly in the central and southern regions – formerly the domains of Champa and Khmer cultures, influenced by Indian traditions – the imprint of Confucianism appears less pronounced. Nevertheless, it is essential to acknowledge Vietnam's traditional societal fabric as inherently Confucian. Keith Taylor characterized contemporary Vietnam as a "Confucian village country", underscoring the deep-rooted influence of Confucian principles within its societal framework (Taylor 1998). Undeniably, the fusion of Confucianism with indigenous elements forms the cultural dynamism of Vietnam. More than a century ago, Pham Quynh's statement resonates powerfully: "As long as the Tale of Kieu remains, so too will the Vietnamese language. As long as the Vietnamese language endures, so too will the survival of the nation". (Pham Quynh2020). Confucianism and indigenous elements remain irreplaceable cornerstones within Vietnam. Present-day Vietnamese society heavily relies on Confucian principles. While Western values introduced during the colonial period have significantly benefited Vietnam's socio-economic development, they haven't entirely filled the void created by the decline of Confucianism in matters concerning morality, culture, and spirituality. Rather than delving into debates regarding the extent of Confucianism's necessity in contemporary Vietnamese society, it's crucial to acknowledge that Confucianism persists as one of the fundamental spiritual underpinnings. The maxim "If the top is not righteous, the bottom will certainly become chaotic" accurately describes the crisis of the current Vietnamese society, partially stemming from the lack of earnest adherence to core Confucian values, evident in both familial and societal realms.

The relationship between Confucianism and science, as understood in the Western context, is intricate. Regarding the worldview, it's evident that Confucianism, categorized as a secular belief system, bears numerous resemblances to scientific interpretations concerning the nature of our surroundings, dissociated from mystical or supernatural interpretations. Both Confucianism and Western science direct their focus towards the tangible issues within the present world, displaying little concern for transcendental matters related to the afterlife. Additionally, both share a common aim centered on promoting human well-being and contentment. Matters such as warfare and impoverishment lie beyond the scope of interest for both Confucianism and science. While Confucianism doesn't emphasize natural sciences, it would be illogical to perceive a contradiction between the compassionate principles of Confucianism and mathematical or physical formulas and equations. Both can coexist without conflict, as the ethical and philosophical underpinnings of Confucianism don't inherently oppose scientific discoveries or theories.

Certainly, within the Confucian cultural milieu, the fundamental reexamination of the role of God or the Supreme Being amidst the context of the fourth industrial revolution – similar to what's observed in the West and some other cultures – is not a pressing necessity. The stark opposition between materialism and idealism, theism and atheism, monotheism and polytheism, or even between religion and secularism, has been a defining characteristic in the extensive history of Western thought. This dichotomy has often been a catalyst for numerous wars and conflicts. However, within Confucian society, even with the introduction of Western ideologies, this paradigm isn't a central concern. This distinction significantly sets apart the relationship between religion and science in East Asia from that in the West. Confucianism's worldview doesn't engage in the same polarized debates or conflicts surrounding the nature of divinity, human existence, or the dichotomy between religious and secular thought. The absence of such intense opposition marks a notable divergence in how religion and science coexist and interact within these cultural spheres.

Indeed, Confucianism doesn't seamlessly align with Western science. Confucian society operated on a hierarchical structure delineating Confucian scholars, peasants, workers, and merchants (學者、農民、工人、商人). The elite class, predominantly led by the intellectual class, emerged from a stringent academic system underscored by clear value orientations. Loyalty, particularly to the king and the royal family, stood as the foremost virtue, followed by filial piety towards grandparents and ancestors. There existed distinct gender value hierarchies, where men prioritized filial piety while women were expected to prioritize virtue. The pursuit of scholarly excellence aimed at becoming a mandarin, emphasizing administrative duties rather than a lifelong dedication to scholarly pursuits and knowledge exploration. This setup differs significantly from Western scientific intellectuals, who often stemmed from aristocratic backgrounds, enjoyed greater freedom of thought, pursued educational improvement, and harbored aspirations to enhance societal knowledge. In Confucian society, the elite class lacked an independent position relative to the court and didn't assume a role in social criticism, thus not resembling the modern conception of an intelligentsia. Confucian ideals didn't embrace concepts such as freedom of thought, democracy, or equality, nor did they foster the inclination of intellectuals towards independence from authority, as observed in the West. Tran Quoc Vuong's perspective highlights that the communist intelligentsia mirrors previous Confucian intellectuals, both subservient to the leadership of the Communist Party without room for independent thought. Consequently, Vietnam features intellectuals rather than an intelligentsia in the modern sense – a distinction marked by the absence of a class exhibiting the independence and critical tendencies typically associated with the Western concept of an intelligentsia (Tran 2020).

In a totalitarian Confucian society, Western scientific thought typically faces challenges in taking root. However, in Vietnam, the introduction of Western science occurred during the colonial period, a time when the Confucian monarchy's ruling influence had waned. Moreover, within the highly tolerant cultural landscape of Southeast Asia, a serious conflict between Confucian values and those introduced by Western science since the colonial era isn't readily apparent. Before the French arrived in Vietnam, the nation functioned as an absolute Confucian monarchy. With the advent of the French, they brought not just Western science and technology but also introduced capitalist methods of production. This period marked a significant shift in the societal landscape, intertwining traditional Confucian values with the modern advancements and economic structures introduced by the colonial powers. The coexistence of these ideologies in Vietnam's cultural fabric reveals a more nuanced relationship between Confucian values and Western scientific thought than might be expected in a more rigidly traditional Confucian society (Tran Bich San). The weakening of Confucianism during the colonial period wasn't solely attributed to the necessity of advancing Western science. Primarily, it stemmed from the colonial government's incomplete implementation of the 1905 law of separation within the country. Despite advocating for a secular state model that to some extent separated the state from religion, the full enforcement of this separation didn't materialize. This dynamic played a pivotal role in diminishing the stronghold of Confucianism during that period. The impediment to scientific development in both Western and East Asian contexts isn't solely rooted in the conflict between religion and science, although in the West, such conflicts, particularly between Christianity and science, have occasionally escalated into atrocities. Notably, the "Galileo case" stands as a tragic episode illustrating this conflict within Western history. However, the relationship between Confucianism and Western science isn't devoid of its own dramatic elements, albeit in a different context.

Attributing the lack of pre-colonial scientific development in East Asia entirely to Confucianism would be a misinterpretation. The agrarian production prevalent in pre-colonial East Asia didn't necessitate extensive scientific advancement. In Confucian societies, the emphasis on agriculture over commerce, as epitomized by the concept of "respect agriculture, despise commerce", played a role in this orientation. However, this alone didn't solely dictate the millennium-long dominance of subsistence agriculture in certain East Asian societies. The surge of scientific progress and the concurrent geographical discoveries in post-medieval Europe shared a common impetus: capitalist-driven production geared towards profit and surplus value (expressed in the formula Money – Goods – Money Plus). This capitalist pursuit of profit propelled the quest for markets to sell goods, as well as the expansion of markets for production materials. Early powerful capitalist nations found European territories limited in meeting these demands, prompting geographical explorations and eventually leading to the colonization of other continents.

Absolutely, in pre-colonial Vietnam, self-sustaining production didn't necessitate extensive scientific development. The advent of capitalist commodity production introduced by the French truly laid the groundwork for scientific advancement in the Western sense within the country. During the colonial era, the fusion of Western ideas with traditional Confucian values led to the emergence of a Western-educated intellectual class alongside the traditional Confucian class. Despite the enduring legacy of the Temple of Literature, the establishment of Indochina University by the French in 1906 in Hanoi marked a significant milestone. This institution, serving as the forerunner of today's Hanoi National University, was the first university in Vietnam constructed on the model of Western universities.

In the context of the fourth industrial revolution, several Confucian concepts require adaptation and evolution. The traditional Confucian perspective, exemplified by the idealized society of Yao and Shun, contrasts starkly with the contemporary views of development and prosperity. The ongoing scientific and technological revolution is profoundly altering multiple facets of our lives in unprecedented ways. Concepts like "for the sake of agriculture is for the sake of the village, for trade is for its sake", rooted in agriculture as the fundamental focus, are more fitting for agrarian societies. The hierarchical relationships inherent in Confucian autocracy – king-subject, mandarin-servant, father-son – find limited applicability in diverse social models. Confucian education, primarily centered on moral and ethical doctrines and delivered through an analytical teaching style, often proves unsuitable in modern contexts. Even the tradition of venerating teachers, while commendable, sometimes hampers the independent and creative thoughts of successive generations of students, highlighting the need for greater flexibility in its application in today's society. Confucian educational philosophy diverges from the learner-centered approach of Western educational philosophy. Furthermore, Confucius's traditional vision of a harmonious universal world contrasts significantly with the realities of our globalized world today.

The historical introduction and integration of Western science into Vietnamese society since the colonial era highlight the coexistence sought between the Confucian monarchy and Confucian values in general with Western scientific advancements over the past two centuries. This coexistence, albeit at times coercive, reflects a pursuit of harmonious interaction between these ideological realms. Given this historical context, there's every reason to believe that the fourth industrial revolution and Confucian values can indeed find a path to peaceful coexistence.

The advent of the fourth industrial revolution brings forth significant changes, notably in the realm of artificial intelligence (AI). AI's capabilities are poised to replace many tasks traditionally performed by individuals while augmenting human abilities. However, alongside its advancements, there exist considerable challenges, particularly concerning the potential for AI to spiral out of control. It's evident that AI stands as the culmination of the Western cultural tradition valuing humanity's dominance over nature, presenting itself as a double-edged sword with immense power and potential risks. The precarious nature of AI is further exacerbated by the latent threat of nuclear war. Recently, United Nations Secretary-General Antonio Guterres expressed grave concern about the use of AI in warfare: "if AI became primarily a weapon to launch cyberattacks, generate deepfakes, or for spreading disinformation and hate speech, it would have very serious consequences for global peace and security". (Gutteres 2023)

The Confucian ideology emphasizes that despite human creativity, individuals are inherently bound by the limits imposed by Heaven and the natural world. While humans possess creative capacities, these capabilities cannot surpass the confines set by the order of Heaven and the natural order. There remains an inherent wisdom within the domain of God. The responsibilities of humans belong to them, distinct from the realm of divine duties; they cannot be assumed by humans on behalf of God. This notion highlights the importance of aligning artificial intelligence with human welfare, necessitating a return to Confucian principles centered on humanity and ethical conduct. Confucius aptly expressed this concept by stating, "Those who transgress the natural order will not find solace, irrespective of the deity they implore for intervention". (Confucius 1950, 39) In Confucianism, individuals are not entirely passive; rather, they are urged to understand the boundaries of their capabilities. While acknowledging the ingenuity of humans, there's a recognition that many have aspired to surpass the realm of Heaven. However, there's a cautionary note that transgressing the limits set by Heaven will inevitably lead to repercussions. This sentiment is encapsulated in the Confucian adage: "People devise plans, but their fruition is contingent upon the will of Heaven". The Vietnamese adage aligns with this view, emphasizing that any scientific or technological progress is akin to a "double-edged sword". Alongside the opportunities it unveils, enhancing labor efficiency and allowing more personal time, it also poses inherent risks.

However, this advancement brings forth the challenge of regulation and control. It serves as a cautionary reminder that the fourth industrial revolution, particularly with the integration of AI, necessitates an awareness of specific boundaries within human governance. Failure to adhere to these boundaries could result in humanity facing severe consequences, akin to the proverbial "his stick beating his own back". The lessons drawn from historical events, such as the remorse felt by scientists involved in the development of the atomic bomb following its use in Japan by the US, as well as the present-day concerns regarding climate change, consistently echo this reminder to humanity. Within the context of the fourth industrial revolution, Confucian concepts like the Mandate of Heaven maintain relevance. It's crucial to note that the reference to Heaven in Confucianism does not denote a supreme Creator akin to God in theological or religious terms. Misattributing Confucianism to either a materialistic or idealistic standpoint would be a misconception, as it holds distinct philosophical underpinnings. According to Confucianism, the rise or fall of a dynasty hinges on whether it upholds or forfeits the Mandate of Heaven. Similarly, in daily life, we often confront circumstances that surpass human control and foresight. While humans act and endeavor, their triumphs or setbacks aren't solely determined by human agency but also by divine will. As the saying goes, "Human plans are not always in line with Heaven's intentions". In this context, Heaven serves a moral role akin to God in Immanuel Kant's ethical framework, acting as a restraint to prevent human transgressions and avert a cycle of wrongdoing. It functions as both a boon, supporting righteous human conduct, and a retribution for irreverent behavior. Heaven embodies a supernatural force, an enigma, an insurmountable limit for humans. Deliberate attempts to surpass this limit may be deemed sinful or morally misguided, signifying a departure from one's rightful place in the order of things.

The potential linkage between the Confucian understanding of humanity and the performance of Artificial Intelligence exemplifies the adaptation of Confucian principles to contemporary society. However, certain traditional Confucian norms, like reverence for the elderly, appear to have diminished relevance in the context of the fourth industrial revolution. This era increasingly necessitates the leveraging of the younger generation's creative prowess and dynamism. This adaptation must be context-specific. In domains aligned with direct production adhering to scientific and technological paradigms, priority should be accorded to the younger generation, given their adeptness in technological manipulations. Conversely, in macro-level management roles, leaders benefit from accumulated experiences, wisdom, and contemplative insights – a concept akin to the East Asian adage that likens the potency of older ginger to the advantages of the elderly. The developmental trajectory observed in East Asian newly industrialized nations underscores the indispensable role played by the middle and older generations. Their amalgamation of experience, valor, and sagacity harmonizes with the innovative capacities of the younger cohort, contributing significantly to the region's remarkable progress.

The tradition of emphasizing the alignment of the human spirit with nature likely positions Vietnam and other nations rooted in the Confucian cultural tradition to possess a heightened awareness compared to many Western countries. In Confucian-influenced societies, the emphasis on harmony with nature has ingrained a distinctive perspective. While Western traditions promote noble and universal values like freedom, democracy, and equal rights, their expressions often appear unconventional or excessive through an Asian lens. The characteristics attributed to a Confucian ruler still retain relevance in contemporary society.

> "I have enough knowledge to understand the way to govern the people according to the Holy Sage, but I don't have enough humane to keep it. Even if I gain it, I will lose it. I have enough knowledge to understand the way to govern the people according to Saints, I have enough humanity to preserve, but when I come to the people, I do not have a dignified appearance, and the people do not respect me. If I have enough knowledge to understand the way to govern the people according to the Holy sage, I have enough humane to protect and approach the people, I have a dignified appearance, but I do not follow etiquette to govern the people, then I am not worthy to be called perfect ruler. So if we want to become a perfect ruler, we should have all the virtues: wisdom, humane, page, and ritual". (Confucius 1950, 251–253)

The utilization of scientific and technological advancements by composed and contemplative Asians, guided by a belief in the significance of measured progress rather than a relentless pursuit of rapid success, appears to present a potentially safer or less precarious approach in the future. This contrasts with Western tendencies that historically tend to overemphasize human creativity and assert human dominance over the world.

The cautionary note highlighted by L. Cadiere regarding the waning influence of Confucianism within Vietnamese society and the subsequent infiltration of Western values into the void left by Confucianism appears to be an undeniable trend. Examining this from a theoretical standpoint, the fourth industrial revolution exerts a dual impact on this trend. On one hand, this revolution encourages individualism and fosters reliance on digital technologies, prompting a drift away from the foundational relationship structures inherent in traditional Confucian society. The divergence between the East Asian agrarian Confucian society centered around familial institutions and the Western post-industrial societal model becomes more pronounced. Conversely, as previously discussed, the fourth industrial revolution necessitates the preservation and promotion of certain core Confucian values. Disregarding these values seems to amplify the negative aspects and adverse consequences stemming from the fourth industrial revolution. Policymakers must acknowledge this interplay and seek a harmonious nexus between Confucianism and the revolution.

Of course, some Confucian concepts are no longer relevant to today's society. One of them is the patriarchal lifestyle, respecting men and disrespecting women. Phrases like "having a son is significant, having ten daughters is inconsequential" no longer hold relevance in addressing the evolving gender equality issues in contemporary society. Vietnam has seen considerable progress in addressing gender inequality, notably after 1945 with the advent of Marxist ideology and the leadership of the communists. These movements emphasized gender equality, a stark departure from the Confucian societal norms that often relegated women to subordinate positions, adhering to principles like "follow the father at home, the husband when married, and the son when widowed". It's important to note that these notions stem more from Song Confucianism rather than the foundational teachings of Confucius. However, navigating the quest for women's liberation raises a critical question: is there a limit to this liberation, considering it contradicts certain Confucian principles? Establishing a connection between Confucianism and the contemporary status of women becomes crucial in this discourse.

The influence of Confucianism remains ambivalent within the framework of the fourth industrial revolution. While certain fundamental Confucian values retain efficacy in contemporary societal dynamics, dismissing Confucianism entirely would be an oversight. Nevertheless, certain tenets of Confucianism necessitate adaptation and modification to align with present circumstances.

Weber posited that in East Asia, unlike the West where secular and religious ethics coexist, only religious morality prevails. This observation appears fitting for both traditional and contemporary Vietnamese society. Consequently, despite the Vietnamese authorities' efforts to propagate Marxist-Leninist ethics and Ho Chi Minh's moral principles over recent decades, the tangible outcomes have been limited. The post-colonial, communist-inspired societal transformations, characterized by the active dissemination of Marxism and materialism, have notably contributed to the erosion of Confucianism, thereby exacerbating this issue. Amidst the context of social secularization and the infiltration of Western culture and ideologies over the past two centuries, it becomes evident that attributing the present Vietnamese moral framework solely to Confucian norms would be oversimplifying. While numerous moral values from the West have been embraced by the Vietnamese populace, they do not seem poised to supplant Confucian ethics.

6. Concluding Remarks

When examining Vietnamese Confucian society within the framework of the fourth industrial revolution, several notable observations emerge.

Firstly, the introduction of the fourth industrial revolution into Confucian society encounters a range of complexities and obstacles. The inherent clash between Confucian societal principles and Western scientific ideals presents a formidable challenge. Confucian society historically operated within a structured framework of absolute monarchy, characterized by the stratification of scholars, peasants, workers, and merchants. This structure does not readily align with the prerequisites of freedom of thought, creativity, and the notion of societal equality espoused by Western science. Emphasizing a social persona rather than the individual, Confucian society contrasts sharply with the emphasis on individual rights advocated by Western science. Moreover, the societal principles of Confucianism, including the emphasis on selflessness in relationships, the patriarchal hierarchy, and the reverence for familial institutions, pose significant barriers to accommodating Western-influenced concepts. The societal norms rooted in Confucianism, such as the prioritization of familial and hierarchical values, encounter discord with the contemporary trends imported from the West, such as pre-marital relationships, movements for gender equality, and the consumer-driven culture that contradicts traditional values. Indeed, the ritualistic and value-based disparities between Confucian society and Western society represent formidable barriers that resist easy reconciliation or integration.

Vietnam remains deeply rooted in Confucian values, which, despite their diminishing influence, continue to serve as essential pillars and spiritual cornerstones of Vietnamese culture and society. However, the emergence of the fourth industrial revolution presents numerous challenges to a traditional Confucian society, ones that cannot be swiftly resolved.

Secondly, a comprehensive examination reveals that the Confucian principle of humanity, along with various ethical and political standards that underpin traditional Vietnamese society, continues to evolve across different societal strata, actively promoting values within contemporary Vietnamese culture. The concept of humanity, a fundamental tenet of Confucianism, appears to possess enduring, universal worth. The stark contrast it draws between virtue and vice, good and evil, remains perpetually relevant. Notably, there exists a significant convergence between Confucius' notion of humanity and the compassion and benevolence espoused by Christ towards humanity. This convergence denotes a meeting ground transcending temporal and spatial boundaries, where great figures from disparate backgrounds intersect. Despite geographical and cultural disparities, essential similarities persist, forming the basis for Ho Chi Minh's self-identification as a student of both philosophies.

Additionally, other core facets of Confucianism – such as the principles of ritual, significance, sagacity, and belief – persist in propagating their values across various strata of society. These concepts continue to adapt and evolve to align with the contemporary social landscape. Notably, certain Confucian ideas, such as the interconnectedness between Heaven, Earth, and Humanity that emphasize humanity as an integral part of nature, advocate the necessity of harmonizing human existence with the natural world. This perspective, acknowledging the limitations of human capacity to supersede the forces of nature, proves markedly pertinent, particularly amidst ongoing debates surrounding the ethical boundaries of artificial intelligence (AI). In essence, the foundational categories of Confucianism remain relevant and adaptable, even necessitating adjustments to suit present circumstances. Conceptions within Confucianism that starkly clash with modern societal norms have gradually waned since the colonial era, leaving minimal impact on contemporary society.

Thirdly, the advent of Western science and the fourth industrial revolution coincided with the waning influence of Confucianism in several East Asian nations. This interaction exerted a dual impact on both Western science and the fourth industrial revolution. On one hand, it mitigated the severity of conflicts between Confucian principles and Western scientific ideologies. Colonial-era Vietnamese society embraced Western science as a novel influence, encapsulated in the adage "Western wind blows East wind", symbolizing the ascendancy of Western values over traditional Eastern ones. The discernible absence of substantial Eastern cultural imprints in Ho Chi Minh's Declaration of Independence signifies that late colonial Vietnamese society acknowledged and embraced the prevalence and integration of numerous Western values as an inherent reality.

However, this emergence also sparks a crucial inquiry: Can Western values adequately replace the void left by Confucianism? Efforts to disseminate communist ideologies, characterized by the radical tenets of Lenin, Stalin, and Mao Zedong, alongside the deliberate erosion of traditional values through anti-feudal movements since the 1950s, led to societal regression. Vietnam faced a series of crises encompassing socioeconomic, cultural, and moral realms, resulting in enduring consequences for Vietnamese society today. The current socio-ethical decline and crises in Vietnam stem, in part, from the insufficient consideration of essential aspects of humanity, exacerbating the vacuum created by the decline of Confucianism. This underscores that while new values imported from the West attempt to bridge this gap, they cannot wholly compensate for the loss. This underscores the finite extent of Western values' influence on Vietnamese culture and society. Vietnam cannot unreservedly adopt the model of France, the United States, or any other Western nation due to the limitations imposed by its cultural and historical context.

Fourthly, Considerations must encompass Vietnam's dual cultural identity as both a Confucian East Asian and Southeast Asian nation. The cultural landscape in Vietnam demonstrates a distinctive manifestation of Confucianism, moderated by an openness to indigenous cultural nuances, distinguishing it from the more stringent forms observed in China and the Korean peninsula. Notably, the historical standing of Vietnamese women within family structures and society has exhibited greater influence compared to their counterparts in aforementioned Confucian-dominant societies. Consequently, the anti-Confucian movements in 20th-century Vietnam did not escalate to the extreme levels witnessed during China's tumultuous "cultural revolution". The Southeast Asian context, characterized by its indigenous facets, tends to temper foreign ideological and religious doctrines through a lens of "customary entry". The expression of Hinduism among the Cham people in Vietnam and Bali, Indonesia, diverges significantly from its practice in India. Similarly, Catholicism in Vietnam gradually assimilated with ancestor worship following prolonged controversies. The introduction of Islam into the region has not manifested as radically as witnessed in the Middle East and North Africa, thereby mitigating the emergence of international terrorism within Southeast Asia. In this milieu, Confucianism in Vietnam adopted a more accommodative and tolerant stance, steering away from the rigidity often associated with its origins. This adaptability extends to subsequent communist movements. The indigenous factor, while serving as an auxiliary element, plays a pivotal role in mitigating conflicts between Confucianism and Western scientific advancements. Consequently, it fosters an environment conducive to synthesizing the traditional Confucian heritage with modernity, prompting a shift in focus towards evaluating the efficacy and functionality of

Confucianism in contemporary society rather than fixating on its potential adverse implications.

Fifthly, inevitably, the advent of the fourth industrial revolution is poised to amplify the sway of Western culture and scientific ideals in Vietnam, potentially eroding many tenets of Confucianism and traditional Vietnamese culture. Over recent decades, Vietnamese society has grappled with a palpable crisis, particularly evident in its cultural and spiritual domains. While Western values have propelled progress towards societal equity, economic advancement, and material prosperity for the majority, they have not adequately compensated for the diminishing strengths of Confucianism, thereby exacerbating the societal void.

The overarching query arises: to what extent is the cultural influence of Western values and ideologies restricted within this nation? The impetus of the fourth industrial revolution further intensifies this dynamic. Vietnamese policymakers must acknowledge this reality to formulate responsive strategies, navigating the challenges posed by rapid scientific and technological advancements while preserving and elevating the enduring values of Confucianism that remain pertinent to society. There exists a critical imperative to establish an optimal synergy between the scientific ethos inherent in Western technology and the humanistic essence embedded within the nation's traditional culture. Amidst the pursuit and utilization of modern scientific achievements, it remains imperative to consistently address and mitigate the adverse repercussions inherent in this progress. This paradox underscores a fundamental facet of life – one where the benefits of progress necessitate vigilant management of its accompanying drawbacks.

The above analysis strongly suggests the fallacy of deeming Confucianism irreconcilable with Western science or the advent of the fourth industrial revolution. Over the past century, Western scientific principles have taken root in Vietnam, and despite the inevitable clashes between Confucianism and Western scientific values, they have managed to coexist harmoniously. Presently, as the fourth industrial revolution steadily becomes an undeniable reality, the prevailing situation is not entirely bleak. A Confucian-based society retains the capacity to function and establish connections with the ongoing fourth industrial revolution.

To summarize, the Confucian perspective on human values remains relevant within the landscape of the fourth industrial revolution. Confucianism exhibits a nuanced stance, embracing both favorable and unfavorable aspects of this technological shift. Despite the trend toward secularization and the burgeoning impact of various Western values, Confucian ethics continue to hold an irreplaceable position in Vietnam. It would be erroneous to perceive Confucianism merely as an impediment to progress suitable solely for an agrarian society, while the fourth industrial revolution represents an entirely contrary force laden solely with negative implications for Confucian societies.

References

Cadiere, L. 2010. *Croyances et pratiques religieuses des Vietnamiens*. Translated to Vietnamese by Do Trinh Hue, vol. 1. Huế: Publishing House Thuận Hóa.

Confucius. 1950. *Analects*. Translated by Đoan Trung Con. Saigon: Tri Duc Tong Tho.

Guterres, A. 2023. Speech on Artificial Intelligence at the UNO Security Council on 18 July, 2023. [online].https://turkiye.un.org/en/239867-guterres-calls-ai-bridges-divides-rather-pushing-us-apart

Hồ Chí Minh. 1998. Tuyênngônđộclập (Independence Declaration). In: *Communist Party of Vietnam, Documents Collected, vol. 7*. Hanoi: Publishing House National Politics.

Huọu, T.D. 1994. *Đếnhiệntạitừtruyềnthống* [To Present from the Tradition]. Hanoi: Vietnam National University Hanoi Press.

Lao Tsu. 2010. Tao Te Chinh. Translated by Nguyễn Hiến Lê. Hồ Chí Minh City: Publishing House Tônghọp.

Pham, Q. 2020. Kyniệm 200 nămngàymấtthihào Nguyễn Du (1820–2020). Nguoidothi.net. Available at: https://nguoidothi.net.vn/lich-su-mot-cau-noi-25168.html

Rhodes, A. 1994. Histoire du royaume de Tunquin. Translated to Vietnamese by Hồng Nhuệ. Ho Chi Minh City: Ho Chi Minh City House Publishing.

Taylor, K.W. 1998. Vietnamese Studies in North America, Keynote Speech No.2. Paper presented at the First International Conference on Vietnamese Studies, Hanoi.

Trần, B.S. 2018. *Thicuvàgiáodục Việt Nam thòi Phápthuộc* [Vietnamese Exams and Education in Colonial Time].[online].https://nghiencuuquocte.org/2018/06/17/thi-cu-va-giao-duc-viet-nam-thoi-phap-thuoc

Trần, Q.V. 2003. *Vănhóa Việt Nam tìmtòivàsuyngẫm* [Vietnamese Culture: Some Observations]. Hanoi: Publishing House Van hoc.

Trần, Q.V. 2020. *Nỗiámanhtùquákhú* [Obsessions from the Past]. [online].https://vanhocsaigon.com/noi-am-anh-cua-qua-khu-tran-quoc-vuong/

Weber, M. 1988. Die Wirtschaftsethik der Weltreligionen. Konfuzianismus und Taoismus. In: *Gesamelte Aufsätze zur Religionssoziologie, Band I*. 9 Auflage. Tübingen: J.C.B Mohr.

Woodside, A. 1971. *Vietnam and the Chinese Model. A Comparative Study of Nguyễn and Ching Civil Government in the First Half of the Nineteenth Century*. Cambridge, MA: Harvard University Press.

Ho Chi Minh's Thought on Human Develoipment in Contrast to Transhumanism

Hoa Thi Kim Do

1. Introduction

The complexity of human experience has been debated philosophically, socio-politically, and technologically throughout history. It has been formed by our increasing understanding of humans, enriched by many intellectuals and innovators. Two opposing ideologies – humanism, represented by Ho Chi Minh's profound views, and transhumanism, a futurist ideology that envisions a technologically enhanced human future – have widened this discourse. Although they have different perspectives, these two ideologies offer a fascinating look at human growth, identity, and our collective future.

Vietnamese revolutionary leader Ho Chi Minh (1890–1969) was a major player in 20th-century global politics. His leadership and beliefs helped Vietnam gain independence from French colonial authority and defined its post-colonial sociopolitical structure. Humanism underpinned Ho Chi Minh's philosophy of holistic, ethical development of individuals and society. Ho Chi Minh Thought emphasized morality, intellectual growth, and social justice. It was inspired by Confucian ideals, Marxist-Leninist ideas, and Vietnamese culture and philosophy.

While science and technology advanced, transhumanism evolved in the late 20th century as a radical response. The futurist philosophy promotes using technology to improve human physiological and cognitive skills, overcome biological restrictions, and better the human situation. It envisions a future where technology can reverse aging, cure diseases, and boost

IQ, strength, and sensory perception. Transhumanism raises deep ethical, intellectual, and sociological problems about human nature.

Comparing Ho Chi Minh's humanism and transhumanism is a critical discourse that can illuminate human development's changing ideas. Ho Chi Minh's humanism ideology praises human agency in social progress and promotes holistic human development by emphasizing morality, intellectual growth, and social justice. Transhumanism's vision of a technologically advanced future challenges us to rethink human potential and species evolution. These opposing views give a rich backdrop for contemplating human identity, human enhancement's ethics, and our future goals. A thorough grasp of these beliefs is essential as we face a technology revolution that could reshape humanity. We want to start a conversation on human development's sociopolitical, ethical, and philosophical aspects by examining Ho Chi Minh's humanism and transhumanism's similarities and differences. This comparative study aims to illuminate the intricacies of human enhancement and the future of mankind and build a sophisticated, multidimensional understanding that can lead our collective journey.

2. Transhumanism and its implications

Transhumanism, as a philosophical and intellectual movement, posits that humans can and should use technology to enhance their biological capabilities. This notion extends beyond just physical enhancements, encompassing cognitive and sensory augmentations, and even the prospect of immortality. As such, transhumanism challenges the traditional biological constraints of human existence, opening a Pandora's box of possibilities. Today, we see transhumanist principles in action in various forms, from prosthetic limbs and cochlear implants to more controversial developments like genetic engineering and neural implants.

While these advancements hold the promise of transcending human limitations and ailments, they also raise complex ethical issues. For instance, questions regarding accessibility and equality emerge, pondering whether these enhancements would only be available to the wealthy, thereby widening socio-economic disparities. Moreover, philosophical dilemmas arise around the notion of human identity, questioning if an extensively modified human would still retain their humanity, or if they would evolve into a distinct, posthuman entity.

3. Theoretical and practical basis for forming Ho Chi Minh's thought on human development

Ho Chi Minh's deep understanding of human development was shaped by an intricate blend of personal, cultural, and political influences. His anthropological perspective combined Vietnam's rich cultural heritage and religious ethics – namely Confucianism, Buddhism, and Taoism – with the principles of Marxism-Leninism and Western doctrines of freedom, equality, and fraternity.

The Vietnamese cultural tradition, established over thousands of years, has always emphasized the development of human personality, particularly under the influences of Buddhism, Taoism, and Confucianism. Key virtues from these traditions include "Mercy" in Buddhism, "Refinement" in Taoism, and "Jen" (or "Ren") in Confucianism. These virtues converge in the cultural traditions of the Vietnamese people. "Jen" signifies human nature, compassion, and love for all beings, and is highly respected and honored. It refers not merely to human nature, but to people in their social relationships, characterized by dignity, virtue, morality, and empathy.

Born into a traditional Confucian family, Ho Chi Minh was raised with a strong emphasis on the development of 'Jen' – humanity and compassion – as the core purpose of family life. He had traveled extensively before becoming the esteemed president of Vietnam. These experiences significantly contributed to shaping his intellect and personality, distinguishing him from his contemporaries. Ho Chi Minh was particularly influenced by Western values, including freedom, democracy, human rights, and philanthropy. This influence is prominently reflected in the 1945 Declaration of Independence, where Ho Chi Minh cited Thomas Jefferson: "We hold these truths to be self-evident, that all men are created equal, that they are endowed by their Creator with certain unalienable Rights, that among these are Life, Liberty and the Pursuit of Happiness". He also referenced the 1789 French Declaration of the Rights of Man and of the Citizen: "All men are born free and with equal rights, and must always remain free and have equal rights". Ho Chi Minh then asserted, "These are truths that no one can deny" (Ho Chi Minh, 2011, vol. 4, 1). Such core values inspired Ho Chi Minh to strive towards modernity, envisioning a world where people could truly thrive.

Moreover, Ho Chi Minh paid special attention to the Marxist-Leninist theory of human: "Human nature is not an abstraction. In its reality, human nature is the sum total of social relations association"(Marx & Engel 1995, vol. 3, 11). This is also the basic foundation for Ho Chi Minh to actively develop people in relationships.

Chi Minh's profound understanding of human growth was influenced by the socio-political climate of the day. He seen the agony and exile of Vietnamese people while serving as a revolutionary leader. Ho Chi Minh was deeply affected by the daily depictions of Vietnamese people suffering under the colonial authority and being persecuted. He commented:

> "A whole abyss separates Europeans from indigenous people. Europeans enjoy all freedom and reign as absolute masters; As for the natives, they were muzzled and led on a leash, with only the right to obey and not to complain; because if he dared to object, he would be declared a traitor" and that "the natives were bound hand and foot, having to endure the whims and despotism of the French rulers and the greed of the remnants of those who were their obedient servants" (Ho Chi Minh 2011, vol. 1, 11–12).

Those images inspired Ho Chi Minh's enthusiasm for the country and the people of Vietnam. Therefore, Ho Chi Minh considered the cause of human liberation and development of the Vietnamese nation as the center of the country's progress.

The central idea of Ho Chi Minh's philosophy appears to be the subject of both national and human liberty. Ho Chi Minh believed that the liberation of the Vietnamese country from such oppressive forces was a necessary condition for comprehensive development, as there was human growth during Vietnam's colonial era, when the Vietnamese people were subjected to various forms of oppression. His concept of emancipation encompassed not only political and economic freedom but also intellectual and spiritual awakening. Maybe for this reason, some Comintern members misinterpreted and condemned Ho Chi Minh, while some of his fellows in the Indochinese Communist Party saw him as a symbol of "nationalism" and "rightist deviationism" (Ministry of Education and Training 2021, 57). But reality has shown that Ho Chi Minh's theory was accurate. Beyond only wanting to be free of colonial control, his ultimate ambition was to create a free, just, and equal society in which every individual might reach their full potential and advance the common good.

4. The condition for human development in Ho Chi Minh's thought

The context for human development, as envisioned by Ho Chi Minh, had several defining characteristics.

Foremost, independence and sovereignty were considered essential preconditions. He believed that only in a free and independent nation could individuals fully exercise their rights and fulfill their potential. He used to say: "I have only one desire, the ultimate desire, to make our country completely independent, our people completely free, all compatriots have food, clothes, everyone can study"(Ho Chi Minh 2011, vol. 4, 187). According to Ho Chi Minh, liberating people entails freeing them from the chains that bind them and from the calamities caused by hunger and ignorance. He believed that human dignity is only attainable when individuals are liberated from slavery and oppression. Comprehensive development can only occur when people live in an independent country and enjoy freedom. Driven by this noble ideal, he famously declared, "Nothing is more precious than independence and freedom" (Ho Chi Minh 2011, vol. 15, 130). This statement encapsulates Ho Chi Minh's humanistic and humanitarian philosophy, significantly contributing to the philosophical discourse on human development.

Secondly, Ho Chi Minh emphasized the importance of a healthy cultural environment. He believed that culture plays an important role in shaping human character and behavior. In his view, a healthy cultural environment fosters morality, promotes intellectual development, and fosters a sense of social responsibility. With a policy of using culture to illuminate the path for the nation, Ho Chi Minh emphasized the development of a culture that both preserves and enhances the valuable aspects of national heritage while incorporating the finest elements of global human culture to achieve the strategic goal of "growing people".

Furthermore, Ho Chi Minh underscored the necessity of social justice, viewing its implementation as a vital condition for human perfection. He envisioned a society where all individuals have equal access to development opportunities across all facets of life, irrespective of their economic or social status. To highlight the importance of social justice, he quoted an ancient thinker: "Not afraid of lack, only afraid of injustice; not afraid of poverty, only afraid of people's discontent" (Ho Chi Minh 2011, vol. 15,

224). He believed that fair practices are essential for creating an environment conducive to development and contribution.

Additionally, Ho Chi Minh stressed the significance of a nurturing and mutually supportive community. The strength of solidarity and community cohesion, he argued, are crucial conditions for human development. This idea is encapsulated in his poem:

"Solidarity, Solidarity, Great Solidarity, / Success, Success, Great Success" (Ho Chi Minh, 2011 vol. 13, 119). Here, Ho Chi Minh suggested that unity fosters success, emphasizing the power of collective action and mutual support in facilitating human development. Thanks to solidarity, all resolutions become reality.

Lastly, he highlighted the importance of economic stability and development. In his view, economic progress serves not as an end in itself, but as a means to facilitate human development by providing individuals with the resources necessary to achieve their goals and aspirations. Essential material conditions, such as sufficient food, clothing, and shelter, are the fundamental requirements for human development. Following the success of the August Revolution, he promptly advocated for immediate action: "We have to do immediately these following: 1. Make the people have food, 2. Make the people have clothes, 3. Make the people have a place to live. 4. Make the people educated" (Ho Chi Minh 2011, vol. 4, 175).

Ho Chi Minh's ideology for human development thus offers a comprehensive and nuanced understanding of the human condition, one that encompasses physical, intellectual, and moral dimensions. It invites us to reflect on the societal, cultural, and economic contexts that facilitate human development and to explore the transformative potential of liberation, education, and social equity in fostering holistic human growth.

5. Ho Chi Minh's conception of the ideal human

Ho Chi Minh's philosophy was a synthesis of traditional and modern ideas, where a person is not just a biological entity but also a social and moral being whose development must be comprehensive, encompassing physical, intellectual, and moral or mental aspects.

Firstly, Ho Chi Minh's conception of the ideal human was deeply integrated into his broader ideology of societal development and transformation. His aim was to build a prosperous society free from oppression and exploitation, which he identified as a socialist society. He envisioned the creation of a "new socialist man" and emphasized, "To build socialism, first of all, we need socialist people" (Ho Chi Minh 2011, Vol. 13, 66). Similar to the philosopher Plato, who believed that the nature of a society reflects the character of its people, Ho Chi Minh aspired to foster a society where individuals possessed high moral qualities and professional capabilities and were devoted to serving the people, society, and the nation. He described the socialist person as one embodying noble moral qualities and selfless service, stating: "A socialist person is a person with morality, thriftiness, integrity, public-mindedness, and impartiality, wholeheartedly serving the people, serving the revolution", (Ho Chi Minh 2011, Vol. 14, 66). This vision was a fundamental aspect of his socialist ideology, which prioritized collective welfare over individual interests.

Furthermore, Ho Chi Minh viewed the ideal human as more than a product of biological evolution; they were also a result of ethical cultivation and social conditioning. Regarding ethics, he promoted the virtues of Diligence (CÂN), Frugality (KIỆM), Integrity (LIÊM), and Righteousness (CHÍNH), which he considered essential human qualities. He poetically expressed this framework:

> "There are four seasons in the heaven (world): Spring, Summer, Autumn, and Winter. The earth has four directions: East, West, South, and North. People have four virtues: Diligence (CÂN), frugality (KIỆM), Integrity (LIÊM), Righteousness (CHÍNH). Lack of a season, the heaven would be incomplete. Without a direction, it would not be the earth. Missing one virtue, the man would not be a true human" (Ho Chi Minh 2011, vol. 6, 117).

5.1 Ho Chi Minh on the concept of CÂN

It is difficult to find adequate English words that can cover the concepts that Ho Chi Minh originally intended. For example, the concept of "CÂN"(Ho Chi Minh 2011, vol. 6, 118–121), as presented by Ho Chi Minh, embodies elements of diligence, perseverance, industriousness, and meticulousness. However, no single English word encompasses all these aspects to fully represent the richness and depth of "CÂN". The closest English terms would be "diligence" or "perseverance", but it should be noted that these words do not completely capture the broad spectrum of meanings embedded in "CÂN". In the context of Ho Chi Minh's ideology, "CÂN" is a comprehensive concept that not only denotes hard work and persistence but also includes the idea of careful planning, consistent effort, and a commitment to long-term and sustainable progress.

This term is also underlined by the belief that there is no obstacle that cannot be overcome by hard work and perseverance. Ho Chi Minh's emphasis on "CÂN" aligns with his humanistic philosophy that values hard work and the pursuit of personal and societal development. He believes that the outcome of any endeavor, regardless of its complexity, can be favorable if approached with diligence. This principle extends to intellectual pursuits, as diligent learning accelerates knowledge acquisition, and diligent contemplation leads to innovative ideas.

Furthermore, Ho Chi Minh stresses that "CÂN" is not about working to the point of exhaustion, but rather about maintaining a steady and sustainable level of effort. It's about cultivating a sense of responsibility and industriousness that can drive long-term personal and societal progress.

In the broader context of our paper, Ho Chi Minh's emphasis on "CÂN" serves as a counterpoint to transhumanist perspectives. While transhumanism seeks to overcome human limitations through technological enhancements, Ho Chi Minh's philosophy highlights the intrinsic human capacity for diligence and the potential for holistic development through effort and persistence. It underscores the idea that the essence of being human is not solely about physical or intellectual capabilities but also about values, such as diligence, that shape character and contribute to societal progress.

5.2 Ho Chi Minh on the concept of KIỆM

The concept of "KIỆM" (Ho Chi Minh 2011, vol. 6, 122–125) as expressed by Ho Chi Minh in his philosophy can best be translated into English as "frugality". However, it should be noted that this term encompasses not only the traditional sense of frugality as careful management of resources and avoidance of waste, but also extends to the idea of efficient time usage and the balanced execution of tasks. It is the practice of exercising restraint and discipline to achieve greater societal and national goals. In his writings, Ho Chi Minh emphasized that "KIỆM" does not imply stinginess but is a thoughtful and disciplined approach to the consumption and usage of resources. This is not merely an individual virtue. It is also a collective obligation aimed at societal progress and national prosperity.

In Ho Chi Minh's view, "KIỆM" extends beyond the mere saving of physical resources. It includes efficient use of time and a careful approach to planning and executing tasks. He advised against procrastination and delay, viewing these as forms of wastefulness. Time, in his perspective, was as valuable as gold and could not be recaptured once lost. Importantly, Ho Chi Minh stressed the balance between "CÂN" (diligence) and "KIỆM"(frugality). These two concepts, in his view, are like the two legs of a person, both essential and complementary. Diligence without frugality could lead to wastefulness, while frugality without diligence could lead to stagnation. His teachings underscore the importance of balancing diligence with frugality, emphasizing the interdependence of these two virtues in fostering sustainable development and societal progress.

5.3 Ho Chi Minh on the concept of LIÊM

"LIÊM", as described by Ho Chi Minh(Ho Chi Minh 2011, vol. 6, 126–128), implies incorruptibility, honesty, fairness, and the absence of greed. It also encompasses the idea of acting in the best interests of the nation and its people, and not merely for personal gain. Ho Chi Minh expands upon the concept of "LIÊM", which he defines as incorruptibility and the absence of greed. The term's definition has evolved over time. In the past, under a feudal regime, "LIÊM" referred narrowly to officials who did not exploit their populace. However, in the context of the Democratic Republic, the scope of "LIÊM" broadens to encompass all citizens, akin to loyalty to the nation and filial piety towards all people, not just one's own parents.

He explained the concept of "LIÊM" is closely tied to "KIỆM" (frugality) and "CÂN" (diligence). Frugality is seen as a prerequisite for incorruptibility, as extravagance can breed greed. Varieties of greed are all categorized as violations of "LIÊM".This includes officials exploiting their power for personal gain, merchants engaging in dishonest trading practices, usurers exploiting the poor, farmers unfairly monopolizing water resources, craftsmen overcharging during times of hardship, and operators of gambling profiting at others' expense.

He emphasized "LIÊM" is also violated by those who undermine more capable individuals to protect their own status and reputation, avoid necessary tasks due to fear of hardship or danger, or retreat in the face of the enemy due to fear of death. Such actions are in direct contradiction to the principle of "LIÊM" and can lead to criminal acts of theft. In this context, any form of corruption, whether public or private, direct or indirect, is equated to theft. As Confucius and Mencius say, a person without "LIÊM" is worse than an animal, and if everyone is greedy, the country will be in danger.

5.4 Ho Chi Minh on the concept of CHÍNH

In Ho Chi Minh's philosophy, the term "CHÍNH" (Ho Chi Minh 2011, vol. 6, 129–131) encapsulates a complex set of moral virtues. It conveys the principles of righteousness, honesty, and uprightness. Therefore, the English word that would most closely encapsulate the meaning of "CHÍNH" in Ho Chi Minh's teachings is "Righteousness". However, it is important to note that "CHÍNH" (Righteousness) in this context extends beyond mere moral rectitude. It also encompasses diligence, thrift, integrity, sincerity, humility, and unity. It signifies a holistic and righteous approach to oneself, others, and one's work. Thus, Ho Chi Minh's concept of "CHÍNH" is a comprehensive moral and ethical philosophy that underpins an individual's conduct in society.

Ho Chi Minh's philosophy on "CHÍNH" (Righteousness) is integral to his vision for the Vietnamese people, and it plays a crucial role in the moral and ethical development of the society. His writings express the concept of "CHÍNH" as a manifestation of an individual's incorruptibility, straightforwardness, and adherence to a moral and ethical path. According to him, "CHÍNH" is the culmination of the principles of Diligence (CÂN), Frugality (KIỆM), and Integrity (LIÊM), and forms the fruit of these foundational elements. Therefore, "CHÍNH" is about cultivating a character that is diligent, thrifty, and has integrity. This results in a society that is strong both materially and spiritually, paving the way for a prosperous and progressive nation.

These four virtues were not arbitrary virtues but carefully selected attributes that Ho Chi Minh believed were fundamental to building a just, equitable, and prosperous society. It is apparent that Ho Chi Minh inherited the moral ideology of Confucianism and developed it in line with the needs of a new society. In it, humans must first know how to cultivate themselves, manage their household, rule the country, so that they might become able to institute peace in the world.

In addition, Ho Chi Minh's philosophy underscores the importance of introspection and self-improvement, encouraging individuals to constantly strive for progress, self-criticize, and welcome criticism from others. Moreover, in terms of sociality, the ideal human, in Ho Chi Minh's view, was not an isolated entity but an integral part of society. This person was envisioned as a contributing member of a collective entity, reinforcing Ho Chi Minh's belief in the inseparability of individual and societal development. The ideal human, therefore, was not merely a recipient of societal benefits but an active participant in the collective journey towards societal progress and transformation.

Ho Chi Minh posited that an individual's social behavior can be analyzed on three fronts: their relationship with themselves, their relationship with others, and their relationship with their work (Ho Chi Minh 2011, vol. 6, 129). Thus, when dealing with oneself, it is crucial to avoid arrogance and complacency, as they lead to stagnation. The emphasis is placed on the importance of continuously striving for progress, as lack of progress leads to regression. In dealing with others, Ho Chi Minh underscored the importance of sincerity, humility, and unity. He encouraged respect for all, regardless of their social status, and advocated for the practice of benevolence and love. As far as people's relationship with their work was concerned, Ho Chi Minh promoted the prioritization of national interests over personal or familial ones. He emphasized the importance of meticulous planning, dedication, and commitment to the task at hand, regardless of its magnitude. He encouraged the avoidance of any harmful deeds, no matter how small they might have seemed, and the pursuit of beneficial deeds, no matter how trivial they might appear.

In addition, Ho Chi Minh's ideal human was one who was in harmony with their natural and social environments. He believed in the principle of sustainability and highlighted the importance of living in a manner that respects the natural environment and contributes to its preservation. Nature is an indispensable part of human life, being in a close relationship with humans. Therefore, Ho Chi Minh always encouraged people to appreciate what belongs to nature, protect nature, and live in harmony with nature. This view led Ho Chi Minh to initiate the "Tree Planting Tet" movement: "Spring is the Tree Planting Tet, making the country more and more Spring; [...] This costs little but benefits a lot". (Ho Chi Minh 2011, Vol. 14, 445).

Furthermore, Ho Chi Minh believed that the ideal human should be a lifelong learner. He emphasized the importance of continuous learning and intellectual growth, viewing them as critical components of human development. He envisioned an ideal human who would continually strive to acquire new knowledge, skills and experiences, and use them to contribute to societal progress. As Ho Chi Minh said: "Learn to work, to be human, to be an officer. Learn to serve the Union, to serve the class and the people, to serve the Fatherland and humanity" (Ho Chi Minh 2011, Vol. 6, 208).

Finally, Ho Chi Minh's ideal human was one who maintained a balance between material and spiritual development. He cautioned against excessive materialism and advocated for a lifestyle that combined material prosperity with spiritual richness. This perspective underscored his belief in the importance of holistic human development that harmonizes physical well-being with intellectual growth and moral refinement.

Ho Chi Minh's conception of the ideal human thus provides a comprehensive and nuanced model of humanity that intertwines moral virtues, social responsibility, intellectual growth, and environmental consciousness. It presents a vision of human development that is integrative, sustainable, and oriented towards the collective good. It invites us to reflect on the potential of each individual to contribute to societal progress and to consider the societal conditions that facilitate the realization of this potential.

6. Ho Chi Minh's holistic approach to human development

The vision of human development, as Ho Chi Minh pointed out, is not limited to physical or economic progress. It combines intellectual development, moral improvement and liberation from mental and physical oppression. For Ho Chi Minh, human development is a comprehensive process including physical, intellectual and spiritual development.

Regarding physical fitness, Ho Chi Minh emphasized the importance of physical exercise and health, advocating regular exercise and a healthy lifestyle. Because according to Ho Chi Minh: "Preserving democracy, building the country, creating new life, everything requires good health to succeed" and "each healthy person, that is, contributing to the whole strength of country" (Ho Chi Minh 2011, Vol. 4, 241). According to Ho Chi Minh",If the people are strong, the country will be prosperous" (Ho Chi Minh 2011, Vol. 4, 241). Because having health means having everything, only health can give people a happy life, the ability to work, fight and study well. He advised every citizen: "Every day when you wake up, do a little exercise. Exercise every day, blood circulation, full spirit, that is health... "(Ho Chi Minh 2011, Vol. 4, 241).

In terms of intellectual development, Ho Chi Minh was clearly aware of the importance of developing human intelligence, calling on the Vietnamese people to seek knowledge and cultivate wisdom. This emphasis on education is evident in efforts to eradicate illiteracy and promote education in post-colonial Vietnam. He said: "For the sake of ten years, we must plant trees, for the benefit of a hundred years, we must plant people, we must train good citizens and good cadres for the country"(Ho Chi Minh 2011, Vol. 11, 528). Education is also an incubator factor to create a healthy culture. Education is considered a basic catalyst for human development. According to Ho Chi Minh, a good educational environment will produce virtuous and talented people. Therefore, Ho Chi Minh advocated for building an education system that not only imparts knowledge and skills but also fosters morality and responsibility. Since morality was perceived as the core of the culture, Ho Chi Minh constantly reminded the mission of ideal education that included moral education. Such education can result in "good citizens, good workers, good soldiers, good cadres for the country"(Ho Chi Minh 2011, Vol. 8, 448).

Ho Chi Minh believed that moral virtues were not innate but were cultivated through education and social influence. Ho Chi Minh's articles and speeches such as "Prison Diary", "Declaration of Independence", and "Correcting the Way of Working" all consistently emphasized these principles. For example, in the poem "In Prison", he wrote: "Everyone sleeps like an honest person / Waking up to distinguish the wicked and the meek; / Kindness, evil is not cassava, / Much of it is due to education" (Ho Chi Minh 2011, Vol. 3, 413). These lines emphasize Ho Chi Minh's belief in the transformative power of education and the cultivation of moral qualities in the fine traditions of the nation and humanity.

He also recognized the importance of a healthy and supportive environment in facilitating this development, stating that the improvement of societal conditions was a prerequisite for the betterment of the human spirit.

Our investigation leads us to recognize that Ho Chi Minh's vision of human development was not simply an abstraction; it was and continues to be an achievable humanistic model that can be realized through a combination of individual effort, social support and favorable conditions. This vision is expressed through Ho Chi Minh's policies and reforms to nurture good qualities in the Vietnamese people. For example, he promoted educational programs that combined professional training with moral education, and he advocated for policies that promoted social justice and cultural enrichment. Moreover, Ho Chi Minh's understanding of the natural cycle of life and death further shaped his perspective on human development. He saw life and death as natural phenomena and emphasized the importance of leading a fulfilling and meaningful life over the pursuit of immortality. His ideology, therefore, contrasts starkly with the transhumanist pursuit of immortality and limitless enhancement.

7. Ho Chi Minh's Humanism vs. Transhumanism: A Comparative Analysis

Exploring the differences and similarities between Ho Chi Minh's humanism and transhumanism provides a fascinating panorama of contrasting visions on human development and enhancement. Both ideologies, despite their distinct points of departure, grapple with the age-old question of what it means to be human, how humanity can and should evolve.

Ho Chi Minh's humanism on the one hand, and transhumanismand Transhumanism on the other, present alternative paths to human development. Ho Chi Minh's humanistic perspective emphasizes the holistic development of individuals, encompassing not just physical and intellectual growth, but moral and spiritual enrichment as well. His philosophy underscores the intrinsic value of human life within its natural life cycle, emphasizing the cultivation of moral virtues and a meaningful life over mere biological survival or boundless enhancements.

In contrast, transhumanism envisions a future where human capabilities are extended far beyond our current biological limitations, facilitated by the integration of advanced technology into the human body and mind. The core tenet of transhumanism, which embraces the possibility of limitless human enhancement and even immortality, stands in stark contrast to Ho Chi Minh's acceptance of life's natural cycle and the importance of living a virtuous, meaningful life within that cycle. While transhumanism highlights the potential for human beings to transcend their biological boundaries, Ho Chi Minh's humanism emphasizes moral and intellectual development. The virtues of diligence, thrift, integrity, and righteousness, which Ho Chi Minh revered, underscore the importance of moral qualities in human development, contrasted against transhumanism's focus on biological and technological enhancement.

Another significant divergence between the two ideologies lies in their respective views on the relationship between the individual and society. Transhumanism, with its roots in individualistic Western societies, tends to emphasize individual autonomy and the right to enhance one's capabilities without societal restraint. It champions the pursuit of personal development and self-realization, often via technological augmentation. On the other hand, Ho Chi Minh's humanism advocates for a communal approach to human development. His vision places the community at the core, emphasizing the development of individuals who contribute to societal progress and uphold communal values. The ideal human, in Ho Chi Minh's view, is not an isolated entity but a participatory member of society, actively contributing to the collective welfare.

8. Ethical and Societal Implications

The comparison of transhumanism with humanism according to Ho Chi Minh raises a number of important ethical and sociological issues. Through the prisms of these two opposing ideologies, we can analyze how we perceive society norms, human nature, and the moral issues that will inevitably influence humanity's destiny.

Ho Chi Minh's socioculturally informed humanistic philosophy advances an understanding of human evolution that transcends intellectual or physical advancement. It places a strong emphasis on moral qualities, social values, and holistic development, which makes us think carefully about the kind of society we want to build, the values we want to inculcate in others, and the methods we want to use to promote holistic human development. It brings up significant moral issues, like: What are the fundamental principles that ought to direct human progress? What part do cultural norms and institutions play in fostering these ideals in society? What steps can we take to guarantee the holistic and balanced development of humankind?

Furthermore, Ho Chi Minh's humanism highlights the need of building a just society in which people have the chance to develop and give back to the community. It raises concerns about society structure, resource allocation, and social responsibility by promoting social frameworks that uphold justice, equality, and mutual assistance.

On the other hand, the ideology of transhumanism brings to the surface a distinct set of ethical and societal considerations. The vision of a future where human capabilities can be enhanced through technology raises critical questions about access to and control over these advanced technologies. As these enhancements could provide significant advantages, who gets to decide who has access to them and under what conditions? Could this lead to increased socio-economic disparities, with the enhanced 'transhumans' gaining an unfair advantage over those who are 'merely' human?

Transhumanism also questions established ideas about what it means to be human and who we are. What does it mean to be human if we can alter our bodies and minds considerably? How much change is too much before we stop being human and begin to change into something else? Significant philosophical and ethical issues concerning one's own identity, the worth of human life, and the meaning of humanity are brought up by this. Hence the need to think carefully about the moral and societal ramifications of these beliefs. They compel us to reconsider our conceptions of human evolution and augmentation, as well as how society is structured and the moral issues that are involved.

9. Conclusion

Though varied and even conflicting, Ho Chi Minh's humanism and transhumanism give a compelling look at human evolution and advancement. They inspire introspection and comprehensive study of our shared human path, predicting our species' fate at the crossroads of natural and technological transformation. Attention is crucial. Ho Chi Minh's humanism supports socio-cultural values, morality, and intellect and honors human agency in society evolution. It promotes comprehensive development and individual-society betterment. His worldview emphasizes community, integrity, and righteousness in human development. His ideas encourage us to critique societal systems and promote human evolution. His social justice advocacy inspires society today.

Transhumanism, which uses technology to overcome biological constraints, challenges us to reevaluate what is possible for humanity. It inspires us to go beyond our comfort zones and discover unexplored territory in human betterment. Because of unequal access to enhancing technology and the effects of considerable human alteration on our species, it also raises ethical concerns such as socioeconomic injustice. Although its technological advancements portend growth, we should be cautious of its drawbacks.

References

Mac, C. and P. Angghen [K. Marx – F. Engel]. 1995. *Completed Works*. Vol. 3, Hanoi: National Political Publishing House.

Ho Chi Minh. 2011. *Completed Works*. Vol. 1. Hanoi: National Political Publishing House.

Ho Chi Minh. 2011. *Completed Works*. Vol. 3. Hanoi: National Political Publishing House.

Ho Chi Minh. 2011. *Completed Works*. Vol. 4. Hanoi: National Political Publishing House.

Ho Chi Minh. 2011. *Completed Works*. Vol. 6. Hanoi: National Political Publishing House.

Ho Chi Minh. 2011. *Completed Works*. Vol. 8. Hanoi: National Political Publishing House.

Ho Chi Minh. 2011. *Completed Works*. Vol. 11. Hanoi: National Political Publishing House.

Ho Chi Minh. 2011. *Completed Works*. Vol. 12. Hanoi: National Political Publishing House.

Ho Chi Minh. 2011. *Completed Works*. Vol. 13. Hanoi: National Political Publishing House.

Ho Chi Minh. 2011. *Completed Works*. Vol. 14. Hanoi: National Political Publishing House.

Ho Chi Minh. 2011. *Completed Works*. Vol. 15. Hanoi: National Political Publishing House.

Ministry of Education and Training. 2021. Ho Chi Minh ideology textbook. Hanoi: National Political Publishing House.

New Age and Romantism, Transhumanism and Enlightenment: The Importance of Transcendence and Authencity

Bojan Žalec

1. Introduction

This paper is part of a broader project of exploring modernity and secularization: their genesis, traps, hardships, catastrophes, as well as achievements. In this context, I also dealt with metaphysical, theological, anthropological, existential, cultural and religious aspects of violence (Žalec 2014; 2016; 2017a; 2020b). Many important thinkers have explained the origins of violence (in modern times) from these points of view (Taylor 2007, 646–710; Bellinger 2001). I will highlight two in particular. Georges Bataille explained it by the loss of intimacy (Bataille 1989; Dyrek 2004), which occurred earlier, but in modern times, the immersion in the world of things and work has reached special intensity. Leszek Kołakowski wrote about the revenge of the sacred (Kołakowski 1990, 63ff; Hagedorn 2017, 611–612), which was "abolished" in modern times. Both pointed out the existential source of violence and its connection to the sacred. The sacred, however, is a matter of the transcendence that the Enlightenment, as Horkheimer and Adorno found in the Dialectic of the Enlightenment, sought to eliminate to get rid of anxiety (Horkheimer and Adorno 2002, 11). In this paper, I argue that extreme transhumanism is a modern threat to respect for transcendence.

Within the framework of modernity, two moments have developed that cannot be understood separately: Enlightenment and Romanticism. Both are crucial to understanding violence. Also, the ideal of authenticity, which is the central ideal of our modern Western moral grammar and an important negative factor of violence, is the child of romanticism (Taylor 1991, 25).

In what follows, I will consider authenticity in the context of New Age and transhumanism. The first can be understood as a form of neo-Romanticism, and the second as a form of neo-Enlightenment. I will sketch an argument for the thesis that (extreme) transhumanism unlike the New Age is a threat to modern Western moral and political (liberal democratic) grammar, as there is no basis in it for respecting the value of authenticity.

2. Secularity and authenticity

Based on the findings of Charles Taylor, one of the most credible researchers and hermeneutic interpreters of our time, we can say that the current age of Western society has two key characteristics: secularism and the ideal of authenticity (Taylor 1991; 2007; Žalec 2019c). Taylor defined the secular era as an era in which exclusive humanism became a practical possibility and a sociologically relevant mass phenomenon (Taylor 2007, 19). Exclusive humanism is the understanding that does not refer to or take into account anything that is beyond human prosperity (Taylor 2007, 18). The ideal of authenticity means loyalty to oneself. It means the tendency to become what and who we are. This ideal is appropriate for our age in which moral grammar is marked by a distinction between ethics and morality. Ethics deals with the good or the good life, and morality speaks to what is right or just. In modern times, philosophy can no longer judge directly what a good life is. It limits itself to a meta-level and deals only with the formal properties of self-understanding processes. In this respect, it is characterized by a posture of restraint, and this posture is difficult to criticize or refuse. (Habermas 2003, 4; Žalec 2019b, 633; 2021, 53) The ideal of authenticity is formal (Junker-Kenny 2011, 124; Žalec 2021, 54). It can be used for worldviews that are completely different in content, even incompatible, or contradictory. Thus, for example, both an atheist and a theist can achieve an authentic life. Therefore, the ideal of authenticity is acceptable for our age and its moral grammar, as it does not violate the division into morality and ethics that is an integral part of this grammar.

Another characteristic of the secular age is that in it, worldviews, due to mutual interaction, have become fragile (Taylor 2007, 303) in the sense that people are aware that their views may be wrong. The fragility of worldviews in the secular age, observed by Taylor, may increase the sensitivity of members of secular society in some respects, their openness and tolerance, as they are aware that their views may be wrong. It also brings anxiety in Kierkegaard's sense of the word (Kierkegaard 1980; Žalec 2014, 445). Anxiety in this sense is a feeling of (existential) insecurity. It involves the awareness that we can walk different paths, that we can choose path A or B or C, etc., but we are not sure if we have, existentially speaking, made the right decision. This feeling of insecurity is a source of anxiety. Man is already inherentlya being of anxiety, because he is aware that he can go the different existential paths, and the fact that he can go the wrong way. Throughout history, we have witnessed a great attempt to overcome anxiety. As already mentioned, Horkheimer and Adorno in The Dialectic of the Enlightenment characterized the Enlightenment project as an attempt to get rid of anxiety by eliminating transcendence.

In the modern technological age, technology puts us in front of various options from which to choose. Those choices are not insignificant but concern the very foundations of man, society and the environment. In many ways, they can be downright fatal. For example, the possibility of liberal eugenics. It can be understood as a form of transhumanism, as will be seen later in this paper. Jürgen Habermas (Habermas 2003; Žalec 2019b; 640; 2021, 57–58) pointed out its incompatibility with modern Western moral grammar. By the term liberal eugenics, I mean prenatal interventions in the embryo genome to enhance a person's abilities, e.g. in terms of mathematical ability (at the expense of some other abilities, such as athletics). Habermas has convincingly shown that such interventions are incompatible with modern Western morality, as they threaten or even block the possibility that a programmed person may develop into an autonomous, equal and responsible member of community. (Habermas 2003, 77–78, 81–82, 92, 94–95; Žalec 2019b, 637; 2021, 57–58) But such individuals are the foundation of modern free Western democracy. We can say that from the point of view of the moral grammar of modern Western society, there is a contradiction in liberal eugenics. On the one hand, its proponents invoke the principle of radical autonomy and "freedom" of man as one of the main building blocks of modern Western moral grammar. On the other hand, liberal eugenics threatens or even undermines this very grammar.

3. New Age and Transhumanism

New Age covers a diverse range of phenomena. (Beckers 1998; Goljevšček 1992; Sire 2002, 144) It is characterized by eclecticism and syncretism (Sire 2002, 152). The thinking of the religions of the New Age is eclectic – drawn from various sources – and syncretistic – because it seeks to combine all religious thought and doctrine to the lowest common denominator. (Beckers 1998, 144) New Age is an umbrella term, but we could also say that it is a concept of family resemblance in Wittgenstein's sense of the word, which means that its content is a set of properties. Still, none of the subsets of these properties provides either the necessary or sufficient conditions that a certain phenomenon must meet to fall under the New Age concept. Another feature of the term New Age is its fuzziness. By stereotyping, we mean that a sparrow is a more typical specimen of a bird than a penguin. The notion of a bird is therefore a fuzzy notion. The fact that New Age is a fuzzy concept therefore means that some examples of the New Age and some characteristics are more stereotypical of the New Age than others and can be attributed to a higher degree of belonging to the concept of New Age than others. A feature that has a high degree of modern stereotyping is the emphasis on or advocacy of "non-institutional" religiosity. Non-institutional religiosity is also a feature that Ulrich Beck (Beck 2010, 100ff) highlights as a feature of contemporary Western religiosity. Another very stereotypical feature of the New Age is the emphasis on techniques, and as a third, I can mention a kind of neo-Gnosticism. (Goljevšček 1992; Beckers 1998, 145)

Like the New Age, transhumanism is an expression that we cannot define clearly. The first reason is the fact that transhumanism is by no means a homogeneous movement, but a diverse orientation (Žalec (ed.) 2019; Petkovšek and Žalec (eds.) 1921; Helmus 2020; Sturm 2021; Dittrich 2021; Gasser 2021). Transhumanism seeks to improve or enhance one's health, reduce or eliminate suffering, achieve extraordinary abilities, inhabit other planets, achieve immortality, and so on. All its representatives promise and advocate the improvement of man through modern science, technology or pharmacology, but differ in how radically they want to change man or even surpass him, abolish or relinquish him, how they understand this change or abolishment or relinquishment, what they consider possible and ethically permissible etc. Certainly, their views contain many ambiguities, as well as traps and dangers that require an answer from both ethical and religious points of view.

We can notice the affinity between transhumanism and the New Age in various respects. We can consider it its successor, which more than the New Age corresponds to the modern technological age and the mentality and intoxication of humanity with modern technological achievements. On the one hand, we can observe some "romantic" elements in the New Age, but on the other hand, we could talk about transhumanism as a kind of neo-Enlightenment. Like the Enlightenment, transhumanism promises to significantly reduce or even eliminate the limitations of man and his suffering. In any case, transhumanism is related to the Enlightenment orientation: "Transhumanism, in its continuous scientific optimism and thinking of progress […], is related to Enlightenment tendencies, which see in the rational penetration/analysis of nature the path to its manageability and improvement of human living conditions". (Sturm 2021, 431)

In this paper, I focus on extreme transhumanism. It is a position that promises and seeks to end virtually all human limitations and suffering. These limitations encompass physical limitations, including understanding the body as unnecessary or even undesirable, and even immortality. Extreme transhumanism sees no value in human "limitations" and suffering. In its basic orientation, it is therefore incompatible with the central message of world religions.[1] While radical transhumanism argues that the path to human happiness is to remove man's limitations as much as possible, the message of world religions is that the path to salvation leads precisely through man's acceptance of these limitations. (Osredkar 2019; 2021) Since this acceptance also means the acceptance of suffering, the views of extreme transhumanism and world religions are opposed to suffering.[2]

There is a similarity between the Enlightenment and extreme transhumanism. Both the Enlightenment and the transhumanists promised and advocated the removal of man's limitations and his prosperity. Exaggeration in removing restrictions, however, has had catastrophic effects. The

1 With this term, I refer to Hinduism, Buddhism, the Jewish religion, Christianity, and Islam. On the question of Confucianism as a world religion, see Sun 2013.

2 On the importance of the acceptance of suffering, in the context of world religions and broader, see Koslowski (ed.) 2001; Bowker 1970; Samuelson 2018; Trakakis 2018; Osredkar 2019, 666; Žalec 2020d; 2020e.

ultimate removal of limitation is the abolition of transcendence, which, however, has proven to be the abolition of respect for humanity. Extreme transhumanism promises an elimination of transcendence and strives to abolish it, which in turn means paving the way for a new catastrophe. Another similarity between the dangerous forms of the Enlightenment and transhumanism is that both forms are a version of exclusive humanism in Taylor's sense. In extreme forms of transhumanism, human prosperity paradoxically means transcending humanity, or abolition of it, because it is best for human, their greatest prosperity, or even their purpose following the "nature" that they tend to transcend.

Let us return to exclusive humanism. The effects of the Enlightenment and the dangers of extreme transhumanism point to the dangerous potential that exclusive humanism carries within itself. This potential is "abolition" or disregard for transcendence. Maybe we can paradoxically say that we work for human when we are not concerned just about human, or even more, when human is not our priority, even though we love them. Such was the position of Kierkegaard, who taught that we must love people, but our priority must be God (Kierkegaard 1995, 149, 448; Žalec 2017b, 81; Žalec 2020a, 57ff). We must love God more than any human being and more than anything else (Žalec 2018, 4–6). This is, following Kierkegaard, the proper path to true human prosperity. It is not necessary for a human to be an ardent believer to be aware of the importance of transcendence for the good of humans. An example of this is the "atheist" Adorno.

There are similarities between the New Age and transhumanism. Like certain forms of transhumanism, those forms of the New Age that contain Gnosticism or overemphasis on the (power) of techniques are incompatible with world religions, especially monotheistic ones. Therefore, we can say that, despite the important differences between the two, both the New Age and extreme transhumanism, in one way or another, reject or exclude the essential components of world religions. New Age also includes popular ideas about the radical change of human nature, the development of human consciousness, the arrival of a new man and a New Age, the development of a new, higher species than man, the quantum leap in human progress, and so on. (Sire 2002, 164ff) From this point of view, extreme transhumanism sounds almost like a transformed New Age, a new "New Age" suitable for the mindset and taste of a man of the technological age. A new offer in the same genre, but more "scientifically" wrapped, more suited to scientific consciousness, just as the New Age was extremely popular, and its stronger connection with naturalism helped it to be more attractive to the modern Westerner than pure Eastern mysticism, from which New Age has otherwise taken much (Sire 2002, 152).

However, as already mentioned, there are also significant differences between transhumanism and the New Age that are important for the topic of this article. As already mentioned, the ideal of authenticity is the child of 18th-century romanticism. Because of their "romantic" nature, the forms of the New Age were able to find space for the ideal of authenticity; moreover, some even emphasized it. On the contrary, transhumanism cannot give any real weight to the ideal of authenticity, it is superfluous, meaningless or incomprehensible in its horizons, and there is no basis for it.

Let us compare New Age and transhumanism in terms of the threat to the modern moral grammar of Western society and free democracy. We can say that transhumanism is more dangerous for it than New Age, although transhumanism may put an even larger emphasis on the values of liberal democracy, especially their libertarian interpretation. The reason for this greater danger of transhumanism is precisely the absence of the ideal of authenticity in transhumanism on the one hand and the presence of this in the New Age on the other.

4. The importance of the value of authenticity and the task of religious communities and institutions

The ideal of authenticity is not only an ideal with great political potential but also religious potential. Indeed, in the case of religions of (post-)axial age or world religions, authenticity is a condition for true religiosity. An undermining of the ideal of authenticity undermines not only modern Western morality but also genuine religiosity. In this sense, transhumanism is a greater challenge for traditional religious communities than New Age. New Age is incompatible with world religions for several reasons, for example for the sake of neo-Gnosis. In addition, it partly contributed to the spread of misconceptions about the importance of the institutionalization of religion (Goljevšček 1992, 23–24). We could continue. In the direction of transhumanism, as in the New Age, we can recognize the characteristics of Gnosticism. This is true, for example, of those forms of it that belittle the importance of the body. In this regard, these forms can be described as techno-gnosticism. Some forms of transhumanism, like some forms of New Age (Beckers 1998, 151), are hostile to traditional forms of religiosity. In short, there are quite a few similarities between New Age and transhumanism. However, as I have already pointed out, there is a fundamental difference between New Age and transhumanism, at least in its extreme forms: unlike in New Age, there is no place for the value of authenticity.

What follows from the above about the tasks and the mission of religion and religious communities and institutions in the modern world? It is certainly imperative that they are aware of the main features of the modern situation to function properly. They must first be aware that a return to a pre-modern state of genuine pre-secular spirituality and religiosity is not possible. Second, they must be aware that secular society is the result of a long historical transformation that began in the 16th century (Taylor 2007), and that both atheists and theists in the West are "products" of this same development and, "under the skin", "siblings". (Taylor 2007, 675; Abbey 2017, 228) This fraternity can be a basis for dialogue, solidarity, or at least fair cooperation (Žalec 2020c). As far as authenticity is concerned, religious communities and institutions should be aware that modern man requires an approach that is consistent with this ideal. Such an approach must be more sensitive, empathetic and reflective than in the past. Only in this way can churches and religious communities keep in touch with the people of the modern world. (Žalec 2019c, 46) In addition to all this, they must be aware, and act accordingly, that their task is not only to adapt to a culture of authenticity but also to protect and cultivate the ideal of authenticity. This is a key moment in the struggle to preserve humanity in the sense of *humanitas*. This is our most fundamental task, which is especially difficult and responsible in the technological age of digitization and AI.

5. Conclusion

Transhumanism is similar to its historical predecessor, the Enlightenment. The Enlightenment also proclaimed itself an advocate of man and the basic building blocks of our modern Western moral grammar, and some of them were formulated and enforced for the first time by the Enlightenment. On the other hand, the Enlightenment allowed for phenomena that were opposed to those that the proponents of the Enlightenment would have desired. The same can be said of (extreme) transhumanism: following its program and ideas could have catastrophic consequences for man. The very absence of the value of authenticity is extremely dangerous from the point of view of modern Western moral grammar, and the fundamental and greatest danger is the disrespect for transcendence, which, like certain forms of enlightenment, is manifested by extreme transhumanism.

References

Abbey, R. 2017. Siblings under the skin: Charles Taylor on religious believers and non-believers in *A Secular Age*. In: A. Carrol and R. Norman (eds.),Religion and Atheism: Beyond the Divide, London & New York: Routledge, pp. 221–231.

Bataille, G. 1989. Theory of Religion. New York: Zone Books.

Beck, U. 2010. A God of One's Own: Religion's Capacity for Peace and Potential for Violence. Cambridge: Polity Press.

Beckers, H.-J. 1998. Novodobskagibanja [New Age movements]. In: V. Škafar (ed.), Verstva, sekte in novodobskagibanja. Celje: Mohorjevadružba, pp. 144–151.

Bellinger, C. K. 2001. The Genealogy of Violence: Reflection on Creation, Freedom and Evil. New York: Oxford University Press.

Bowker, J. 1970. Problems of Suffering in the Religions of the World. Cambridge: Cambridge University Press.

Dittrich, T. S. 2021. Transhumanistisches Glückstreben und christliche Heilshoffnung. Ein Vergleich. Zeitschrift für Theologie und Philosophie, 143(3): 452–474.

Dyrek, Z. 2004. Bataille on Immanent and Transcendent Violence. Bulletin de la Société Américaine de Philosophie de Langue Français, 14(2): 29–49.

Gasser, G. 2021. Leibliche Existenz und die Vision des Mind-Uploading. Zeitschrift für Theologie und Philosophie 143(3): 365–387.

Goljevšček, A. 1992. New Age in krščanstvo [New Age and Christianity]. Koper: Ognjišče.

Habermas, J. 2003. The Future of Human Nature. Cambridge: Polity Pres.

Hagedorn, L. 2017. Spectres of Secularism – Remarks on (the Loss of) Religion and its Implications. Bogoslovnivestnik 77(3–4): 601–613.

Helmus, C. 2020. Transhumanismus – Der neue (Unter-)Gang des Menschen? Das Menschenbild des Transhumanismus und seine Herausforderungen für die Theologische Anthropologie. Regensburg: Friedrich Pustet.

Horkheimer, M. and Adorno, T. W. 2002. Dialectic of Enlightenment. Stanford: Stanford University Press.

Junker-Kenny, M. 2011. Habermas and Theology. London, New York: T&T Clark International.

Kierkegaard, S. 1980. The Concept of Anxiety. Princeton: Princeton University Press.

Kierkegaard, S. 1995. Works of Love. Princeton: Princeton University Press.

Kołakowski, L. 1990. Modernity on Endless Trial. Chicago: The University of Chicago Press.

Koslowski, P. (ed.). 2001. The Origin and the Overcoming of Evil and Suffering in The World Religions. Dodrecht: Kluwer Academic Publishers.

Osredkar, M. J. 2019. Religijakotizziv za transhumanizem [Religion as a challenge to transhumanism]. Bogoslovnivestnik 79(3): 657–668.

Osredkar, M. J. 2019. Resignation as the foundation of life. In: R. Petkovšek and B. Žalec (eds), Transhumanism as a Challenge for Ethics and Religion, Zürich: Lit Verlag, pp. 165–172.

Petkovšek, R. and Žalec, B. (eds). 2021. Transhumanism as a Challenge for Ethics and Religion. Zürich: Lit Verlag.

Samuelson, S. 2018. Seven Ways of Looking at Pointless Suffering: What Philosophy Can Tell Us About the Hardest Mystery of All. Chicago and London: Chicago University Press.

Sire, J. W. 2002. Izazovsvjetonazora: pregledtemeljnihsvjetonazora [orig. The Universe Next Door]. Zagreb: STEPress.

Sturm, W. 2021. Transhumanismus und Digitalisierung. Theologisch-anthropologische Perspektiven. Zeitschrift für Theologie und Philosophie 143(3): 425–451.

Sun, A. 2013. Confucianism as a World Religion: Contested Histories and Contemporary Realities. Princeton: Princeton University Press.

Taylor, C. 1991. The Ethics of Authenticity. Cambridge and London: Harvard University Press.

Taylor, C. 2007. A Secular Age. Cambridge, MA & London, England: The Belknap of Harvard University Press.

Trakakis, N. N. 2018. The Problem of Evil: Eight Views in Dialogue. Oxford: Oxford University Press.

Žalec, B. 2014. Nazism and Stalinism in the Light of Kierkegaard's Thought. Filozofia 69(5): 443–450.

Žalec, B. 2016. Human refusal of the basic truth about self as the origin of violence. In: R. Petkovšek and B. Žalec (eds), Truth and Compassion: Lessons from the Past and Premonitions of the Future, Zürich: Lit Verlag, pp. 29–39, 171–172.

Žalec, B. 2017a. Radical Islamism and Totalitarianism. In: V. Strahovnik and B. Žalec (eds), Religion, Violence, and Ideology: Reflections on the Challenges of Postmodern World, Zürich: Lit Verlag, pp. 23–34, 101–102.

Žalec, B. 2017b. The relevance of Kierkegaard for political thought: violence and the divine command. European Journal of Science and Theology, 13(3): 75–87.

Žalec, B. 2018. Kierkegaard and the ethics of sacrifice as part of the ethics of love. European Journal of Science and Theology, 14(3): 1–11.

Žalec, B. 2019a. Between secularity and post-secularity: critical appraisal of Charles Taylor's account. Bogoslovnivestnik, 79(2): 411–423.

Žalec, B. 2019b. Liberalna evgenika kotuničeval katemeljev morale [Liberal eugenics as a destroyer of morality]. Bogoslovnivestnik 79(3): 629–641.

Žalec, B. 2019c. Charles Taylor on religion in a modern cultural frame: secularity and authenticity. In: R. Petkovšek and B. Žalec (eds), Religion as a Factor of Intercultural Dialogue, Zürich: Lit Verlag, pp. 39–48, 193.

Žalec, B. (ed.). 2019. Transhumanizem [Transhumanism]. Bogoslovnivestnik, 79(3) (special issue).

Žalec, B. 2020a. Kierkegaard o ljubezni in preizkušnjah: krščanska antropologija tesnobe, nasilja in trpljenja [Kierkegaard on Love and Afflictions: A Christian Anthropology of Anxiety, Violence, and Suffering]. Ljubljana: KUD Apokalipsa and Srednjeevropskiraziskovalniinštitut Søren Kierkegaard.

Žalec, B. 2020b. Islamophobia as a False Image of Islam and a Negative Factor of Intercultural Dialogue. In: M. Godawa and B. Žalec (eds), Krakow: The Pontifical University of John Paul II in Krakow.

Žalec, B. 2020c. Fair cooperation and dialogue with the other as a rational attitude: the grammarian account of authenticity. Annales. Series historia et sociologia, 30(3): 383–394.

Žalec, B. 2020d. Kierkegaard on the beneficial yoke of suffering. XLinguae 13(3): 3–12.

Žalec, B. 2020e. Kierkegaard on the joyful anxiety and suffering. In R. Petkovšek and B. Žalec (eds), Ethical Implications of One God: The Significance of Monotheism, Zürich: Lit Verlag, pp. 41–52, 184–185.

Žalec, B. 2021. Liberal eugenics as a destroyer of moral agents: Habermas' critique. In: R. Petkovšek and B. Žalec (eds), Transhumanism as a Challenge for Ethics and Religion, Zürich: Lit Verlag, pp. 53–59, 215.

ENGAGED BUDDHISM TOWARD TRANSHUMANISM

Ha Thanh Pham and Hai Hoang Nguyen

1. Introduction

The desire to acquire new powers, such as strength, intelligence, well-being, and longevity, appeared through myths, religions, and beliefs at the dawn of humankind's civilization. Like the civilizations of Egypt, Greece, and Mesopotamia, Vietnam has many myths and legends that express the expectation for rapid development and superior power. The fairy tale about Saint Giong, one of the only four Vietnamese immortals, is a prime example of a superhuman helping people save the country. When a strong enemy threatens, the country needs exceptional individuals. From a boy of about three years old, in a short time, Saint Giong became a tall man, more potent than many others, using iron horses and iron weapons to transform into a superhuman to defeat foreign invaders. Then he flew to the sky. Even so, people still thought he was immortal. Saint Giong appeared as early as Vietnam gained independence from the Chinese in the 11th century. The transformation of Saint Giong from a mythological symbol to a national symbol of heroism in anti-invader history was recorded in many documents during the Tran dynasty (1225–1400) (Lê Tắc 1400; Trần Trọng Kim 1920). The Giong Festival, one of Vietnam's most important festivals, was recognized as UNESCO's intangible cultural heritage in 2010 (Dinh 2020).

Transhumanist desire is not limited to religions, beliefs, or imaginations. People's constant efforts in developing science and technology have changed our perceptions. By the 19th century, with the birth of Darwin's theory of evolution, it was realized that human was not the last step of the evolutionary process and could be enhanced further than we are today.

In the 20th century, with modern science and technology advances, it was believed that they could be used to improve the human body.

Transhumanism is a philosophical movement that advocates using technology to increase lifespan, physical health, intelligence, and emotional well-being. Many scientists consider philosopher Friedrich Nietzsche the first person who inspired transhumanism through his thought of transcending man. However, he attributed that progress to individual efforts rather than technology. Perhaps the first person to introduce the concept of superhumanity was Julian Huxley in 1957, who put it in a speech about the possibility of using technology to enhance human abilities (Huxley2015, 15):

> "The human species can, if it wishes, transcend itself – not just sporadically, an individual here in one way, an individual there in another way, but in its entirety, as humanity. We need a name for this new belief. Perhaps transhumanism will serve: man remaining man, but transcending himself, by realizing new possibilities of and for his human nature".

In 1983, Max More (1998)formulated the Extropy principles to guide the development of transhumanism.[1] There he wrote: "We see humanity as a transitory stage in the evolutionary development of intelligence. We advocate using science to accelerate our move from human to a transhuman or posthuman condition".Thus, Extropians argue that man is only an intermediate process of intelligence through which technology can reach a posthuman state. In 1998, Nick Bostrom and David Pearce established the World Transhumanist Association, now known as Humanity+, integrating a philosophical movement with disciplines such as computer science, artificial intelligence, and nanotechnology. The advancement of biotechnology, particularly gene editing applied to human embryos to produce individuals with exceptional abilities, has sparked ethical debates concerning transhumanism.

Transhumanists posit that contemporary strides in science and technology enable humanity to transcend its current intellectual confines, bypassing the slow pace of biological evolution. They advocate for a judicious embrace of technological innovations, not as entities to be feared, but as

[1] Extropy is an antonym of entropy. It is symbolized by a progressive increase in order, organization, vitality, energy, life, human intelligence, and the capacity for adaptive change.

instrumental tools designed to augment human capabilities and welfare. In his declaration of superhumanity, Nick Bostrom argues that superhumanity is not limited to humans on Earth and can transform humans into interplanetary beings. Instead of banning it, we should turn technology to human advantage, including its application to reproduction. Technology does not only apply to humans but can, in principle, apply to all sentience, such as artificial intelligence, humans, posthumans, and non-humans. To avoid negative consequences in the future, people need to establish forums for dialogue to debate issues that need to be solved responsibly (Bostrom 2005).

Opposition to transhumanism stems from a multitude of concerns, encompassing ethical, religious, and socio-economic dimensions. The advent of advanced technologies, while promising in terms of enhancing physical capabilities, simultaneously poses risks to human dignity and autonomy. Ethical and religious objections frequently surface as primary considerations, highlighting the moral quandaries associated with technological augmentation. Additionally, a stark disparity emerges between those who possess the means to access such technologies and those who do not, thereby exacerbating social inequalities and creating an insurmountable divide among different societal factions. The personal and environmental impact of technology adoption warrants critical examination, as it harbors the potential to deplete natural resources and inflict irreversible damage upon the Earth. Particularly alarming is the partial comprehension of technology by the populace, which may precipitate unforeseen and irreparable consequences for future generations.

The discourse on transhumanism, particularly when examined through the lens of various religious perspectives, bifurcates into factions both endorsing and opposing the movement. Certain religious viewpoints advocate for transhumanism as a conduit for human progression, while others critique it as an affront to natural order and an intrusion upon the domain of the supernatural. Contentious debates frequently revolve around the nature of human self-conception, the dynamics of human interrelations, the connection with other life forms, the broader interaction with the environment, the cosmos, and the realm of the supernatural. This discourse specifically delves into the contemplation of transhumanism from a Buddhist standpoint, offering a nuanced exploration of its alignment or conflict with Buddhist doctrines and ethical principles.

Buddhism, initiated by Siddartha Gautama more than 2500 years ago, is the dominant religion in Cambodia, China, Japan, Korea, Laos, Sri Lanka, Thailand, and Vietnam. Although diverse and with many schools, Buddhism uses suffering (dukkha) as the core concept. The most important features are the liberation of suffering to reach the state of Nirvana and the principle of dependent origination. Therefore, the studies on transhumanism and Buddhism all take these concepts as the basis. Most of the studies on transhumanism say that Buddhism supports transhumanism.

The state of Nirvana, the ultimate goal of Buddhism, is a state that can only be experienced directly and cannot be described through the ordinary senses, representing spiritual enlightenment and liberation from the cycle of birth, death, and rebirth (samsara). Transhumanists believe that the Nirvana state is posthuman and superhuman. Therefore, Buddhism and transhumanism have the same purpose: the desire for people to have a better life in the future without suffering. Nirvana may be an abstract concept, but some Mahayana schools, such as Pure Land and Tantric Buddhism, give a specific goal and are often used by transhumanism as an analogy to superhuman or posthuman.

Suffering and liberation from suffering are standard features of Buddhism. The Eightfold path, the right way (Dharma) to cease suffering, focuses on morality, concentration, and wisdom. Buddhist practice mainly requires spiritual and psychological efforts. Buddhism emphasizes moderate physical training to complement intellectual and spiritual development. Advances in neuroscience and psychology have elucidated brain functions, benefiting both Buddhists and transhumanists. Nonetheless, a divergence exists: meditation emphasizes the present, while transhumanism is future-oriented (Evans 2014). If the Eightfold Path in Buddhism is viewed as a liberation tool, technology could potentially augment physical and mental capacities. Thus, Buddhists may pursue enlightenment with technological support, integrating self-cultivation with scientific advancements.

The principle of dependent origination is one of the basic principles of Buddhism. This principle holds that all things and phenomena have a cause and will lead to an effect on other things and phenomena. An essential representation of dependent origination is that a thing has no permanent, unchanging, and independent self, no-self (anatman). The origin of suffering is the constantly changing desires for the self, explained by neuroscience research. The feeling of satisfaction and happiness does not last long. It comes quickly and goes quickly. People are always looking for a feeling of pleasure and then disappointed with that feeling. This is the suffering of change, the mental aspect of suffering.

However, some studies argue that Buddhist concepts do not fully support transhumanism. Buddhism's goal is Nirvana, an abstract, positivist concept that destroys all personal desires, while the goal of transhumanism is particular and highly personal. The nature of impermanence in Buddhism holds that things constantly change, contradicting transhumanism's desire to be immortal. The concept of no-self contradicts the progress of the ego of transhumanism. Transhumanism comes from the desire to improve the ego of the West, where the distinction between the self and the outside world is evident.

One of the authors who believe that Buddhism supports transhumanism is James Hughes (Hughes 2019). He argued that humans in Abrahamic religions were created sacred but immutable, while humans in Buddhism regularly evolved into gods and superhumans. Furthermore, Buddhism is not against using spiritual technology or medicine to live longer. Western scientists removed the superstitious elements of Buddhism to work together on meditation methods to improve emotional control, compassion, and change of consciousness. James Hughes put forward the idea of Cyborg Buddha, which presumed that transhumanism and the Buddhist tradition have a common goal of liberation from suffering and affirm that every human being can achieve liberation through his own efforts. Thanks to the support of technology, the liberated state of people in the future is Cyborg Buddha. The future of Buddhism combines Buddhist wisdom with technology, intellectual and physical growth. He also thinks that his idea may face many ethical and spiritual questions. He emphasizes the balance between the goals of transhumanism and ethical and social justice.

Benjamin Ross used suffering and dependent origination concepts to evaluate transhumanism (Ross 2020). The author argued that Buddhism and transhumanism recognize suffering because of impermanence. A pleasant sensation passes as quickly as it appears. Therefore, if people are constantly craving gratification, they will invariably suffer. However, Buddhism and transhumanism differ on how to deal with the problem. Buddhism emphasizes the destruction of the self, while transhumanism promotes the self through technology. It sounds like two conflicting philosophies, but the author explains that Buddhism is a compensating part of or an alternative solution for transhumanism.

Michael LaTorra identifies himself as a Buddhist Transhumanist (Ross 2020; La Torra 2015) and believes that transhumanism is a modern version of Buddhism. He said that the four noble truths and the eightfold path are essentially inner technologies used to realize the nature of suffering and thereby get rid of suffering. He introduced a Buddhist Transhumanist concept with an analogy between transhumanism and Buddhism. He drew a comparison between the Mahayana Buddhist concept of skilled means, which advocates the utilization of any expedient method to attain spiritual objectives, and the application of contemporary technology in the modern era. He showed that technology is also a skillful means of attaining liberation.

In what follows, we will examine the intersection of transhumanism with Buddhist thought, juxtaposing key Buddhist tenets against the backdrop of recent scientific progress. This examination will reveal varying degrees of receptivity towards transhumanist ideas across different Buddhist traditions, including Meditation, Pure Land, and Tantric Buddhism. Additionally, the discourse will extend to an examination of the interplay between neuroscience and genetic technology and foundational Buddhist principles, offering a comprehensive insight into their synergies and divergences.

2. Buddhism

2.1 Hinduism

According to plate tectonic theory, the collision of the Indian and Asian plates around 52 million years ago resulted in the formation of the Himalayas and the Tibetan Plateau, creating a natural demarcation between the Indian subcontinent and its northern neighbors (Rowley 1996). Around 66–70 thousand years ago, early Homo sapiens arrived in this region, later evolving into the Dravidian populations of the East and South and the Austro-Asiatic speakers of the central areas (Kumar et al. 2008). This area is also the cradle of the Indus Valley Civilization, dating back to 7000 BCE (Mark 2012).

Ancient India has two famous rivers originating in the Himalayas and flowing in opposite directions: the Indus and Ganges. The Indus River is more than 1500 km long and flows southwest to the Gulf of Oman (Mark 2012). In Sanskrit, Sindhu means river or sea. This word is used to call the Indus River. When the Persians entered the land of India, they called this river Hindus, and the northern part of India Hindustan (the land of rivers). Indians today identify themselves as Hindus. The Ganges River is 2500 km long and flows southeast, crossing northern India and Bangladesh to pour into the Bay of Bengal (Kumar 2017). The river was named after the Hindu goddess Ganga in ancient texts and art. Because of its origin in the Himalayas, the river has an inexhaustible water source from this mountain range's snow and ice. The basin of the Ganges River is the most densely populated in the world.

Originating from the Sintashta culture in the southern Urals, Aryans are believed to have entered India around the 18th century BCE (Beckwith 2009, 50). Contrary to the notion of an invasion, some scholarly theories propose that the Aryans' movement into India constituted a migration. Then when faced with resistance from the natives, they turned the migration into an invasion. They soon captured the northern part of India, advancing East of the Indus and along the Ganges until they took possession of all the land of Hindustan. There is no evidence of wars, so most scientists now believe that the Aryan incursions were peaceful, and over time they gradually merged with the natives.

The Aryans brought the Sanskrit language along with their religious system given in the Vedas. From here, India began a new civilization, the Vedic civilization. The Vedas were originally from the Aryans and later absorbed many aspects of the religions of the Indus valley civilization. Thus, for the Vedic to become a religion, the Vedic scriptures, originally of the Aryans, absorbed many of the beliefs of the Indus Valley civilization and became complete around the 12th century BCE.

A distinctive characteristic that distinguishes Indian civilization from others is the enduring caste system, historically entrenched and persisting into the present. In Sanskrit, the term "varna", often translated as "caste", literally means "color". This linguistic nuance suggests a possible origin story where the lighter-skinned Aryans, migrating southward, encountered the darker-skinned indigenous populations. The ensuing social stratification and discrimination against the natives might have given rise to the caste system.

There are four main castes:

1. Brahmana refers to priests and scholars who must care for the soul, the quintessential part of man. This is the highest caste.
2. The Kshatriya consists of princes and warriors who must look after the country and maintain social order.
3. Vaishya indicates farmers and merchants with the task of labor and production to create wealth in society. They also have to pay taxes and serve as soldiers for the state.
4. The Shudra is laborers whose duty was to serve the upper castes unconditionally. They were not allowed to participate in religious ceremonies other than worshiping deities exclusive for their caste.

   In addition to the four castes, there is an outcast and untouchable class called the Paria, today also known as the Dalit, who are only allowed to do the lowest things in society.

For such a caste society to be stable in the long term, the structure of the society needs to be made religious so that everyone in the society voluntarily conforms. Those regulations were incorporated into Hinduism. Hinduism is not a term referring to a religion as it is commonly understood. However, Hinduism refers to a group of indigenous traditions and beliefs in India that have many similarities and divergences. Some traditions have survived almost intact for thousands of years to the present day. It can be said that Hinduism is a way of life and undergoes many changes over time. Transformative shifts within the religious landscape of ancient India gave rise to distinct religious traditions such as Buddhism and Jainism. These changes, while sufficient to catalyze the emergence of new faiths, also precipitated internal transformations within Hinduism itself. Consequently, Hinduism evolved to encompass a diverse array of philosophical perspectives, including atheistic and monotheistic branches. In 1995, the Supreme Court of India wrote the following:

> "[Hinduism] does not worship any one God; it does not subscribe to any one dogma; it does not believe in any one philosophic concept; it does not follow any one set of religious rites or performances; in fact, it does not appear to satisfy the narrow traditional features of any religion or creed. It may broadly be described as a way of life and nothing more". (Rautray 2016)

In 2016, after many debates for a change of opinion, the Supreme Court of India voted and upheld the above statement and emphasized that "Hindutva was not a religion, but a way of life and a state of mind" (Rautray 2016).

2.2 Buddhism

Emerging from the philosophical and spiritual milieu of Hinduism, Buddhism inherited a multitude of values from its precursor. Both Hinduism and Buddhism share several core concepts, including the belief in the cyclical nature of existence (samsara), the governing principles of karma, adherence to a righteous path (Dharma), and the ultimate goal of liberation (moksha). While both traditions advocate practices such as meditation, yoga, and the use of mantras, the specific techniques and underlying principles exhibit notable distinctions.

Karma in Sanskrit means "action" or "deed". While karma is often associated with Eastern religions, the concept can be found worldwide in many different cultures and belief systems. Karma is not necessarily a punishment or reward but a natural consequence of one's actions. Some people believe in "instant karma", where the consequences of one's actions are immediately felt, while Hinduism and Buddhism believe in a more long-term view of karma, where the effects may not be felt until later or in future life. Karma can also be seen as a way to encourage positive behavior and discourage negative behavior since one's actions will ultimately affect their well-being and those around them. The hierarchical worldview of Hinduism puts Brahman as the ultimate reality and highest rank, followed by humans, animals, plants, and things.

Despite shared origins, Buddhism significantly diverges from Hinduism in several aspects, notably in its foundational history. Hinduism, lacking a singular founding figure, is a confluence of indigenous religious traditions of India. In contrast, Buddhism was established by an individual, Siddhartha Gautama, known as the Buddha. Hinduism acknowledges a supreme reality, Brahman, manifesting through myriad deities, and posits that the universe was created by this ultimate entity. Buddhism, however, does not subscribe to the notion of a creator; it asserts that the universe is governed by impersonal, objective laws, devoid of divine orchestration. Consequently, Hinduism places a greater emphasis on ritualistic practices, whereas Buddhism prioritizes ethical conduct and personal enlightenment.

Hinduism is characterized by a structured caste system, wherein the doctrine of karma dictates the soul's experiences across various incarnations. In stark contrast, Buddhism repudiates the caste system, advocating for the eradication of social stratification among individuals and emphasizing the interconnectedness of all beings, thereby diminishing the distinctions between humans and other forms of life. Humans and animals all have a Buddha nature, the ability to be liberated of living beings. Humans have many advantages over animals. Therefore, human life is vital for practicing Dharma. This is a significant difference between Buddhism and Hinduism, and other religions. The breakdown of caste was revolutionary in a society where class distinctions were very significant. Sentient beings can directly cultivate their selves to achieve the goal of liberation without requiring a special Brahman to do this. Both have liberation as theirgoal, but liberation in Hinduism is the unification of the individual soul with the universal soul (Brahman). Buddhist liberation is the liberation from the cycle of samsara to an entirely new state of Nirvana.

Human is essential but not supreme, not perfect; the human is merely a stage in a chain of evolution. Within the Abrahamic religious traditions, it is posited that humans are created in the image of an omnipotent deity, imbuing them with an inherent sense of immutability and perfection. In contrast, Buddhism assigns a more modest role to humanity, viewing it as one of numerous existential states through which an individual may traverse en route to Nirvana. While humans are considered to possess certain advantages in the practice of Dharma, their status is not regarded as ultimate. Consequently, the extension of human lifespan holds significant importance, facilitating the pursuit and realization of spiritual objectives.

This critical point makes a significant difference between the East and the West. The West places the position of humans at the center of the universe, but the East, not only Hinduism and Buddhism but also Taoism, places humans in a much more modest position within the universe.[2] The difference is very significant. It has affected the entire history and development process of humanity. Western civilization often elevates anthropocentrism, positioning human interests and perspectives at the apex of its value system. In stark contrast, Buddhism articulates a view of humanity

---

2 Confucianism is not considered a religion in a true sense but as a moral system, so we will not discuss it here.

as merely one element within the extensive continuum of evolution. This perspective necessitates the acknowledgment of humans as integral components of a vast web of interrelations with other sentient beings, underscoring the imperative to consider our existence within the broader context of all life forms.

Another difference is the recognition of suffering as the key to human beings through the Four Noble Truths. The ultimate goal of Buddhism is liberation from samsara, liberation from rebirth, and the attainment of Nirvana. Buddhism recognizes suffering as the key to human existence.

There are three kinds of suffering:

1. Physical suffering expressed by birth, old age, sickness, and death. This refers to the physical suffering that all beings experience, such as pain, illness, and loss.
2. Mental suffering expressed by the constant change of desire. This refers to the suffering that arises from change, impermanence, and the inevitable decay and death of all things.
3. Suffering because of ignorance refers to the illusion of suffering that arises from the conditioned nature of existence, the endless cycle of birth, death, and rebirth, and the endless cycle of a separate self.

When we talk about physical suffering, we refer to the common sense of this concept. According to Buddhism, there are four main kinds of physical suffering, considered as the basis of samsaric life. These are the sufferings of birth, old age, sickness, and death. Therefore, Buddhism holds that while we are still in samsara, all kinds of suffering are inevitable. Life can be described as existence in the cycle of birth and death and the interval between the two. There is indeed a variety of sufferings associated with sickness and old age. We will see later that pain is a protective mechanism for life and living beings' survival. Without pain, the body as an individual self is unlikely to survive for a long time and therefore cannot pass on this characteristic to the next generations. Pain is associated with existence, associated with life, associated with samsara.

The second suffering is mental. Human's biggest problem lies in constantly changing desires. Failure to achieve the desired goal will cause suffering. However, even when the desire is fulfilled, the pleasure passes quickly. People will have other, often more extravagant desires. This process keeps going on. Not achieving what one expects will be painful, but achieving the expectation will also bring suffering.

Neuroscience has shown that some chemicals, neurotransmitters released at synapses-junctions between one neuron and another, are responsible for emotions. All of our sensations are interpretations of the brain in the presence of those chemicals. Dopamine is an important neurotransmitter, for example. It occurs in the brain's reward system when achieving a desire or having a particular stimulus. Dopamine plays a role in stimulating the body to pursue a goal. However, the body also has a mechanism to regulate this chemical to create the next motivation. When achieving the expectation, dopamine is released, creating pleasure (Bressan and Crippa 2005). However, very quickly, the amount of dopamine returns to a normal state, and the body cannot be excited forever. Upon subsequent encounters with a previously desired stimulus, the produced dopamine levels diminish compared to initial exposure, leading to lessened excitement. This necessitates heightened stimuli to achieve equivalent dopamine release, underpinning the psychological discontent stemming from perpetual dissatisfaction.

The third type of suffering, also known as ignorance, is due to not realizing the nature of things as impermanence, suffering, and not-self (known as the three marks of existence). Ignorance does not recognize the existence of dependent origination, a principle that illuminates all things, which manifests itself in three aspects (Dalai Lama 1998):

1. All things and events come only from the interaction between various causes and conditions, the law of causality.
2. All things and events can be understood based on the concept that many parts compose a whole, and wholeness depends upon the parts.
3. All things and events arise solely from the mere coming together of many factors which make them up. Therefore, nothing has any independent and intrinsic identity of its own. That is the emptiness of all things.

In the sutras, the Buddha often repeats: "whoever understands the dependent-arising [dependent-origination] nature of reality will understand the Dharma, and whoever understands the Dharma will understand the Buddha"(Shulman 2008). If we approach Buddha's words from the perspective of Nagarjuna's Madhyamaka teachings, we can arrive at the most comprehensive understanding of their profound meaning. According to Nagarjuna[3] in Buddha's words, there are three meanings:

---

3 Nagarjuna was a highly influential Buddhist philosopher and thinker who lived in

First, the understanding of dependent origination, which is very common in all schools of Buddhism, interprets the above Buddha's words in terms of interdependence for the arising of meaning. This principle means that the existence of all things and events in the universe is merely the result of the interaction between many causes and conditions. This rules out two possibilities. The first posits the spontaneous emergence of phenomena devoid of causality, and the second suggests the creation of entities by a supernatural agent. Both scenarios are deemed untenable.

Second, the principle of dependent origination can be understood in terms of the constituent elements and the whole. All physical objects can be perceived by how the components constitute a complete entity and by the notion of "whole" or "wholeness", which depends on the existence of the components. Such dependence exists explicitly in the physical world. Similarly, nonphysical entities, such as consciousness, can also be considered in sequences of the time continuum: a whole idea's perception is grounded in successive actions to form a stream of thought. So, when we look at the universe in this way, we not only see that every conditioned thing is created dependently, but we also understand that the entire phenomenal world is also formed according to the principle of dependent origination.

Third, according to the principle of dependent origination, all phenomena – the whole of reality – exist only due to the simultaneous combination of all its constituent elements. When analyzing things in perception by breaking them down into their constituent elements, we will understand that everything is formed with complete dependence on other factors. Therefore, nothing has an independent or separate self. Whatever character we ascribe to things depends on the interaction between our perception and reality. However, this does not mean that things do not exist. Buddhism does not teach nihilism. Things do exist but are not self-sustaining independent entities.

2.3 Buddhism in Vietnam

Buddhism came to Vietnam in two periods and in two different ways. The first period is around the 2nd century from India, and the second is around

India during the 2nd century CE. He is considered one of the most important figures in the development of Mahayana Buddhism and is revered as a great philosopher and scholar.

the 6th century from China. Some documents show that by the end of the second century, there was already an important and prosperous Buddhist center called Luy Lau in Vietnam. This place included an area now in Bac Ninh province, north of Hanoi capital (Nguyen 2008, 17). For ordinary people, Buddhism penetrated and mixed with indigenous beliefs without reaction or obstacles. The Vietnamese traditionally venerated deities associated with the Sun, rivers, mountains, animals, and fertility rituals. However, Buddhism faced the challenge of assimilating within a socio-political milieu dominated by Confucianist principles, heavily influenced by Chinese culture, particularly among the ruling elite.

In the 6th century, Buddhism was introduced to Vietnam from China, bearing resemblances to the form of Chinese Buddhism prevalent during that era. Despite being classified within the Mahayana tradition, Vietnamese Buddhism exhibits distinct characteristics. Notably, its canonical texts encompass both pre-Mahayana and Mahayana elements, reflective of the period in which Mahayana Buddhism was crystallizing and its scriptures were inclusive of both strands (Harvey 2013).

When Vietnam gained independence from China in 938, Buddhism became the dominant religion and heavily interfered with the country's governance. Here, the so-called Vietnamese Engaged Buddhism was used to refer to the intervention of this religion in Vietnamese society. Until about the 15th century, when the Le Dynasty used Confucianism to govern the nation, Buddhism functioned as the religion of the ordinary people.

Mahayana Buddhism in Vietnam has three schools: Meditation, Pure Land, and Tantric Buddhism. The most documented school is Meditation. Chinese Meditation Buddhism, founded by Bodhidharma, came to Vietnam three times. The first time was at the end of the 6th century by an Indian monk, Vinitaruci. Two other times were in the 9th century by Chinese monks VôNgôn Thông and ThaoĐuòng. They were the initial three Vietnamese Meditation Schools, which then united into Trúc Lâm Meditation School in the 13th century by Trần Nhân Tông (Thich Tam Duc 2022).

Meditation Buddhism mainly relies on self-practice through meditation. In the context of Vietnamese Engaged Meditation Buddhism, the practice extends beyond the confines of pagodas, permeating the daily lives of individuals and even influencing the governance of the country by emperors. After three victories over the Mongolian army, King Trần Nhân

“居塵樂道且隨緣
饑則飡兮困則眠
家中有宝休寻覓
对鏡無心莫問禪”

“Ở đ̀oivuiđạohãytùyduyên,
Đóiđ̂́enthìăn, mệtnguliền.
Trong nhàcóbáuthôitìmkiếm,
Đ̂́oicaanhvôtâmchóhoithiền”.

“Be happy with the right path
in accordance with the circumstances,
Eat when hungry, sleep when tired.
Valuables are at home, do not seek them elsewhere,
Empty thought when seeing things
does not need meditation”.

Tông unified the contemporary branches of Meditation Buddhism to become the Trúc Lâm Yên Tu school with an important philosophy: living is meditating, living in life is Nirvana (Thich Tam Duc 2022).

Unlike Meditation Buddhism, other schools seek help from outside. Pure Land Buddhism prays to Amitabha Buddha through the continuous recitation of Namo-Amitabha. The goal is to reach the realm of the bliss of Amitabha Buddha. Pure Land Buddhism does not require complicated practice like Meditation Buddhism but is practical and straightforward, so many Vietnamese people follow it. Tantric Buddhism uses other external forces through recitation and mantras. This school does not exist independently in Vietnam because it is often mixed with Meditation Buddhism and indigenous beliefs.

Pure Land Buddhism considers the recitation of Amitabha Buddha as a form of meditation to reach the Pure Land, a realm of bliss and enlightenment. Pure Land is not a definite place but an enlightened state of mind. Pure land is also not the goal of spiritual practice but only the last realm to be reborn before liberation. Depending on personal vows, one can reach Nirvana or be reborn along the Bodhisattva path to save others.[4] Pure Land Buddhism promotes the collaborative practice: the more Buddhists practice together, the faster they will attain enlightenment.

---

4 A Bodhisattva voluntarily delays their complete enlightenment to assist others in their spiritual journey by staying in samsara.

Tantric Buddhism uses esoteric practices and techniques to attain liberation in just one lifetime. This school is considered the fastest and most advanced compared to other schools. Tantra emphasizes the use of mantra recitations, symbolic images, and mandalas.[5] The principle is to attain liberation with the help of other forces outside oneself.

The pursuit of external assistance to expedite the attainment of liberation aligns closely with the ethos of transhumanism. Should technology be regarded as an ancillary force conducive to spiritual practice, its integration could be harmonized with the Buddhist concept of skillful means (Sanskrit: upaya). This principle pertains to the nuanced aspect of navigating the Buddhist path towards liberation, characterized by deliberate, intentional actions informed by a nuanced understanding of their ultimate direction.

3. Human enhancement by biotechnology from the Buddhist perspective

There are many technologies to enhance human capacity. Here we refer to one of the most important technologies as biotechnology. Human enhancement through biotechnology can be achieved through gene modification and gene editing. Gene modification involves altering or adding genes to an individual's DNA, while gene editing involves precisely cutting and modifying specific genes. Both methods could enhance physical and cognitive abilities.

3.1 Accelerating evolution with technology

All human traits are the outcomes of one or many genes. In biology, how many years does it take to get a new gene in humans? The answer is not straightforward because the occurrence of a gene is proportional to the number of mutations, which depends not only on time but also on the population. Let us consider a sea nomad tribe called Bajau living in the islands of Indonesia, capable of diving up to 20 m deep and can hold their breath for up to 13 minutes. In 2018 a team of scientists studied the tribe's genes

5 A mantra is a sacred sound, word, or phrase repeated or chanted as a form of meditation, prayer, or spiritual practice in various religious and spiritual traditions. A mandala is a geometric design or pattern representing the universe.

to see if the ability to hold their breath was linked to genetic variation. When the body holds its breath, the blood vessels in the extremities constrict so that oxygen can flow to vital organs. At this time, the spleen will pump red blood cells carrying 9.6% more oxygen into the blood vessels. The ability to hold the breath is related to the spleen. Ultrasound machines measure the size of Bajau's spleen to be 50% larger than that of a normal person. It was found that a gene called PDE10A, responsible for spleen enlargement, is found only in the Bajau and not in others (Ilardo et al. 2018). This gene is thought to control the thyroid gland to make the spleen bigger and carry more oxygen when diving underwater.

It is estimated that the time for such a new gene to emerge is from a few hundred to a thousand years. Not only do the Bajau have new genes, but people living at high altitudes, such as the Tibetan Plateau, also have genes that adapt their bodies to low oxygen conditions (Ilardo and Nielsen 2018). People in Siberia who live near the Arctic under freezing temperatures also have genes that help them survive. Studies of English people over 100 generations from 2000 to 3000 years ago show that new genes take only a few dozen to hundreds of years to emerge. Humans have been evolving and seem to be evolving faster (Yair et al. 2016). In contrast to the rapid advancements achievable through contemporary genetic technologies, which span mere weeks to a few years, biological evolution unfolds at a markedly slower pace when juxtaposed with technological progression. So, if we can edit or modify genes, we can shorten the evolutionary time to have a desired trait without waiting a long time for natural selection. That is the crux of transhumanism.

Meditation Buddhism emphasizes the individual's responsibility in the process of enlightenment and encourages the cultivation of inner wisdom through practices such as meditation and mindfulness rather than relying on external forces. However, some schools incorporate external forces, such as Pure Land and Tantric practices. The acceptance of technology as a tool for advancing Buddhist practice can be accepted. Technology can enhance the practice by providing access to teachings, facilitating communication with other practitioners, and aiding in meditation. Others may view technology as a distraction or barrier to deepening their spiritual practice. Technology can improve human intelligence and thus help people realize the three marks of existence and quickly achieve results on the path of practice. In that respect, Buddhism advocates using technology to increase human potential.

3.2 Genetically Modified Organism

Humans make genetically modified food by altering the plant's DNA using genetic engineering techniques. The most popular method today is recombinant DNA technology, which takes a gene from one organism to insert it into another organism's gene, usually a food plant. First, one must identify the required characteristic, such as pest, herbicide, antiviral resistance, or rich nutrients. The corresponding gene will then be isolated from different organisms such as plants, bacteria, or viruses. After isolating and separating the above gene, people must insert the gene into the plant that wants to change. Gene guns, electroporation, or Agrobacterium-mediated transformation are commonly used for gene insertion.

Gene gun consists of metal particles made of gold or tungsten, on the surface of which the isolated gene is attached. These particles are shot into cells and tissues with a high-pressure Helium gas beam. The metallic particles carrying the gene will penetrate the membrane to enter the cell. One can use electroporation, where high-voltage electrical pulses are applied to cells creating holes for isolated genes to enter cells and tissues. The scientists also used a naturally occurring bacterium called Agrobacterium tumefaciens to transfer genes into plants. This bacterium can insert a fragment of its gene into plant cells to create tumors. Agrobacterium-mediated transformation is a popular method for generating transgenic plants.

In most cases, the expected gene is not isolated but attached to a vector, an intermediate entity that carries the gene into a cell. In addition to the desired gene segment, vectors have genetic elements such as promoters and selectable markers to express genes into proteins. A plasmid is a commonly used vector (Kumar et al. 1991). The plasmid is a circular DNA molecule widely found in bacteria and is replicated independently of the bacterial DNA. The vectors are introduced into the host cell by bacteria or yeast, thereby entering the host cell.

For example, ringspot on Carica papaya is a viral disease spread by several aphid species and is virtually incurable. This disease caused the papaya to be wiped out in Hawaii in the 1990s. Some other papaya species have genes resistant to the virus mentioned above, but they cannot be transferred to Hawaiian papayas, so people must use genetic engineering technology (Azad, Amin, and Sidik 2014). The first step is isolating the interest gene using biological techniques such as polymerase chain reaction (PCR) or restriction enzyme digestion. This is the stage of locating and cloning genes out of DNA from virus-resistant papaya plants. This gene is carried by metal particles to bombard the host cell of Carica papaya, making the plant resistant to the virus.

Many countries, such as the United States, Canada, and Brazil, accept genetically modified (GM) foods. For example, in 2020, GM soybean, cotton, and corn acreage in the United States accounted for 94%, 96%, and 92%, respectively (U.S. Department of Agriculture 2022). Thus, most of the area for planting these three types of trees is genetically modified plants. People have gradually accepted GM foods as common ingredients in their meals. If we accept genetic modification in other organisms, then Buddhists may have grounds to accept genetic modification in humans.

3.3 Gene Editing Technique

Technological evolution is many times faster than biological evolution, allowing humans to become superhuman in the future. Humans can use a gene editing technique called CRISPR (Clustered Regularly Interspaced Short Palindromic Repeats) to edit genes precisely as desired. For humans, gene editing technology has only been developed in the last few decades. However, for organisms, especially bacteria, CRISPR is the oldest molecular biological weapon used against the entry of viruses. When a virus attacks a bacterium, it transfers its DNA into the bacterium and uses the material of the bacterium to copy itself. The bacterium's protection is cutting the viral DNA with a protein called Cas9. How does a bacterium recognize a virus without the senses or brain to remember its enemies?

A virus has many characteristics, such as shape, size, protein, DNA, or RNA (later, we call it DNA). However, bacteria do not have specialized organs such as senses to recognize, so bacteria will use viral DNA to identify them. The viral genome length ranges from 0.859 to 2473 thousand base pairs (BP) (Campillo-Balderas, Lazcano, and Becerra 2015). Each BP is a pair of A-T or G-C nucleotides. Thus, the DNA of a virus ranges from nearly a thousand to more than two million base pairs. Bacteria do not need to use many base pairs to identify a virus. Only a few tens of BP are enough. If the number of BP is too small, for example, a few base pairs, the probability that different viruses overlap is high. However, if there are too many, it is a waste of resources. That is why, in most cases, the length to recognize guide DNA is only about 21–72 BP, which is enough for specificity, an average of 32 BP (Barrangou and Marraffini 2014).

When a virus invades a bacterium, the bacterium cuts a segment of the virus genome with an enzyme Cas to insert it into its gene, in what later came to be known as CRISPR. CRISPR is a family of DNA sequences found in prokaryotes such as bacteria and archaea. It consists of a DNA segment repeated many times, called a repeat. Between the repeats are spacers where a piece of viral DNA is recorded. Remembering viral genes is how bacteria remember their enemies. This memory is permanent and can be passed on to the next generations.

When a virus attacks bacteria, the viral DNA fragments stored in CRISPR are transcribed into RNA and attached to the Cas9 (CRISPR-associated) enzyme to form a ribonucleoprotein complex. This complex checks the viral DNA to see if one of the viruses that have attacked the bacteria before will have a matching code called guide RNA. If this happens, Cas9 will act as a pair of scissors to cut the virus' DNA, making the ability to clone no longer work. When DNA is cut, it can regenerate, but the recovery by random connection with other BP will not be able to make the correct command, so the gene will become inactivated.

It is the most primitive immune system in the history of biology, appearing in prokaryotic cells. Thus, the bacteria used a piece of viral DNA to recognize and remember by their DNA of themselves. When they reencountered this virus, the bacteria would recognize it using the memorized DNA fragment. If it is a virus, the bacteria use a memorized DNA-binding Cas9 protein called guide DNA to cut the viral DNA to inactivate it.

In 2012, Jennifer Doudna and Emmanuelle Charpentier used CRISPR-Cas9 as programmable scissors that could manipulate each base (Jinek et al. 2012; Doudna and Charpentier 2014). Two scientists have shown that molecular scissors can also cut all organisms' DNA at a pre-determined position. The DNA cut site is recognized through the programmed DNA guide. People can edit each base when DNA is cut by attaching pre-designed DNA fragments. Thanks to this, scientists can edit the genes of any organism. The discovery of these two scientists started from a purely fundamental study of the immune system of bacteria (for which they earned the Nobel Prize in chemistry in 2020) but soon became an effective tool for practical applications. The importance of research is reflected in the number of related publications that have increased exponentially in the last few years. In just eight years, from basic research, applied studies of this technique have been developed to cure genetic diseases such as β-thalassemia or sickle cell disease (Doudna 2020).

Many consider this discovery one of the most important discoveries in the history of biology because humans understand the mechanism of evolution at the most basic level and can also manipulate and interfere with the process. If natural selection randomly changes genes, some changes are suitable for the new environment that is retained and passed on to future generations. The fact that people can understand secrets and master tools that can edit genes is a tremendous human revolution. Gene editing can shorten the time needed to get a trait from a few hundred or a few thousand years to weeks. That is the scientific basis for the transhumanists to use to create superhumans.

3.4 Debates regarding Biotechnology

Many people oppose transhumanism because people are transcendent, ignoring the risk factors and ethical issues in using technology. If human capacity enhancement is controversial, it seems easier to accept human deficiencies. For example, sickle cell anemia, an inherited disease involving the dysfunction of red blood cells in the blood, was the first to be diagnosed as a gene-related disease found mainly in black patients. Human blood consists of four components: red blood cells, white blood cells, platelets, and plasma. Red blood cells carry oxygen from the lungs to the organs and take carbon dioxide from the organs to the lungs. Oxygen transport is done through a protein called hemoglobin. Hemoglobin is made up of two proteins called alpha-globin and beta-globin. The balance between the two types of globin produces normal hemoglobin in humans.

Sickle cell disease is caused by a mutation in a beta-globin-producing gene called HBB that comes from a single defect in which -GAG- is replaced by -GTG- (Newby et al. 2021). This gene produces abnormal hemoglobin that can be stuck together by polymerization, and as a result, red blood cells, instead of having a flattened sphere, have a sickle shape. Sickle cells do not carry oxygen and are prone to deformation that causes blood vessel blockages, chronic pain, organ failure, and premature death. This disease has been well-studied in medicine for a long time, and the primary treatment is blood transfusion. Recently, with the development of the gene-editing technique CRISPR, people have used gene-edited cell therapy. Scientists take stem cells[6] from the patient's body, then replace T with A in the HBB gene to create normal red blood cells, and then reinfuse the patient. Scientists classify cells into kinds: germ cells, referring to sperm and egg cells, and somatic cells, referring to the other cells. Those applications are for somatic cells only. Research on germ cells is just stated. For example, the CRISPR technique for fetuses allows the adult hemoglobin (S) suppressor gene to be switched off and replaced with unmutated fetal (F) hemoglobin.

Sickle cell anemia is an example of the development of technology. Natural selection may need thousands of years to fix this disease. In contrast, the gene-editing technique CRISPR can interfere with DNA to cure in months. This is one of the prime examples because the cause of the disease comes from a single failure of a single gene. With other genetic diseases, when the cause comes from many genes, the treatment will be much more complicated.

From a technical and social perspective, there are many obstacles to using gene editing technology with humans. Within the human genome, comprising approximately 20–30 thousand genes, our comprehension of the functions and interrelations among these genes remains limited. Consequently, it is challenging to precisely forecast the outcomes of the gene editing process. Furthermore, only about 1.5–2.0% of the total human 3.1 billion BP are directly involved in protein coding (Reichetzeder 2021). The function of the remaining BP still needs to be determined. Some have suggested that about 15% of BP belongs to the genes that regulate protein-coding genes. For the most part, the function of the human genome is still unknown. Therefore, modifying human genes while the relationship between genes is not fully understood is risky and can cause unpredictable consequences and risks.

Gene editing is not always accurate, either. There is always the possibility of editing the wrong gene (off-target effect), changing genes we do

6 Stem cells are undifferentiated cells that have the remarkable ability to develop into various specialized cell types in the body. They are characterized by their capacity for self-renewal and their potential to differentiate into different cell lineages.

not want to edit. Studies show that the frequency of off-target gene editing can be more than 50% with CRISPR-Cas9 technology (Zhang et al. 2015). This can result in new diseases that are difficult to treat.

After gene editing, it must be delivered to cells and tissues. This is also a challenge because the body's immune system treats gene therapy as a foreign object and attacks it. This reduces effectiveness and can cause damage. Most importantly, the long-term effects/consequences from an individual or species point of view of gene editing still need to be clarified, especially concerning the individual's overall and long-term relationship with the community.

Moreover, limited knowledge might lead to gene editing that homogenizes traits, thereby diminishing biodiversity. However, gene editing also holds promise for conservation, potentially bolstering the resilience of endangered species to diseases. In agriculture, genetically modified foods aim to have high yields and be rich in nutrients, pests, pesticides, herbicides, and disease resistance. An example of a genetically modified food is Bt corn, which has been genetically modified to produce a protein called Bacillus thuringiensis (Bt), which is toxic to the European corn borer. Bt acts as a natural insecticide to protect corn, reducing the use of pesticides. Bt was approved by the United States in 1996 and has become the most-grown maize in the world. According to the International Service for the Acquisition of Agri-biotech Applications (ISAAA), in 2019, the world planted 19.8 million hectares. This example shows that the reduction of biodiversity caused by the application of technology as desired by humans may put biodiversity in danger. Therefore, when a disease arrives, it will be a disaster.

An example is the Cavendish banana. It is very popularly grown, accounting for 47% of the world's bananas, because of its advantages, including large, delicious, sweet, beautiful yellow fruits. It is one of the most consumed fruits in the world. This banana was cloned, so when a disease attacked it, it could not resist. A virus called Tropical Race 4 (TR4) could make this banana species extinct (Ploetz 2021). Since all banana plants are genetically similar, the TR4 virus that infects one plant can infect all others. Currently, people are researching to save this banana species. If the Cavendish banana went extinct, it would not be the first time. In the late 19th century, a banana species called Gros Michel was also popular, but in the 1950s, it became extinct due to Panama disease caused by a toxic fungus that lived in the soil.

From a social perspective, gene editing raises the issue of fairness in access to technology. Presently, the complexity and high cost of gene therapy render it accessible only to a financially privileged few, engendering significant social inequities and widening societal divides. The immediate benefits conferred by gene editing may not necessarily translate into long-term advantages, casting doubt on the overall efficacy and desirability of such interventions.Natural selection takes hundreds, thousands of years to adjust a particular gene, while humans only need a few years of research. The two time periods are so far apart that it is doubtful that the gene-edited subject can fully adapt to the surrounding environment.

From the Buddhist point of view, human is only one stage in nature's long process of attaining liberation. We can invoke here an analogy with the evolutionary process, where humans are in a long chain link with other creatures. Using biotechnology to overcome human sufferings such as sickle cell anemia could easily be embraced by the Buddhist goal of eliminating suffering. The disease comes from only a single gene, so if it is modified, it is unlikely that the other genes will be affected much. However, sickle cell anemia is an infrequent case involving only one gene. Other diseases relate to many genes and the relationships between them. Therefore, the use of biotechnology needs to be studied carefully.

The utilization of technology for curing human diseases is widely accepted, whereas its application for augmenting human capabilities is met with considerable debate. This issue transcends mere technical challenges, necessitating a comprehensive understanding; moreover, the pursuit of enhancement does not inherently justify its implementation. Throughout history, humans have done many things that at first seemed promising but then turned out to be very harmful. This is especially the case in genetic engineering for germline cells,[7] which can be passed on to the next generation and lead to irreversible changes. Looking ahead, should the objectives pursued by humanity prove misguided, the possibility of reversion may be non-existent. Buddhism does not categorically forbid the employment of

[7] Germline cells, also known as germ cells, are a specialized type of cells that give rise to eggs in females and sperms in males. These cells are responsible for the transmission of genetic information from one generation to the next through sexual reproduction.

such technologies; rather, it advises a measured and thoughtful approach to their application.

3.5 Longevity

The vital goal of transhumanism is to prolong lifespan. From the Buddhist point of view, how important is the lifespan? The goal of Buddhism is liberation from samsara, liberation from reincarnation, and attainment of Nirvana. The human body is a tool for practicing the right path Dharma, where wisdom, compassion, and mindfulness help liberate. Within the philosophical framework of Buddhism, longevity is valued not as an end in itself but as a means conducive to awakening. Consequently, while extended lifespan is not deemed crucial to Buddhist doctrine, the human life span is nonetheless regarded as a precious opportunity for achieving enlightenment. This perspective is reflected in the veneration of Bodhisattva Amitayus, who symbolizes longevity, underscoring the importance of a prolonged life for spiritual cultivation and the attainment of enlightenment.[8]

Buddhism does not see longevity as an ultimate goal but as a skillful means. If life is too short, there is not enough time to practice, but if life is too long without practice, there is no meaning. The issue of longevity is discussed in some Mahayana sutras, especially the Buddha's life span of 80 years, which is said to be short compared to other bodhisattvas such as Vipasyin, which is 84,000 years, Krakucchanda 60,000 years, Kanakamuni 30,000 years.[9] The explanations suggest that the Buddha's lifespan is limitless and immeasurable. The temporal span of eighty years represents merely a tangible expression of the eternal and boundless nature of the Buddha. This finite embodiment serves as a skillful means, a deliberate adaptation intended to aid sentient beings by way of the Buddha's reward body. The actual life span of the Buddha is the life span in the concealed form which is limitless and immeasurable. Thus, longevity is also important in the Buddhist scriptures but is not the purpose of this religion (Guang

[8] Amitayus, is a significant figure in Buddhist cosmology, particularly within the Pure Land tradition. Amitayus is regarded as a Buddha or enlightened being associated with infinite life and boundless light.

[9] Vipasyin, Krakucchanda, and Kanakamuni are the past Buddhas in Buddhist cosmology. According to Buddhist scriptures, a succession of Buddhas arise throughout the eons to guide beings towards enlightenment and liberation from suffering.

Xing, 2002). Buddhism emphasizes wisdom and compassion for life that will improve physical and mental health.

In this context, Buddhism advocates for the type of longevity envisioned by transhumanism, provided it is accompanied by an ethical and intellectual approach to living.

3.6 Mental enhancement

Buddhism emphasizes that physical enhancement must be linked to mental improvement because physical strength is a means for mental activity in the way of practicing. Mental activity is more important than physical strength. That fact is reflected in all sects of Buddhism. For example, Vietnamese Meditation Buddhism focuses on the direct experience rather than studying the scriptures. By directly experiencing reality, a practitioner increases wisdom and practices wisdom in everyday activities.

One of the purposes of meditation is to understand the self, the true expectation of the mind and the body. Understanding oneself is fundamental to Buddhism and some Eastern religions, such as Taoism. Meditation facilitates an individual's recognition of themselves as an integral part of the expansive cosmos.

Now we will elaborate on the importance of understanding ourselves in a modern world.

In civilized life, one thing that is inseparable from each person is probably a smartphone. In 2020, 66% of the world's population will use 5.22 billion units (Kemp 2021). Each smartphone stores personal information such as photos, messages, location, email, contacts, etc. According to the World Economic Forum, each internet user spends 2 hours and 27 minutes on average daily surfing social media (Buchholz 2022). While surfing the net, personal information is constantly being collected and monitored. Time spent on social media is increasing, and in many places, that time is much larger than the time spent with loved ones such as spouses and children.

Smartphones help people remember much information. A study of Whistleout on 425 Americans found that 50% of respondents only remember 1–5 phone numbers, 21% of whom only remember their own phone numbers (Long 2022). If in the past, people had to remember information such as telephone numbers, contact names, meeting times, etc., now that task has been transferred to smartphones, iCloud, and artificial intelligence of multinational corporations. The only thing a person must remember is the username and password of his/her account. In other words, the human mind has gone beyond its physical body. Memory is only a part of the mind, which has been extended to the world and becoming part of the common data of humanity. With large amounts of data, humans must advise machines whenever making decisions. Sooner or later, machines will make decisions on behalf of humans. Therefore, humans are giving machines the most vital capacity to make decisions. In history, humans have created the most terrible weapons, such as nuclear weapons, which can destroy human civilization. However, nuclear weapons are tools and cannot make decisions. Now, when data is so large that humans must use the analysis of machines, the decision-making ability of humans will be deprived.

The proliferation of smartphones has led to the widespread adoption of virtual assistants or artificial intelligence (AI) systems designed to aid users as required. These AI-based virtual assistants, through continuous user interaction and the accumulation of extensive personal data, may attain a level of understanding of human behaviors and preferences that surpasses our own introspective capabilities. This emergent reality raises profound questions regarding the intrinsic value of human judgment, traditionally underpinned by emotional and rational dimensions. The classic psychological dilemma, known as the trolley problem (Lieberman et al., 2019), exemplifies the significant influence of emotions on human decision-making processes, even within identical scenarios. This interplay often precipitates a cognitive dissonance, with the most pronounced conflict manifesting between logical reasoning and emotional response – wherein reason typically offers a long-term perspective, whereas emotion tends to prioritize immediate outcomes.

AI is different from humans. It has no emotions, which is a significant advantage of AI that, indeed, in the future, humans will have to consult regularly. If everyone depends on AI, what role do humans play? Should the right to make decisions also depend on others? This is an important point of how meditation can help people. Artificial intelligence can only help based on objective data and algorithms. Algorithms are available. The more data, the more accurate the decision will be. Nevertheless, meditation brings subjective information and helps people experience it directly. To put it shortly, amidst ongoing scientific endeavors to elucidate the genesis of consciousness, meditation emerges as a pivotal practice for augmenting human value relative to machines. The journey of self-discovery facilitated by meditation serves to preserve and enhance intrinsic human values, distinguishing the human experience from mechanistic functions.

Meditation is a mindfulness intervention, considered as psychotherapy, using breathing exercises and body awareness to treat psychological disorders such as reducing stress, emotional regulation, cognitive flexibility, and self-awareness. Regular meditation can effectively reduce stress, anxiety, and harmful effects of stress on the mind and body. Meditation can also help individuals develop better emotional regulation, which can be beneficial in managing difficult emotions such as anger, sadness, or anxiety. Regular practice allows individuals to observe their thoughts and feelings with greater detachment and develop skillful reactions. Some research shows that meditation can help improve mental flexibility by switching between different ways of thinking and solving problems. This can be beneficial in many contexts, including work, school, and personal relationships. Meditation can also help individuals develop self-awareness, which can benefit personal growth and development. Through practice, individuals can learn to observe their thoughts and feelings more objectively and better understand their thinking and behavioral patterns.

Among three Buddhist schools in Vietnam, Tantric has the most pro-transhumanist views owing to the wish to be liberated in just one human lifetime. Following Tantric school, Pure Land also requires Amitabha Buddha's aid by reciting his name. If asking for help from external forces is accepted, using technology to increase and promote mental practices to achieve results quickly is entirely acceptable. Meditation Buddhism is based on the practitioners' inner efforts; therefore, this school is the least encouraging of transhumanism.

4. Buddhist concepts from the transhumanist perspective

Dependent origination in Buddhism is displayed through the fact that a self exists but is not considered an independent, permanent, intrinsic entity because it emerges from other things and events. The principle of dependent origination and its manifestation in emptiness is one of the unique principles of Buddhism when compared to other religions. Emptiness is presented through three marks of existence: impermanence, suffering, and non-self (anatman). Impermanence holds that all things and events, including the self, are mutable and constantly changing because their existence comes from many causes and conditions. The world is like a river that keeps flowing. Every moment is a new moment. If we know that ever-changing truth, we will live in the present moment and enjoy the beauty and wonder in each Satna (a short time in Buddhism). Due to the constantly changing nature, while the self (atman) does not realize it, the self always wants the best for its own. Later on, the self will be disappointed about what it has achieved. That is suffering. Atman has no intrinsic nature and is not permanent because it results from causes and conditions. This leads to the third mark of no-self.

4.1 Suffering

Buddhism focuses on suffering. Can transhumanism help people overcome suffering? There are three types of suffering: physical, mental, and ignorance. Physical suffering manifests in birth, old age, illness, and death. Mental suffering is dissatisfaction with all phenomena because things are constantly changing. Ignorance refers to the fact that humans do not recognize the truth but the illusion of reality, which is the cause of all suffering. We will discuss each of them in the following.

Physical suffering is related to pain. Note that not all pain leads to suffering. Although pain is a physical or emotional experience, suffering is our response to that experience. To understand physical pain, we need to talk about the mechanism of pain transmission. The literature often assumes that we already understand pain, but pain is more complex than we thought. Pain is a physiological and psychological experience involving many systems and processes in the human body. The scientific mechanism of pain consists of a network of sensory neurons, neurotransmitters, and brain regions that work together to detect, transmit, and process pain signals. Pain is always an individual experience influenced to varying degrees by biological, psychological, and social factors. According to the International Association for Study of Pain, pain is defined as "an unpleasant sensory and emotional experience associated with or resembling that associated with actual or potential tissue damage". (Raja et al. 2020)

Tissue damage in the body, sometimes called injury and pain, are different phenomena. There are many cases where there is damage, but the brain is not aware of it, and conversely, there is no damage but still feel pain. For example, one of the causes of neuropathic pain is phantom limb pain, which occurs in people with amputated limbs. The person still feels pain in the toes and fingers even when they are gone. The cause is still unclear, but some theories suggest that the nerves that once connected the amputated parts to the brain still send perturbed signals to induce pain. The pain can last long enough to become chronic. In addition to medication or surgery, meditation has been applied to treat this disease to reduce pain and discomfort (Ehde et al. 2000). This example of pain unrelated to trauma can be treated with meditation or psychotherapy.

In contrast, there is tissue damage but no pain, especially in organs without sensory nerves. C cirrhosis is an example of a common disease where liver tissues are damaged and replaced by scar tissues. Because the liver does not have sensory nerves, we do not feel pain when damaged. However, as the disease progresses, symptoms and complications such as jaundice, fatigue, and fluid buildup in the abdomen appear. If left untreated, it affects liver function and is life-threatening.

Can technology help people solve this problem? Should sensory nerves be created in organs that are naturally absent? Pain cannot be inferred solely from the activity of sensory neurons, but through their life experiences, individuals learn the experience of pain. So, in addition to the physical damage, pain also depends on many psychological factors, which is where Buddhism and Western psychology can come in.

When tissue damage or inflammation occurs, specialized sensory neurons called nociceptors are activated. These neurons detect harmful or potentially harmful stimuli, such as heat, pressure, or chemicals, and send signals to the spinal cord and brain. The spinal cord is a relay station for pain signals, transmitting them to different brain regions for processing and interpretation. A critical region in pain perception is the somatosensory cortex, which receives and processes sensory information from various body parts, including pain signals.

A nerve signal is an electrical pulse with a potential close to 100 mV, duration of 3 ms generated by the difference in Na+ and K+ ions inside and outside a nerve cell (Shana Kerr et al. 2023). This signal is transmitted from about ten m/s to hundreds of m/s. Nervous signals do not travel directly from the nociceptors under the skin to the brain but through several layers of neurons. Between neurons, there are synapses where signals must go through. The signals can be stimulated or inhibited by neurotransmitters. The body's regulation to produce pain is these neurotransmitters. Anxiety is caused by adrenaline; euphoria is caused by dopamine; happiness is caused by serotonin, etc. They are chemicals that create human emotions.

Physical suffering is manifested through pain, which serves as an indicator of tissue damage. This is corroborated by neuroscience, which posits pain as an essential defensive mechanism intrinsic to human physiology. Humans cannot survive without pain. However, there are many mismatches between pain and damage: pain without damage and damage without pain. The right path is to avoid those mismatches and find a way to harmonize pain and damage.

4.2 Dependent origination

Dependent origination leads to emptiness, which manifests in all things and events. Let us consider the emptiness in the human body. We will examine from three scales: the individual, the cell, and the DNA. On an individual scale, a 70 kg adult human body has about 30 trillion cells, but 38 trillion bacteria live in our body, known as the microbiome. Some literature uses the word "parasitic" to refer to the microbiome, but here we use the word "endosymbiotic" to say that the existence of bacteria is not only harmful but also beneficial to our bodies. If we count all microorganisms, including viruses, bacteria, and fungi, the number of microbiomes can reach 100 trillion (more than the number of our cells) with a biomass of about 3 kg (Di Simone et al. 2023). They are mainly living in the intestinal tract and oral cavity.

The microbiome has three critical functions in the human body. The first function is immunity. The microorganisms in the intestinal tract protect the intestine from attack by other microorganisms from the outside and produce vitamins such as B, B12, K, thiamine, and riboflavin. Vitamin K also helps with blood clotting. The second function is digestion. When we eat carbohydrates and starches, the bacteria break them down into shorter molecules by digestive enzymes. Microbiome digests about 10–15% of the food we eat, and in return, they produce short-chain organic substances that our intestines can absorb. Humans can only eat a minimal amount of food without the gut microbiome. The third function is the nervous system. Many scientists recognize microbiome in the gut as the second brain (Ochoa-Repáraz and Kasper 2016). The gut-brain axis is an essential two-way connection between the gut and the brain. Most neurotransmitters are made in the gut and carried to the brain. For example, Enterococcus produces serotonin; Bacillus makes dopamine; Lactobacillus and Bifidobacterium are in charge of gamma-aminobutyric acid (GABA); Lactobacillus releases histamine (Dietert 2016). It can be said that the state of the brain depends a lot on the gut microbiota. Happy gut, happy brain. The human body cannot survive without the microbiome. We, humans and microbiome, live together in an endosymbiotic way.

At the cellular scale, human body cells can be divided into about 200 types, such as muscle cells, nerves, blood cells, etc. Each type has its functions and characteristics. Cells are organized into tissues and organs to work together to perform bodily functions. Despite their diversity, cells all share some of the same components. The cell membrane is the border between the inside and outside and controls cells' metabolism. The cell nucleus contains the genetic material DNA located in the chromosomes. The cytoplasm contains many organelles, such as mitochondria, ribosomes, cytoskeleton, vesicles, etc.

One of the cell organelles is mitochondria, which is considered a bacterium whose DNA, ribosomes, and systems function independently. Mitochondrial DNA (mtDNA) has about 17,000 base pairs, similar to many bacteria, and completely independent of human DNA. Human DNA can be inherited half from the father and the other half from the mother through the maternal line with recombination (where parental DNA is mixed). A child receives the characteristics of both mother and father through the genes carried by DNA. However, mtDNA can only be inherited from the mother. The egg cells contribute most organelles to embryonic development, including mitochondria, so sperms contribute very little. Because mtDNA is inherited through the maternal line without genetic recombination, it plays an important role in studying human evolution. A recent investigation employing mitochondrial DNA (mtDNA) analysis has illuminated a significant epoch in human prehistory, pinpointing a population bottleneck event approximately 200,000 years ago. During this period, humanity had a population bottleneck of only a few thousand individuals living in an area of about 120 thousand km2 in the deserts of southeastern Africa (Rice University 2010).

In the past, mitochondria were considered organelle like any other cell organelle. However, in the 1960s, Lynn Margulis (former name was Lynn Sagan) proposed the endosymbiosis theory that mitochondria in animal cells and chloroplasts in plant cells were once free bacteria eaten or swallowed by ancient eukaryotic cells (Sagan 1967).[10] Nevertheless, somehow, they survive and coexist with the host cell. This theory was initially controversial but is now widely accepted as the origin of mitochondria and chloroplasts. The endosymbiosis theory is used to explain the coexistence of mitochondria in human cells and extended to the branches of biology to help explain the evolutionary process of many organisms.

The role of mitochondria in cells is quite diverse. The most important function is to generate fuel for the cell, which is adenosine triphosphate (ATP), through cellular respiration (Brand et al. 2013). In cellular respiration, the food transported to the cell will be synthesized by mitochondria to produce ATP, commonly known as the cell's energy currency. Cell activities such as muscle contraction, transport of molecules across cell membranes, synthesis of proteins, nucleic acids, fatty acids, and nerve signal transmission all require ATP. The more energy a cell uses, the more mitochondria it has. For example, liver cells have up to 2000 mitochondria, while red blood cells do not have any of them. The second role of mitochondria is to program cell death in apoptosis, where the mitochondria decide which cells must be destroyed, which is extremely important for the life cycle of cells. Mitochondria also regulates the cell's time by controlling the fundamental metabolic processes, including biochemical reactions and the gene expression that underlies them (Diaz-Cuadros 2023). The third role is to absorb Ca2+ ions, which the cell uses when needed. The fourth role is to generate heat using a tissue called brown fat.

With so many vital roles, the cell certainly trusted mitochondria. It is hypothesized that mitochondria were once a prokaryotic bacterium with an aerobic redox advantage that somehow infiltrated a eukaryotic cell and succeeded in endosymbiosis co-existence with the host cell sometime 1.7 to 2 billion years ago (Lane 2009). From an alien organism, mitochondria have become an indispensable component of almost all cells in the human

[10] Eukaryotic and prokaryotic cells are two primary types of cells that differ in their structural and organizational features. Eukaryotic cells have a well-defined nucleus that houses the cell's DNA. Prokaryotic cells lack a true nucleus. Instead, their DNA is located in a region called the nucleoid, which is not enclosed by a nuclear membrane.

body. Without them, cells die. In plant cells, chloroplasts function similarly to mitochondria and are successful endosymbionts.

What about at the molecular scale of DNA? Can DNA be the unique identification of a self? The human genome comprises 23 pairs of chromosomes, with 3.055 billion BP (Nurk et al. 2022). If we stretch a cell's DNA on the human body, we will get a wire 2 nm wide and about 1.1 m long. If we connect all the DNA in the human body, we will get a wire 30 trillion meters long, 200 times larger than the distance from the Earth to the Sun. All traits of an individual, such as hair color, skin color, height, etc., are controlled by one or several genes that are recorded in the DNA.

The human genome project helps us understand the structure of the genome system, which shows that the number of protein-coding genes that humans have is about 20–25 thousand. Humans' genome is 99.9% genetically similar to one another. Of which, 98.8% are like chimpanzees, 90% are like musculus, 36% are like fruit flies, 21% are like roundworms, and 7% are like E-coli. The genetic similarity between humans and other organisms is proof of the past human evolution from other organisms. Genetic studies also reveal when our ancestors diverged from those prehistoric creatures. The interconnectedness between humans and other creatures is displayed by the fact that every human DNA contains the imprints of the entire evolution process. Another way of saying this is that human DNA is the information fossil of the biological process that has occurred on Earth.

It is worth noting that the entire human protein-coding gene represents only 1.5% of the total BP of the whole DNA. Most DNA is non-protein-coding. Part of that is responsible for regulating protein-coding genes. Up to 45% of BP are transposable elements, DNA fragments repeated many times in the human genome. 26% of introns have no coding role. Introns were originally called junk genes, but they were later discovered to play a role in controlling protein-coding genes or altering them to create new genes.

In the human genome, up to 8% of genes are imported from viral genes (Human endogenous retroviruses). RNA viruses can be inserted into the human gene. Most of these genes are inactivated, but some are co-opted into human genes. For example, the ability to give birth and raise offspring in the womb through the placenta rather than eggs is an ability that mammals have acquired from a viral gene called syncytins (Dupressoir, Lavialle, and Heidmann 2012) since hundreds of millions of years ago. It is precisely a gene that the virus uses to penetrate cell membranes and is used by mammals so that the fetus can implant in the uterus (Frank et al. 2022).

How does emptiness affect transhumanism? Above, we have presented emptiness in the human body at the individual, cell, and DNA scales. All of them prove one thing that at any scale, the perception of an independent, permanent, intrinsic self is not correct. That is the no-self in the three marks of existence. Since all humans are interconnected to other elements in the universe, changing a particular characteristic, such as editing a gene to treat disease or increasing a capacity, will unpredictably affect many other things. We need careful studies at all scales because the components are already balanced with others. Any sudden change can disrupt the balance and be very difficult to adjust. The Middle way of Buddhism does not deny the changes but emphasizes that any modification in one part should unexpectedly affect the other parts.

5. Conclusion

Buddhism brought new values to Hinduism: the suffering of sentient beings, the equality between humans and other creatures, the middle pathway for attaining liberation, and the dependent origination principle of all things and events. In Vietnam, Buddhism evolved from a focus on individual enlightenment to a more pronounced engagement with social life. Notably, Trần Nhân Tông advocated for the integration of Buddhist practices into daily activities, emphasizing mindfulness of the Dharma. The advances in biotechnology, such as gene modification and gene editing, allow a much faster shortcut (within weeks or months) to superhumans compared to natural selections (within thousands of years). Buddhism offers varying levels of support for transhumanist objectives, with a spectrum ranging from strong to moderate endorsement. Such goals include the augmentation of intellectual and physical capabilities and the extension of human lifespan. This alignment is primarily grounded in the centrality of wisdom within Buddhist practice. Enhancements in physical capacities and longevity are considered supplementary to the core spiritual pursuits. Moreover, the extent of support for transhumanist ideals differs among the various Buddhist traditions. Among the three prevalent Buddhist traditions in Vietnam, Pure Land and Tantric Buddhism hold particular relevance to the discourse on technology, as it is perceived as a skillful means to facilitate practice. Conversely, the Meditation school is less amenable to such integration. Furthermore, foundational Buddhist tenets, including the concepts of suffering and dependent origination, find resonance within the scientific fields of neuroscience and biology, underscoring a symbiotic relationship between Buddhist philosophy and contemporary scientific understanding. Using scientific advances to enhance the individual capacity of humans can be applied, but with great care, because of the interrelationship between humans and other living things. Will the enhancements eliminate suffering, and will it cause Buddhism to be outdated? This is highly unlikely. Buddhism remains a way to liberation from suffering. Buddhism and Vietnamese-engaged Buddhist schools support the goals of transhumanism at different levels.

References

Azad, Md. A. K., L. Amin & N. M. Sidik. 2014. Gene Technology for Papaya Ringspot Virus Disease Management. *The Scientific World Journal*, vol. 2014, Article ID 768038, 11 pages. https://doi.org/10.1155/2014/768038.

Barrangou, R.& L. A. Marraffini. 2014. CRISPR-Cas Systems: Prokaryotes Upgrade to Adaptive Immunity. *Molecular Cell*, 54(2): 234–44. https://doi.org/10.1016/j.molcel.2014.03.011.

Beckwith, C. I. 2009. *Empires of the Silk road: A history of central Euroasia from the Bronze age to the present*, Princeton University Press.

Bostrom, N. 2005. A History of Transhumanist Thought. *Journal of Evolution and Technology*, 14(1): 1–25. https://ora.ox.ac.uk/objects/uuid:55ab57ec-70d0--4b93-b058--0d7f57167cc2/files/me7362f022f645636ed10948d03a7bfab

Brand, M. D., A. L. Orr, I. V. Perevoshchikova & C. L. Quinlan. 2013. The Role of Mitochondrial Function and Cellular Bioenergetics in Ageing and Disease. *British Journal of Dermatology*, 169(s2): 1–8. https://doi.org/10.1111/bjd.12208.

Bressan, R. A.& J. A. Crippa. 2005. The Role of Dopamine in Reward and Pleasure Behaviour – Review of Data from Preclinical Research. *Acta Psychiatrica Scandinavica*, 111(s427): 14–21. https://doi.org/10.1111/j.1600--0447.2005.00540.x.

Campillo-Balderas, J. A. Lazcano & A. Becerra. 2015. Viral Genome Size Distribution Does Not Correlate with the Antiquity of the Host Lineages. *Frontiers in Ecology and Evolution*, 3. https://www.frontiersin.org/articles/10.3389/fevo.2015.00143.

Dalai Lama. 1998. The Four Noble Truths: Fundamentals of the Buddhist Teachings. Thorsons.

Di Simone, S. K., I. Rudloff, C. A.Nold-Petry, S. C. Forster, & M. F. Nold. 2023. Understanding respiratory microbiome–immune system interactions in health and disease. *Science translational medicine*, 15(678). https://doi.org/10.1126/scitranslmed.abq5126.

Diaz-Cuadros, et al. Metabolic regulation of species-specific developmental rates. *Nature* 613, 550–557 (2023). https://doi.org/10.1038/s41586--022--05574--4

Dinh, H. H. 2020. The Symbol of Saint Gióng and the Gióng Festival in the Historical Context of Vietnam. *Asian Education and Development Studies*, 9(1): 37–45. https://doi.org/10.1108/AEDS-01--2018--0015.

Doudna, J. A. 2020. The Promise and Challenge of Therapeutic Genome Editing. *Nature*, 578(7794): 229–36. https://doi.org/10.1038/s41586--020--1978--5.

Doudna, J. A.& E. Charpentier. 2014. The New Frontier of Genome Engineering with CRISPR-Cas9. *Science*, 346(6213): 1258096. https://doi.org/10.1126/science.1258096.

Dupressoir, A., C.Lavialle & T. Heidmann. 2012. From Ancestral Infectious Retroviruses to Bona Fide Cellular Genes: Role of the Captured Syncytins in Placentation. *Placenta*, 33(9): 663–71. https://www.sciencedirect.com/science/article/pii/S0143400412002044.

Ehde, D. M. et al. 2000. Chronic Phantom Sensations, Phantom Pain, Residual Limb Pain, and Other Regional Pain after Lower Limb Amputation. *Archives of Physical Medicine and Rehabilitation*, 81(8): 1039–44. https://doi.org/10.1053/apmr.2000.7583.

Frank, J. A. et al. 2022. Evolution and Antiviral Activity of a Human Protein of Retroviral Origin. *Science*, 378(6618): 422–28. https://doi.org/10.1126/science.abq7871.

Harvey, P. 2013. *An Introduction to Buddhism: Teachings, History and Practices*. 2nd ed. Cambridge.

Hughes, J. J. 2019. Buddhism and Our Posthuman Future. *Sophia*, 58(4): 653–62. https://doi.org/10.1007/s11841--018--0669--2.

Huxley, Julian (1957). *Transhumanism*. New Bottles for New Wine. London: Chatto & Windus. pp. 13–17. Reprint: Ethics in Progress. 2015. 6(1): 12–16. doi: 10.14746/eip. 2015.1.2.

Ilardo, M. A. et al. 2018. Physiological and Genetic Adaptations to Diving in Sea Nomads. *Cell*, 173(3): 569–580.e15. https://doi.org/10.1016/j.cell.2018.03.054.

Ilardo, M.& R. Nielsen. 2018. Human Adaptation to Extreme Environmental Conditions. *Current Opinion in Genetics & Development*, 53: 77–82. https://www.sciencedirect.com/science/article/pii/S0959437X18300777.

Jinek, M. et al. 2012. A Programmable Dual-RNA–Guided DNA Endonuclease in Adaptive Bacterial Immunity. *Science*, 337(6096): 816. http://science.sciencemag.org/content/337/6096/816.abstract.

Kemp,S. 2021. Global Overview Report (April 25, 2023). https://datareportal.com/reports/digital-2021-global-overview-report.

Kerr, S., E. Weigel, C. Spencer & D. Garton. 2023. Neurons. *Organismal Biology*(June 18, 2023). https://organismalbio.biosci.gatech.edu/chemical-and-electrical-signals/neurons/.

Kumar, D. 2017. River Ganges – Historical, Cultural and Socioeconomic Attributes. *Aquatic Ecosystem Health & Management*, 20(1–2): 8–20. https://doi.org/10.1080/14634988.2017.1304129.

Kumar, P. K. R., H-E. Maschke, K.Friehs & K. Schügerl. 1991. Strategies for Improving Plasmid Stability in Genetically Modified Bacteria in Bioreactors. *Trends in Biotechnology* n 9(1): 279–84. https://www.sciencedirect.com/science/article/pii/0167779991900905.

Lane, N. 2009. On the Origin of Bar Codes: Genetic Sequences in a Cell's Mitochondria Can Be Used to Accurately Determine Species. Could This Be Because They Are Responsible for Creating What They Identify? *Nature*, 462: 272+. https://link.gale.com/apps/doc/A213406385/AONE?u=anon~709d4480&sid=googleScholar&xid=c21239dd.

LaTorra, M. 2015. What Is Buddhist Transhumanism? *Theology and Science*, 13(2): 219–29. https://doi.org/10.1080/14746700.2015.1023993.

Mark, J. J. 2012. Ancient India. *World history encyclopedia* [online]. https://www.worldhistory.org/india/

More, M. 1998. The Extropian Principles, v. 3.0: A Transhumanist Declaration [online]. http://mrob.com/pub/religion/extro_prin.html.

Newby, G. A. et al. 2021. Base Editing of Haematopoietic Stem Cells Rescues Sickle Cell Disease in Mice. *Nature*, 595(7866): 295–302. https://doi.org/10.1038/s41586--021--03609-w.

Nguyen Tai Thu. 2008. *The history of Buddhism in Vietnam*. Institute of Philosophy.

Nurk, S. et al. 2022. The Complete Sequence of a Human Genome. *Science*, 376(6588): 44–53. https://doi.org/10.1126/science.abj6987.

Ochoa-Repáraz, J.& L. H. Kasper. 2016. The Second Brain: Is the Gut Microbiota a Link Between Obesity and Central Nervous System Disorders? *Current Obesity Reports* 5(1): 51–64. https://doi.org/10.1007/s13679--016--0191--1.

Ploetz, R. C. 2021. Gone Bananas? Current and Future Impact of Fusarium Wilt on Production. In: P. Scott, R. Strange, L. Korsten, & M. L.Gullino(eds.), *Plant Diseases and Food Security in the 21st Century*. Cham: Springer International Publishing, 21–32. https://doi.org/10.1007/978--3-030--57899--2_2.

Raja, S. N. et al. 2020. The Revised International Association for the Study of Pain Definition of Pain: Concepts, Challenges, and Compromises. *PAIN*, 161(9). https://journals.lww.com/pain/Fulltext/2020/09000/The_revised_International_Association_for_the.6.aspx.

Rautray, S.2016. Supreme Court in 1995: Stray Slogans Do Not Attract Section 124A Pertaining to Sedition. The Economic Times (Feb 20, 2016). https://economictimes.indiatimes.com/news/politics-and-nation/supreme-court-in-1995-stray-slogans-do-not-attract-section-124a-pertaining-to-sedition/articleshow/51062254.cms?from=mdr

Reichetzeder, C. 2021. Overweight and Obesity in Pregnancy: Their Impact on Epigenetics. *European Journal of Clinical Nutrition*, 75(12): 1710–22. https://doi.org/10.1038/s41430--021--00905--6.

Rice University. 2010. 'Mitochondrial Eve': Mother of All Humans Lived 200,000 Years Ago. Science Daily. https://www.sciencedaily.com/releases/2010/08/100817122405.htm

Rodney D. 2016. *The Human Superorganism: How the Microbiome Is Revolutionizing the Pursuit of a Healthy Life*. Penguin Random House.

Ross, B. 2020. Transhumanism and Buddhist Philosophy: Two Approaches to Suffering. In: *The Philosophy of Transhumanism*. Emerald Publishing Limited, 147–166. https://doi.org/10.1108/978--1-83982--622--120201007.

Sagan, L. 1967. On the Origin of Mitosing Cells. *Journal of Theoretical Biology*, 14(3): 225-IN6. https://www.sciencedirect.com/science/article/pii/0022519367900793.

Shulman, E. 2008. Early Meanings of Dependent-Origination. *Journal of Indian Philosophy*, 36(2): 297.

Thich, Tam Duc. 2022. *The Way to Truc Lam Meditation School in Vietnam*. Vietnam National University Press.

Trần, Trọng Kim. 1920. *Việt Nam SuuLuọc (Abridged Chronicles)*. Hà Nội: Trung Bắc Tân Văn.

U.S. Department of Agriculture. 2022. Adoption of Genetically Engineered Crops in the U.S. [online].(September 14, 2022). https://www.ers.usda.gov/data-products/adoption-of-genetically-engineered-crops-in-the-u-s/

Yair, F. et al. 2016. Detection of Human Adaptation during the Past 2000 Years. *Science*, 354(6313): 760–64. https://doi.org/10.1126/science.aag0776.

Zhang, Xiao-Hui et al. 2015. Off-Target Effects in CRISPR/Cas9-Mediated Genome Engineering. *Molecular Therapy – Nucleic Acids*, 4. https://doi.org/10.1038/mtna.2015.37.

Practical Implications and Future Prospects

Transhumanism in Practice: Societal, Educational, and Ethical Considerations

The Impact of the Fourth Industrial Revolution on Human Life: Perspectives from Vietnam

Hoa Thi Kim Do and Duc Hong Nguyen

1. Introduction

The Fourth Industrial Revolution (4IR), characterized by rapid developments in digital technologies and artificial intelligence (AI), is transforming societies globally (Schwab, 2016). This report critically evaluates a survey among university teachers and students conducted in Hanoi, Vietnam in 2023, elucidating public perspectives on the impact of the 4IR on various aspects of human life.

Methodologically, the survey employed a mixed-methods approach. Quantitative data were collected through Likert-scale questions to measure the level of agreement with a series of statements about the impact of the 4IR. The qualitative data were gathered through open-ended questions, capturing nuanced views and the rationale behind respondent perspectives. The sample size and demographic distribution are not representative of the Vietnamese population but gathered results offer us a preliminary glimpse into the thinking and attitudes of the Vietnamese university students on this important topic.

The study reveals that the majority of respondents, regardless of gender, acknowledge the profound impact of 4IR on human existence. In particular, 82.1% agreed that scientific and technological advancements have significantly reshaped human life, echoing international sentiment.

2. Impact on Human Emotions

AI's capacity to mimic or even enhance human emotional capabilities remains a contentious issue (Picard, 2000). Approximately 50.4% of respondents favored the concept that technology could augment human emotions, while 48.7% opposed it. However, fewer respondents (41.6%) believed AI could replace human empathy, indicating a more cautious stance towards AI's potential to substitute complex human emotions. A gender difference was noted, with males displaying higher skepticism. This aligns with previous research indicating gender-based differences in attitudes towards AI (O'Shaughnessy et al., 2023).

Moving Forward:

Guidelines and policies pertaining to ethics can be developed with consideration for the various viewpoints that are now available regarding the effects of AI on human emotions. Promoting an open discourse between AI engineers, ethicists, psychologists, and the general public is essential to moving forward. Legislators ought to think about enacting rules that guarantee AI's emotional intelligence is created and applied appropriately, guarding against possible abuse and encouraging useful applications. In order to promote acceptance and trust, technologists must place a high priority on transparency. They must clearly explain to users how AI systems interpret and react to emotional cues.

3. Impact on Ethics and Morality

When considering the implications of technology on ethical standards and moral norms, the survey noted a significant level of polarization. The ethical implications of rapid technological advancement form a significant part of the discourse surrounding the 4IR (Boddington, 2017). A slightly higher proportion of respondents (52.2%) felt that advancements in science and technology would erode ethical norms and moral standards, indicating concerns about the potential negative consequences of unrestrained technological growth. This perspective was more prevalent among males, suggesting the need for gender-specific considerations in technological policy development.

Moving Forward:

It is imperative that governments, educators, and technologists give serious consideration to concerns regarding the degradation of moral and ethical standards. All educational levels should implement programs aimed at promoting ethical literacy and a knowledge of the moral implications of 4IR technologies. Creating and enforcing thorough ethical standards for AI development and application is crucial. In order to solve ethical issues and create global AI standards that support ethical coherence across national boundaries, international cooperation should be promoted.

4. Impact on Religious Beliefs

Another key area investigated in the survey was the influence of AI on religious beliefs which is rather complex and multifaceted (Vincenzo et al., 2019). Only one-third of the respondents (32.7%) believed AI could strengthen religious faith. This response was consistent across genders, implying that most people see a clear distinction between technology and religious or spiritual experiences. This suggests that, for the majority, technology and religion occupy separate spheres of human experience.

Moving Forward:

It is crucial to make sure that the development and deployment of AI respects religious and cultural diversity, given the intricate relationship that exists between technology and religious values. The separate domains of technology and religion must be acknowledged and respected by legislators and AI developers. Any attempt to combine these fields ought to be undertaken with caution, morality, and active religious community consultation. In this manner, we can guarantee that religious rituals arc supported by technology without violating religious freedom or unintentionally creating spiritual suffering.

5. Impact on Human Existence and Behaviour

The influence of technology on human existence and behavior is widely acknowledged in academic discourse (Brynjolfsson & McAfee, 2014). Consistently, the majority of respondents agreed that technological developments have influenced human existence and behavior. A significant 82.1% believed technology has altered the way humans exist, reinforcing the profound impact of the 4IR. The average rating of 3.50 for technology's influence on human existence was comparable to the rating of 3.63 for the 4IR's influence on human behavior, demonstrating a consensus on the pervasive influence of technology.

Moving Forward:

There is broad agreement that technology has a profoundly transforming effect on human existence and behavior, necessitating the development of comprehensive strategies that maximize advantages and limit hazards. Regulators should concentrate on enacting laws that promote beneficial technological developments while reducing any potential drawbacks. This involves drafting laws that guarantee fair access to technology, protect privacy, and advance digital literacy. Future studies should look into how technology might be used to improve quality of life, encourage sustainable development, and further societal objectives.

6. Further Considerations

Diverse Perspectives: While our survey delved into the perspectives of individuals based on gender, the views of different socio-economic, age, and occupational groups could offer a more complete picture. Variations in access to technology, technical understanding, or direct experience with AI and 4IR could contribute to these differences. For instance, blue-collar workers might feel threatened due to potential job displacement, while tech entrepreneurs might see the developments as an opportunity for innovation and economic growth (Bessen, 2019). Similarly, older generations might have concerns about privacy and data security, while younger individuals, who have grown up digital natives, might be more accepting of these technologies.

Historical Context: Technology has always been a transformative force in society, often bringing about significant social, economic, and behavioral changes. The Industrial Revolution, for instance, brought about significant shifts in workforce requirements, living conditions, and societal structures (Mokyr, 1990). Similarly, the advent of the internet profoundly changed communication and information access. Learning from these historical events can help society anticipate and prepare for potential challenges and opportunities brought about by AI and 4IR.

Comparative Analysis: Comparative studies across different societies could reveal how cultural, societal, and economic factors shape attitudes towards AI and 4IR. For instance, Asian societies with a high level of societal trust might be more receptive to these technologies compared to societies with greater individualism and privacy concerns (Choung, David, & Ross 2023). Such comparative analyses can inform global policy discussions and help design culturally sensitive strategies for AI and 4IR implementation.

Theoretical Underpinnings: Applying theories from sociology, psychology, and philosophy can provide a deeper understanding of our findings. For instance, the Social Shaping of Technology theory (MacKenzie&Wajcman, 1999) could explain why people perceive the impact of AI and 4IR differently, depending on their social context. Similarly, philosophical theories like Technological Determinism could offer insights into why some participants believe that technology will inevitably reshape human existence.

Practical Implications: Our findings can inform strategies for AI and 4IR implementation. Policymakers could design regulations to address public concerns about privacy and data security, while educators could incorporate AI literacy in curriculums to alleviate fears and misconceptions (Russell et al., 2015). Furthermore, AI developers could engage in ethical design practices to ensure that AI and 4IR technologies are inclusive, transparent, and respect users' rights.

Future Trends: As AI and 4IR continue to evolve, public perceptions are likely to change. Society needs to stay vigilant and adaptive, continuously reevaluating its policies, ethical considerations, and educational curricula. Anticipatory governance and foresight exercises could help in preparing for these changes (Guston, 2014).

AI Literacy: Enhancing AI literacy could be crucial in shaping public opinion. Knowledgeable individuals can make informed decisions and engage in meaningful discussions about the ethical implications of AI and 4IR. Hence, efforts to enhance AI literacy should be an integral part of education and public engagement strategies.

Ethics in AI Design: The concept of "Ethics by Design" in AI development could alleviate many public concerns. This approach involves integrating ethical considerations into all stages of AI development, from conceptualization to deployment (Mittelstadt et al., 2016). It can help ensure that AI systems are fair, transparent, and respect user rights, thus increasing public trust.

Limitations and Opportunities: Our study had several limitations, such as a focus on gender differences and not incorporating age, occupational, or socio-economic factors. Future research could explore these aspects to provide a more comprehensive understanding of public perceptions. Furthermore, future studies could delve into specific aspects of AI and 4IR, such as autonomous vehicles, AI in healthcare, or AI in education, to understand public attitudes towards these specific applications.

7. Conclusion

The survey results clarify the intricate interaction between the alleged advantages and difficulties presented by this unparalleled period of technical progress in Vietnam, therefore illuminating the complicated public attitude towards the Fourth Industrial Revolution (4IR). Especially, the general consciousness tends to believe that the 4IR has the ability to change many aspects of human existence, from emotional to ethical. This perspective is gently, but crucially, laced with a mixture of excitement and worry about the new technological environment and its far-reaching effects on society.

Importantly, public views reflect a complex evaluation of the possible benefits and drawbacks of quick technical advancement; they are neither rigid or absolute. Excitement in the promise of technology to improve human potential coexists with worries about a possible deterioration of moral standards and essentially human characteristics. So, the poll catches the social pulse characterized by a careful concern about the contradictory character of technical advancement.

Significant gender differences in the comprehension and assessment of the effects of the 4IR are also found by the analysis. These gender disparities provide important new information for more study, especially when it comes to views about how AI can replace human empathy and how ethical standards are seen to be undermined. An inclusive technology future will need acknowledging and resolving gender differences in the reaction to and involvement with the 4IR.

Especially remarkable is the almost uniform agreement on the need of regulation. Almost all of the respondents expressed the same wish for people to continue to be in charge of their technical inventions when they said that governance is necessary for the development and use of 4IR technologies. This result should be a crucial signal to regulators and politicians to emphasize the requirement of maintaining social control and ethical compliance as we proceed along the 4IR route.

Though the survey produced some very interesting results, there could be some restrictions on how representative the data are. Because these subgroups had comparatively small sample sizes, the poll did not assess variations in perceptions across a range of demographic factors including age, occupation, religious beliefs, or areas of competence. Thus, a request for greater study to clarify these complex viewpoints is necessary in order to give a more thorough picture of society views on the 4IR. The results of the poll emphasize how, taking into account the intricate fabric of public opinion, the 4IR must be shaped with a deliberate, moral, and inclusive strategy. As Bostrom and Yudkowsky (2014) note, the future of the 4IR age must be socially conscious, ethically aware, and aware of maintaining the essence of humanity in the face of ongoing technical advancement.

References

Bessen, J. E. 2019. AI and Jobs: The Role of Demand. NBER Working Paper No. 24235. Cambridge, MA:National Bureau of Economic Research.

Boddington, P. 2017. Towards a Code of Ethics for Artificial Intelligence. Cham: Springer International Publishing.

Bostrom, N., & Yudkowsky, E. 2014. In: K. Frankish & W.M. Ramsey(Eds.), The Cambridge handbook of artificial intelligence. Cambridge: Cambridge University Press, pp. 316–334.

Brynjolfsson, E., & McAfee, A. 2014. The Second Machine Age: Work, Progress, and Prosperity in a Time of Brilliant Technologies. New York: W.W. Norton & Company.

O'Shaughnessy, M. R., Schiff, D. S., Varshney, L. R., Rozell, C. J., & Davenport, M. A. 2023. What governs attitudes toward artificial intelligence adoption and governance? Science and Public Policy, 50(2): 161–176.

Guston, D. H. 2014. Understanding 'anticipatory governance'. Social Studies of Science, 44(2): 218–242.

Choung, H., David, P., & Ross, A. 2023. Trust in AI and its role in the acceptance of AI technologies. International Journal of Human–Computer Interaction, 39(9): 1727–1739.

MacKenzie, D., & Wajcman, J. 1999. The Social Shaping of Technology. Buckingham:Open University Press.

Mittelstadt, B., Allo, P., Taddeo, M., Wachter, S., &Floridi, L. 2016. The ethics of algorithms: Mapping the debate. Big Data & Society, 3(2): 2053951716679679.

Mokyr, J. 1990. The Lever of Riches: Technological Creativity and Economic Progress. Oxford: Oxford University Press.

Picard, R. W. 2000. Affective Computing. Chicago: MIT Press.

Russell, S., Dewey, D., & Tegmark, M.2015. Research Priorities for Robust and Beneficial Artificial Intelligence. AI Magazine, 36(4), 105–114.

Schwab, K. 2016. The Fourth Industrial Revolution. New York: Crown Publishing Group.

Vincenzo, F., Ma, Y., & Koul, A. 2019. Artificial Intelligence in a Spiritual World: An Evolutionary Perspective. London: Palgrave Macmillan.

THE PLASTICITIES OF HUMAN NATURE: FROM TRIVIAL TO HORRENDOUS

Winfried Löffler

1. "Human Nature" – a precarious notion?

Talk of a "human nature" is precarious in a peculiar way because it is questioned from two directions: On the one hand, it is suspected of being potentially suppressive or authoritarian, of representing an essentialism and a rigid account of the human being that endangers human possibilities for development as well as individual responsibility for our actions. This is the traditional concern of existentialism, but also to some extent of Critical Theory or postmodern thinkers such as Michel Foucault. On the other hand, although there are obvious regularities in human needs, capacities and ways of behavior that would be foolish to ignore, especially regarding our planning and acting, the postulate of a timeless, static "human nature" would be problematic for several reasons. Firstly, it would conflict with scientific knowledge, insofar as evolutionary biology teaches us that human evolutionary change continues. Secondly, examples from the past should be a warning that familiarity and customariness can easily be mistaken for naturalness: The times when, for example, women's suffrage was considered "unnatural" were not too long ago. Proposals of natural law doctrines have been criticized time and again for falling prey to this confusion. And in recent years, a bundle of problematic, right-wing populist and identitarian narratives has gained ground politically, which is actually highly heterogeneous, but whose common denominator seems to include a coding of "(good) naturalness vs. (bad) unnaturalness".[1] Thirdly, there is the question of the source of insights into a purported human nature:

[1] Think, e.g., of anti-vaxxing, especially the rejection m-RNA vaccines (instead, this is often accompanied by an emphatic trust in the strong natural immune system); skepticism on experts and belief in large-scale betrayal by modern media ("common sense

and here the temptation to try to answer questions about nature by merely thinking about definitions or "armchair reasoning" is highly problematic. As an example, gender debates have long been burdened by the prejudice that there simply could not be persons who are not either unambiguously male or unambiguously female – a prejudice that was based on purported *a priori* insights into "human nature".

So, should the concept of human nature perhaps be discarded and abandoned altogether as outdated or too prone to ideology? However, not only the aforementioned regularities in human life speak against such a radical solution, but also the other conditions by which the things set obvious constraints for our actions. In a way, hence, talk about a "nature of things", human beings included, seems to be indispensable. In section 2, therefore, a moderate and plausible proposal of a definition of "nature" in the philosophical sense will be made, on the basis of which it is also possible to analyze and do justice to the plasticities in human nature (sections 3 and 4). Some brief reflections on what might follow from all this for the assessment of "transhumanism" (section 5) conclude the essay.

2. "Human Nature" – a modest proposal of definition

I suggest the following general definition:

> The "Nature of x" = DEF the sum of typical properties, structures, processes, abilities, potentialities, patterns of activities/reactions of x.

---

has it better"); fear of asylum and migration movements as unnatural processes; fear of abolishment of cash as the natural way of payment; fear of genetically manipulated food; belief in the "Great Reset conspiracy", "population exchange" etc.; fear of "gender craze" that questions the purportedly exceptionless and natural male/female dichotomy; fear of "transhumanism"; narratives of (natural) "localism" versus (unnatural) "globalism"; disbelief in anthropogenic climate disaster (and instead, belief in natural climate shifts); preference of alternative/complementary medicine, "traditional European medicine", old esoteric knowledge suppressed by modern artificial medicine etc. – Seen as such, these opinions are actually very heterogeneous in their content. And one is therefore perhaps tempted to assume as a proximate explanation for their bundling that they belong to the propaganda of certain political groups. But this propagandistic bundling would hardly work if there were not certain connections regarding their content. And I suggest that "naturalness versus unnaturalness" is one of these connections.

This definition, of course, immediately suggests the question from which sources one could recognise such a nature of things. That one should not place too much trust in a mere analysis of ideas or in philosophical or theological "decrees" about the nature of man and other things has already been mentioned. Rather, an (in a broader sense neo-Aristotelian[2]) approach that sees practical dealings with things and the empirical sciences that have arisen from them as the main source of our insights into the nature of things seems more purposeful. To take up our example from above: whether or not there are persons who are neither clearly a man nor clearly a woman is an empirical question that is essentially to be answered by some biological or medical sciences, such as genetics, physiology and anatomy.

In order to avoid an ideologization of the notion of nature and a kind of epistemological arrogance or hybris, it seems useful to point out two typical mistakes or confusions that can occur when using the word "nature".

Firstly, "nature" is not to be confused with "fully/comprehensively understood nature". Whoever speaks of the nature of a thing or the nature of a human being does not necessarily claim to have already fully understood this nature. On the contrary, we can usually still learn something about the nature of things, and the primary source for this is the natural sciences. Since science is not resistant to error, it can also happen that we are temporarily mistaken in our judgements about the nature of human beings and are surprised or taught better by later research.

Secondly – and related to this – it is again necessary to warn against obvious confusions: "the familiar/entrenched/usual" – especially when it comes to human nature – does not necessarily have to be "the natural". Human beings and their behavior are to some extent also culturally malleable; and cultural regularities can sometimes be so strong that they are taken for natural (one might recall some professions that used to be considered "naturally inaccessible" for women, but which are now as a matter of course also practiced by women). Moreover, it can happen that certain sections of human nature are seen as particularly striking or characteristic, so that other aspects fade into the background. In this context, it is worth recalling a certain intellectualization that has long characterized the Western

[2] For a broader survey of philosophical nations of "nature" and "human nature" see, e.g. (Roughley 2021).

image of man and made other, more bodily, affective or animalic aspects of it seem irrelevant, embarrassing or even morally problematic.

3. Plasticities in human nature: insights from classical philosophy

However, that the classical philosophical tradition as a whole represented a static image of man is probably based on a cliché or certain interpretations of this tradition. The Aristotelian tradition in particular has intellectual resources to integrate flexibilities and plasticities in the nature of man into its conception of man. Some of these "built-in" flexibilities and potentials for development will be recalled here.

1. For Aristotelian-Scholastic anthropology and ethics, the concept of habitus as "second nature" is crucial.[3] Habitus are acquired, trainable abilities and dispositions of a thing. The "first nature" of a thing (i.e., its essence, or the kind of thing it is) defines which habitus a thing could acquire and which it could not; in this respect, humans are presumably the most "malleable" of all beings, able to acquire a particularly wide range of habitus, from sporting and manual skills to foreign languages and musical virtuosity. They are called "second nature" because they determine the individual's repertoire of agency in much the same way that first nature does. Philosophically important and well-known habitus are the intellectual virtues (like knowledge and prudence) and the moral virtues (like helpfulness and politeness). These virtues (and the intellectual and moral vices opposed to them, such as gullibility and aggressiveness) can be partly influenced by people themselves and cultivated in them, so these virtues and vices are also the subject of moral evaluation. The classical philosophical tradition therefore sees human beings not only as capable of, but also as called to, general intellectual and moral development.
2. Especially in the Christian variants of classical philosophy, this call to further development is also embedded in a larger interpretation: Further development in the life of man is manifestation of a deeper dynamic toward God.[4] If the human being cultivates and realizes its best disposi-

[3] The elaboration of this doctrine – on Aristotelian fundaments – is a product of the Middle Ages. See, e.g., (Nederman 1989–1990).

[4] This idea was especially developed, based on Thomas Aquinas and Kant, by the school of Joseph Maréchal (1878–1944). Up to my knowledge, his opus magnum *Le point*

tions, this is at the same time the best path toward the vision of God in the afterlife.

3. It is little known that, according to the most influential Aristotelian-Scholastic philosopher Thomas Aquinas (1224/5–1274), the lex naturalis / law of nature (ontologically and morally understood, not so much in the modern scientific sense) also has "statistical" character. That is, it is valid for most and only for standard cases, and it can also change in principle.[5]

In sum, then, human nature in the classical view appears to be neither static nor timeless. This is a point where contemporary transhumanists can connect to the classical tradition (whether they do so in a justified or unjustified way is another question, see section 5).[6]

4. Plasticities in human nature: contemporary dimensions

After this look at the classical philosophical tradition, let us consider the plasticities of human nature as seen from today's scientific and medical-technical point of view. (Behind the few keywords, to which I must limit myself here, there are of course broad fields of research with their respective accompanying philosophical discussions).

(1) The permanent evolution of humans has already been mentioned; co-evolution with the symbionts of humans (e.g., in the microbiome of the digestive tract) and the potentials for comparatively fast epigenetic change could be added here. (2) Studies in population genetics have shown that in humans (as in most other organisms) genetic variation within the gene pool of populations is considerably greater than previously suspected. These variations are partly statistically neutralized, but they can also be the source of changes. (3) The huge field of new medical technologies (including occasional genetic interventions also in the therapeutic field) enables new

---

de départ de la métaphysique: leçons sur le développement historique et théorique du problème de la connaissance (Maréchal 1922–47, see especially volume V (1926)) was never translated, but there is a selection: (Maréchal 1970).

5 See (Weingartner 1997).

6 This plasticity and flexibility of human nature is, incidentally, also a point that imago Dei anthropologies must take into account and integrate into their theories: (1) God's immutability does not seem to simply "transfer" to us humans; (2) "Imago Dei" does not imply a non-dynamic account of human nature.

ways and forms of living despite existing health handicaps and has led to a significant statistical prolongation of life in most countries. (4) The field of possible forms of enhancement and optimization of the human body and its conditions has broadened. However, the boundary between therapy and enhancement is still unclear and therefore much discussed: not every state of health or mind that is perceived as undesirable is already a case for therapy. However, it can be observed that the social standards for this can change; this can be seen, among other things, in the discussions about which forms of treatment should be publicly financed (dental braces and plastic surgery measures provide illustrative examples here). (5) There is an increasingly broad spectrum of ways in which people live their lives as a sort of "compounds" of natural and non-natural components. Familiar are cases of people who are dependent on eyeglasses, hearing aids or walking aids, but also, for example, on blood pressure tablets and other permanent medication, without which a longer-term continuation of life would not be possible at all. More recently, there are people with transplanted organs or artificial limbs, insulin pumps, heart pacemakers, "brain pacemakers" in cases of epilepsy, Parkinson and other diseases, cochlea implants etc. (6) Some philosophers would also consider e.g. smartphones (and their use as "extended memory", means of communication etc.) or even our reliance on the stock of knowledge of our social environment as a case of such compounds, but here the connection to the human body is less dense.[7]

All in all, there is a basis to see here certain analogies to a "second nature" in the sense of classical philosophy: A human being living as such a compound extends his possibilities of action, and the use of some of these aids must be learned or can be cultivated and improved. Many of these modifications of human nature are completely unproblematic, at least as far as their anthropological aspects are concerned.[8] However, some extrapola-

---

[7] The exact distinction, however, is surprisingly difficult: after all, eyeglasses, hearing aids and walking sticks are also removable from the body. One might be tempted to say that they serve life functions in a more direct way than, for example, a smartphone; but on the other hand, communication is demonstrably important for health and well-being, so the difference between glasses, hearing aids, and smartphones again seems only gradual.

[8] Some of these devices have costs and also consequences for the lives of their users that are worthy of ethical consideration. For example, there is debate about whether cochlear implants, in addition to their undisputed benefits, may also contribute to deaf people losing certain cultural techniques and connections to their communities.

tions, visions and promises for the future, as they are sometimes expressed, may raise concerns.

5. A short word on transhumanism: Where the problem really lies

The talk of "transhumanism" is in itself problematic and in need of clarification, among other things because the word has been used in the context of populist rhetoric and conspiracy theories to mark an enemy image. Thus, the false impression has been created that we are dealing here with a clearly definable group of doctrines and the people who represent them, i.e., a kind of philosophical school and/or socio-political actors close to it. But this is not true in this simplicity. It is true that the word has been around since the late 1950s, and that since the 1980s there have been some philosophers, scientists, historians and writers (e.g., Nick Bostrom, Ray Kurzweil, Stefan Laurenz Sorgner, Max Tegmark, Yuval Noah Harari etc.) who call themselves transhumanists or sympathize with transhumanist ideas; in professional philosophy they have little overall influence and are (despite of the professional web appearance https://www.humanityplus.org) little noticed. In addition, there are activists who approach the public with more or less eccentric technological and social ideas or technical modifications to their own bodies, for example by staging themselves as "cyborgs", and thus attract a certain amount of media attention. And of course, there are people in various fields of society who de facto propagate transhumanist ideas; the borderline to mere exaggerated ideologies of progress is sometimes fuzzy. Accordingly, one can only delineate a vague doctrinal core of transhumanism; first, it is about the thesis that humans, their bodies and social coexistence could be optimized in various directions by a wide range of technical, medical and other measures. The result of these measures is not only the fight against known problems (such as diseases, aging and scarcity of resources), but also the realization of various ideals and desires, such as the prolongation of life, freedom from pain, combating poverty, more social justice, etc. Secondly, this factual thesis is connected with the normative thesis that such measures would also be ethically demanded, among other things because one could increase happiness and enjoyment of life of humans and reduce existing discriminations.[9] "Transhumanism" is the

9 See the beginning of the "Transhumanist Declaration" of 1998 (under https://www.

name of this thinking insofar as it explicitly also considers and approves of changes in human nature. One can characterize transhumanism as a general emphatic ideology of progress with an underlying ethical concern; such a style of thinking can, of course, be found in broader circles (i.e., beyond avowed "transhumanists"), which is why the impression of a broad, socially powerful movement has been created in some eyes. Some eccentric theses or visions of individual transhumanists have received special media attention and shape the broader public perception of transhumanism to a probably great extent, for example that of copying/uploading the "program" of the human mind onto a sort of huge server for later survival. Leaving aside the complete lack of clarity how such a process could function technically and on which theoretical basis (although the small-scale processes in the brain, for example at the synapses, and also the functions of the large brain regions are comparatively well understood, there is still very little known about the "medium-scale" processes and the emergence of consciousness in the brain), such visions are rather a part of science fiction and do not belong to the core of transhumanism, but they are also used as external attributions to discredit it. The perceived distance of such ideas to entirely absurd conspiracy theories (for example to the thesis that the world is already ruled by "reptiloids") is no longer large.

Nevertheless: Transhumanist views are indeed inherently problematic.[10] The problem, however, is not so much the interventions in human nature that are being considered: As we have seen in the previous sections, there have always been and still are smaller and larger plasticities and modifications in human nature. Some of these are unproblematic, some of them are not. There may be expansions of these plasticities here and there. All that is a gradual problem and must be evaluated in each individual case. There are no simple "sacred boundaries" or fixed "red lines" here; in particular, interventions in the genome constitute, per se, no such red lines.

---

humanityplus.org/the-transhumanist-declaration): "1. Humanity stands to be profoundly affected by science and technology in the future. We envision the possibility of broadening human potential by overcoming aging, cognitive shortcomings, involuntary suffering, and our confinement to planet Earth. – 2. We believe that humanity's potential is still mostly unrealized. There are possible scenarios that lead to wonderful and exceedingly worthwhile enhanced human conditions. [. . .]".

10 See, e.g., the Anti-Transhumanist manifesto by Georg Franck, Sarah Spiekermann et al. (2023).

To declare the genome as an absolute limit would even be an implausible ethical biologism. (Among other things, it should be pointed out that there are already some successful forms of somatic gene therapy, which would then also be reprehensible per se – which is implausible). Some modifications, however, would indeed be horrendous. The problem, however, is not so much the modification of human nature, but the associated uncertainties, dangers, risks and fairness problems. In short, then, the issue is one of ethics (especially social responsibility) rather than metaphysics. Concerns about hard-to-foresee consequences and collateral consequences of new medical and technological possibilities are well founded: They involve not only questions of safety, but also questions of fair cost-sharing for these (often costly) technologies and fair distribution of access to these possibilities-for the people affected now, but also for future generations.

Based on such considerations, the concern that many people intuitively have about genetic interventions can even be partially justified: Because of the complex structure and functioning of the genome, the full consequences of interventions are often not precisely known, but they are irreversible, can be drastic, and may in some cases be passed on to future generations. Thus, they then affect people who were not involved in the decision to use such agents in the first place. And these procedures are costly and raise questions of distributive justice – how access to them could be implemented for all is difficult to see.

So even if transhumanist theses were developed partly out of ethical concerns, they are questionable from an ethical point of view. The implied ethical problems are often obscured behind diffused and apparently humanist visions of progress. This is problematic. The hope of disease control and eradication through genetic manipulation, for example, is in most cases exaggerated: Indeed, the simplistic correlation scheme of "1 trait – 1 section on the DNA" does not apply in most cases. Only relatively few diseases are monogenic, but they are related to a wide variety of DNA regions, which can then also have other functions. Moreover, in the outbreak of diseases, the genetic basis interacts with environmental influences in a complex way. The hope of eliminating diseases through simple genome editing is therefore unfounded in many cases, even in the age of the CRISPR-Cas9 gene scissors. The same applies to physical and mental characteristics that one might want to favour through genetic intervention: these, too, are generally not determined by a single DNA segment. Transhumanist promises of progress should also be critically questioned from another ethical point of view: In some authors, an ideology of quasi-Nietzschean superhumanity is discernible, which blatantly ignores the need for self-restraint and solidarity. To be sure, no one will deny that reducing suffering and enabling people to live as long and as well as possible are in principle ethically good tasks, as is the use of intelligent advanced technologies to achieve these goals. But the elimination of all suffering and the optimization of all life circumstances is arguably an illusion: limitations, failure, and the experience that some desires turn out to be unfulfillable are all part of human life – starting with the knowledge of its temporal finitude. Above all, the effort and the price of such optimizations must always be considered from a socio-ethical point of view: Where transhumanist ideas turn out to be a luxury ideology for the economically privileged, which could not be implemented at all in solidarity for all (one thinks, for example, of the fantasies of stopping the aging process, which would inevitably lead to the overcrowding of the planet) or whose consequential costs are outsourced to other groups of people, there they should be rejected from an ethical point of view.

References

Maréchal, J. 1922–1947. *Le point de départ de la métaphysique: leçons sur le développement historique et théorique du problème de la connaissance* (5 vols.). Bruges-Louvain: Charles Beyaert.

Maréchal, J. 1970. *A Maréchal Reader*, edited and translated by Joseph Donceel. New York: Herder & Herder.

Nederman, C. J. 1989–1990. Nature, Ethics, and the Doctrine of 'Habitus': Aristotelian Moral Psychology in the Twelfth Century. *Traditio* (45): 87–110.

Roughley, N. 2021. Human Nature. *Stanford Encyclopedia of Philosophy*. https://plato.stanford.edu/entries/human-nature/ (accessed September 18, 2023).

Weingartner, P. 1997. Kann sich das natürliche Gesetz ändern? Kommentar zu Thomas v. Aquin, S. Th. I-II, 94.5. In: W. Löffler (ed.), *Dialog und System*. Sankt Augustin: Academia, 197–230.

AN ATTEMPT AT A METAPHYSICAL INTERPRETATION OF POSTHUMANISM

Ion Cordoneanu

1. Introduction

There are already classical authors whose ideas, by the nature of their concerns, are associated with the issue of posthumanism. One of these is Norbert Wiener, who as early as 1964 made a comprehensive and focused statement about the place that technology should occupy in the human world: "As engineering technique becomes more and more able to achieve human purposes, it must become more and more accustomed to formulate human purposes". (Wiener 1966, 64).

After the mid-20th century, academic literature on the impact of technology on human existence becomes increasingly abundant in academia and popular culture, where terms such as "transhumanism" and "posthumanism" inspire many texts on the changing nature of the human condition: "technology is not only spreading to the far corners of the world, it is transforming us. It is changing our understanding of ourselves and challenging the ontological models and the foundational claims that we rely upon to define being human" (Philbeck 2014, 173).

Some assessments of new technologies, and therefore of the scientific theories on which they are based, go so far as to note that "for transhumanists, humanity is gravely and irremediably flawed, but salvation is achievable if we but dedicate ourselves to creating posthumanity" (Levin 2021, 7). In the Romanian space of ideas about the social role of technology and the moral impact it has on man, it is well known that "in the global debate, information technologies are simultaneously mythologized as the answer to the great problems of mankind, but also decried as the beginning of the end of liberal democracies". (Rughiniş 2022, 189, *our translation*).

In this context of controversy and excommunication, philosophy is called upon to contribute an integrative vision of the new position/situation of the human being in relation to technology. That is why some possible evaluations and interpretations could take into account the ideas of Heidegger, "one of the philosophers who had the courage for this kind of disturbance, and it does not stop there – he has pointed out the possibilities for developing a more daring stance toward philosophy, as well as an understanding of the human being. This is why today we can consider Heidegger to be the philosopher who can still inspire us to explore philosophy as something relevant to our own human condition" (Popović 2016, 127).

2. Human nature

When transhumanists argue that the "enhancement of the human species through technology represents the only chance for *Homo sapiens* to avoid being overtaken by the very machines they themselves invented" (Alexandre et al. 2018, 2) and that the unprecedented Promethean project behind technological evolution, which is the source of the most lively debate and contention today, is in fact about human modification, improvement, augmentation, and ultimately overcoming, the narrative is by no means new. Those who criticize or express major fears on this topic follow in the footsteps of Nietzsche, who proclaimed, at the end of the 19th century, "the death of God". In a way, it would even be coherent: God created man and man symbolically killed Him, excluding Him from his own world; now it is man's turn – the creator of artificial intelligence – to be placed in the twilight of his own history to make way for machines that replace not only human strength but also knowledge, intelligence, analysis and reasoning.

Notwithstanding, in the paradigm and project of man's enhancement, it is obvious that Rousseau's definition of man is correct – a definition that is self-sustaining and self-referentially validated by the very paradigm it generates. It must be stated, however, that *Man as a perfectible being* has nothing to do with the religious (not only Christian) ideal of human restoration. It is a definition specific to modernity, a historical era dominated by technology, whose foundations have been known, since the 17th century, as modern natural science. I nonetheless believe that this view on human nature deprives the human being of an entire universe of its own and of its own alone, being entangled in the modern ideal of progress – a myth as any other, a narrative by which the human is reduced to an ideal of reason that demystifies and dissolves man's journey into his own History.

In the context of modernity which is constantly redefining itself by "post" (poststructuralism, postmodernism, postcolonialism, etc.), posthumanism is made apparent by the manifest preoccupation for topics concerned, on the one hand, with the advancement of sciences (ethology, evolutionary biology, cognitive neuroscience, computer sciences, nano- and biotechnologies) and, on the other hand, in Francis Fukuyama's words, "the need to exercise greater political control over the use of science and technology" (Fukuyama 2003, x).

Fukuyama's thesis is that biotechnology poses a significant threat through its potential to alter human nature. The American author sets out from two dystopias that defined the "future and potentialities" of the 20th century, *1984* by George Orwell (1949) and *Brave New World* by Aldous Huxley (1932). According to the American political scientist, Orwell made accurate predictions about technological progress but his political predictions were entirely wrong. By contrast, Huxley's predictions appear to be increasingly concrete, considering the project circumscribed by technological progress: evil is no longer manifest in *Brave New World*, no one is hurt, there is no disease, social conflict, insanity, loneliness, etc., "the people in *Brave New World* may be healthy and happy but they have ceased to be *human beings*" (Fukuyama 2003, 6). If the human being status is traditionally associated with fighting for an ideal, aspiring, loving, making moral decisions and others of the same kind that make up human dignity, these no longer define the existence of the species whose individuals live in an unnatural world "in the most profound sense imaginable because *human nature* has been altered" (Fukuyama 2003, 6). Fukuyama defines posthumanism in close connection with the concept of human nature. Starting from the premise that the latter's role, alongside religion, has been to confer the species stability and define the fundamental human values throughout history, he notes: "Human nature shapes and constraints the possible kinds of political regimes, so a technology powerful enough to reshape what we are will have possibly malign consequences for liberal democracy and the nature of politics itself" (Fukuyama 2003, 7).

3. Free will – a myth

"Twenty-first-century science is undermining the foundations of the liberal order" (Harari 2016, 228) and, with it, the notion of free will that gives sense to the universe. Harari argues that the belief that humans are endowed with free will contradicts the latest findings in contemporary science, even though it made sense 200 centuries ago. Today, geneticists and neuroscientists explain all actions by electrochemical processes, genetic structures, and ancient evolutionary pressures, the former being either deterministic, arbitrary, or a combination – but never free. Harari is categorical:

> "To the best of our scientific understanding, determinism and randomness have divided the entire cake between them, leaving not even a crumb for 'freedom'. The sacred word 'freedom' turns out to be, just like 'soul', an empty term that carries no discernible meaning. Free will exists only in the imaginary stories we humans have invented" (Harari 2016, 229).

There is indeed a fundamental difference in the epistemological approach between "acting according to one's desires" and "choosing desires". According to the new sciences, the mechanism of the emergence of desires is one thing, and action according to desires is something else entirely. Free will, understood as the capacity to act according to one's desires, only makes sense from the latter perspective. Otherwise, the processes at the origin of a desire are determined, or arbitrary, but never free: "The decision to press either the right or left switch certainly reflected the person's choice. Yet it wasn't a free choice. In fact, our belief in free will results from faulty logic. When a biochemical chain reaction makes me desire to press the right switch, I feel that I really want to press the right switch. And this is true. I really want to press it. Yet people erroneously jump to the conclusion that if I want to press it, I *choose* to want to. This is of course false. I don't *choose* my desires. I only *feel* them, and act accordingly" (Harari 2016, 231).

Along with free will, another myth falls into contemporary science: that of the self or soul. This is replaced by the idea of a stream of consciousness that can be manipulated and controlled, and the practical implications are manifold: from medicine to virtuosity to learning mathematics or work efficiency or skills in various other fields, technology is improving at a rapid pace. Harari's prediction for the technological world we already live in?

Free will is no longer constitutive of human nature, but will be a commodity like any other, to be accessed with a simple click and the installation of a helmet: “If and when such manipulations become routine, the supposedly free will of customers will become just another product we can buy”. (Harari 2016, 234).

With the undermining of free will and the self, it is not only the idea of liberalism that suffers but all anthropologies whose foundation is the idea of the unity of the human being, as well as so many other narratives specific to history that have the individual or collective self at their center. At the individual level, everyone tells a story that gives meaning to experiences of all kinds; at the collective level, stories invent nations, gods and money – all of which present-day science and technology reduce to mere fiction: “Medieval crusaders believed that God and heaven provided their lives with meaning. Modern liberals believe that individual free choices provide life with meaning. They are all equally delusional” (Harari 2016, 246–7).

The new science will be translated into technology, economy and everyday life. This phase will inevitably question the structures of society, from beliefs to political institutions and economic values. Liberalism, not only the political and economic paradigm of the 20th century but the integrating anthropological vision, will thus be *threatened by the new technological leap*, with the following practical consequences: “1. Humans will lose their economic and military usefulness hence the economic and political system will stop attaching much value to them, 2. The system will still find value in humans collectively, but not in unique individuals., 3. The system will still find value in some unique individuals, but these will be a new elite of upgraded superhumans rather than the mass of the population” (Harari 2016, 248).

4. A metaphysical “mutation”?

We are faced with a reality and a question. Reality is defined by the technological revolution in which nano- and biotechnologies converge with artificial intelligence and from this convergence comes the possibility of improving the performance of the human body and mind, as well as human augmentation/upgrading. However, before asking whether technology should be allowed to do this (Alexandre et al. 2018, 11), the question must be asked about the essence of technology in order to understand what is, in fact, the "mutation" that is about to take place in human history.

From Heidegger, we get an answer to the question of technology (*Die Frage nach der Technik*, 1953). It must be said that, in this lecture, the German philosopher is concerned with the relationship we have with the essence of modern technology, which is not something of the order of technology – in other words, Heidegger develops a metaphysical analysis of technology, and by technology is meant modern technology as it developed up to the middle of the 20th century. It should also be said that, in my view, the development of technology brings with it a different kind of relationship that man begins to develop, in continuation of the age of technology – a metaphysical "mutation" that I identify in the leap from *modern* technology to *present-day* technology. I will develop this idea in the next section.

According to Heidegger, modern technology is a means to an end – the view is correct and accurate but says nothing of the essence of technology. Heidegger himself noted precisely what concerns us today with regard to technology: we pursue its domination and "the will to mastery becomes all the more urgent the more technology threatens to slip from human control" (Heidegger 1977, 5). Furthermore, we accept that the purpose of technology construed as a tool is an essentially correct one – that of improving the human condition – but, following Heidegger, this still does not show "the essence of technology". Having defined the purpose, we find ourselves in an "empire of causality" – technology, as we have seen, places man in this domination, this position being only the consequence of the way in which, with modern technology, we understood "the causality theory" from the Greeks, restrictively and depleted of the original meaning of the "four modes of being responsible", i.e., in the area of ethics, as error, or in the area of determinism.

One of the distinctions we need to bear in mind between *modern technology* and *present-day technology* is that, in the case of the former, the interaction of the four causes takes place outside man, in the realm of nature. In the contemporary age of technology, on the other hand, man is subject to the impulses and triggers produced by technology.

Heidegger's hermeneutic archaeology brings to light some meanings without which we cannot understand the age we live in – the age of technology. First, what is technology – *techne*?

4.1 Modern technology

The first point Heidegger makes about technology is that it is a name for craft activity and skill, but also for art. The second aspect is that *techne* is accompanied by *episteme*, designating knowledge in a broad sense – knowledge provides the illuminating explanation of skill in a field. Being associated with knowledge, *techne* is a way of *aletheuein*, i.e., of unconcealment of being. This is why Heidegger states that "*techne* is a mode of *aletheuein*. It reveals whatever does not bring itself forth and does not yet lie here before us" (Heidegger 1977, 13).

This is the field of technology that is valid for Greek thought – the field that determines the essence of modern technology based on engine power is quite different. Modern technology is also a way of unconcealing a type of being, generally called nature. This unconcealment specific to modern technology is "a challenging which puts to nature the unreasonable demand that it supply energy that can be extracted and stored as such" (Heidegger 1977, 14). Thus, the domain of being specific to modern technology has the character of constraint, in the sense of insistent demand for delivery (Heidegger covers the characterization of the domain with extraction, transformation, storage, distribution, redistribution, direction, and securing), and what is born out of constraint "is ordered to stand by, to be immediately at hand" (Heidegger 1977, 17), being in a "standing reserve (*Bestand*)". From this perspective, the machine as an instrument of modern technology is not autonomous.

Heidegger's thought is taken further: in the age of modern technology, man himself is subject to the demand to 'supply' himself to the extraction of natural energies, thus he belongs to the "standing reserve" (*Bestand*), even more originally than nature.

What is, in Heidegger's view, the relationship between modern technology and modern natural science, and how does one arrive at this relationship in which modern technology places mathematical natural science in its own service? For this, Heidegger brings into play a concept from Greek philosophy, to which he finds a German equivalent but gives it a meaning of its own. I believe that the closest Greek philosophical term is *logos*, and the German equivalent used by Heidegger to designate the relationship between modern technology and modern science is *Ge-stell* [enframing]. *Logos* is what gathers together, and *Ge-stell* is "the gathering together of that setting-upon which sets upon man, i.e., challenges him forth, to reveal the real, in the mode of ordering, as standing-reserve" (Heidegger 1977, 20). One could indeed regard *Ge-Stell* as the designation of the essence of technology in its gathering together as planning, ordering and arranging of the world. Modern physics is the science on which the modern theory of nature is based – the theory of nature, thus founded, prepares not only the emergence of modern technology but also its essence: the gathering together, with its insistent demand to supply for the unconcealment that is subject to order is already manifest in physics.

The unconcealment of the real as a standing reserve does not take place beyond human activity; to put it otherwise, man is caught in the sphere of this *logos* of modern technology called *Ge-stell*; he is no longer free to choose his relation to this *logos*.

4.2 The age of technology – posthumanism

Technology is not a *pro-traction* from self but from the other; the logos of what is *pro-tracted* is found in another (craftsman, artist, engineer). What is the great "mutation" that takes place, from the perspective of the metaphysical considerations above, with the advent and expansion of technological domination in the domain of the human? In the age of modern technology, production was exterior to man, while with technological advancement, it is within man. The human is subject to the possibility of being dominated by something external yet assimilated – the technological.

The image of the river "built" inside the hydroelectric plant that Heidegger uses to represent the constraint of nature in the sense of the insistent demand to supply itself is, to my mind, a significant metaphor for understanding the relationship between man and technology: the human begins to be walled in and annexed by technology. Moreover, the directing as a main feature of the real towards supply becomes or, better yet, is taken over, in the age of technology, by algorithms. Technology supplies man in the sense that it directs him according to algorithms and determines him to manifest himself (to unconceal) according to the ways and modes of the algorithm.

Technology makes man subject to command so that the latter delivers himself and is always at hand: constantly connected to social media, more effective at the workplace, more subject to social algorithms – which, in

Heideggerian metaphysical terms, is equivalent to saying that, in the age of technology, the "standing reserve" being is not nature but man.

In the age of modern technology, nature represented both supply and resource. Nowadays, man himself becomes a resource and delivers himself as such. Back then, the machine was not autonomous, now man is no longer autonomous either; connected to the point of intimacy and subject to delivery, he is the main resource of the world dominated by technology which, in its turn, is becoming more and more autonomous from the human mode of existence. It is only now that man replaces the machine as a standing reserve but, in his turn, is replaced by technology and becomes a mere resource.

If according to Heidegger, modern technology is not a simple human activity as a revelation that makes the real subject to command (therefore, as a specific mode of unconcealment), then neither is present-day technology a simple human activity. But the technology's mode of revealing the real addresses man directly, who, in his capacity as a "standing reserve", is annexed to the technology-specific algorithms. The modern *Ge-stell* reclaims nature as a standing reserve subject to command. Posthumanist *Ge-stell* reclaims man – the latter is called forth as a constant standing reserve, i.e., subject both to command and algorithm. He is no longer free to choose his relation to the new *logos*, so, what has changed? The difference lies in the fact that, in the age of modern technology, the narrative of freedom, free will, and the self still held strong roots, and that this narrative generated and nurtured economic and political systems and patterns of social organization within a relatively stable macro-historical paradigm. Today, with the demythization that we witness happening to these "fictional characters", the human itself is thought of through the lens of technological determinism.

4.3 How can we rethink freedom in the age of technology?

Man is in the sphere of technological logos and is not free to choose his relationship. In what terms, then, can we rethink freedom, as we have travelled this road from Greek *techne* to modern technology and now to present-day technology? It is again Heidegger who gives us a path to understanding: the journey along this road was accompanied by an "ordering", and the whole of this ordering – itself a logos under whose dominion the real unfolded – is termed "destining" by Heidegger: "Always the destining of revealing holds complete sway over man. But that destining is never a fate that compels. For man becomes truly free only insofar as he belongs to the realm of destining and so becomes one who listens and hears [*Hörender*], and not one who is simply constrained to obey [*Höriger*]" (Heidegger 1977, 25). Listening and hearing, therefore understanding the destining, will place us in its open space, which "in no way confines us to a stultified compulsion to push on blindly with technology or (. . .) to rebel helplessly against it and curse it as the work of the devil" (Heidegger 1977, 25–26). It is a responsibility that remains valid for the future of technology, a future that is not free from the danger of man understanding himself as subject to command and setting his rules within this limitation; or the danger of misinterpreting the essence of technology.

5. Conclusions?

Heidegger anticipates in his own terms, however, the danger with regard to man: that of being taken as a mere standing reserve made up of algorithms and information, i.e., so far removed from his essence. How can man be thought of henceforth, in the age of technology, from the perspective of something enduring and therefore saving? And, above all, what in man can be brought to light as *an event that reveals what is his own* (Ereignis)?

Tom Wolfe announced as early as 1997, in the famous article "Sorry, but your soul just died", the collapse of the foundations: "Since consciousness and thought are entirely physical products of your brain and nervous system – and since your brain arrived fully imprinted at birth – what makes you think you have free will? Where is it going to come from? What "ghost", what "mind", what "self", what "soul", what anything that will not be immediately grabbed by those scornful quotation marks, is going to bubble up your brain stem to give it to you?" (Wolfe 1997).

One can start with the observation that the foundations are shaking and cracking. And yet it is these foundations that have held humanity together until now and told the story of man, accompanying him like the characters without whom the hero could not have met the challenges and overcome the obstacles. What, then, is left to man alone?

Even with the effort that technology remains in the service of man and does not take him over, perhaps what we are looking for lies in human dignity and moral status related to the fact that we are whole and not the sum of the parts. In search of that factor X, "an essential human quality" (Fukuyama 2003, 149) worth of minimum respect, maybe this event will occur when we become aware that the domination of technology could shadow the dignity of the human being as a whole: "Factor X cannot be reduced to the possession of moral choice, or reason, or language, or sociability, or sentience, or emotions, or consciousness, or any other quality that has been put forth as a ground for human dignity. It is all of these qualities coming together in the human whole that make up Factor X" (Fukuyama 2003, 171).

What can we do? In his time, Heidegger saw the critical situation in which we were in the sense that the excess of technology prevented us from finding out what was truly essential about technology. Just as today, when the essence of technology makes us question what we used to consider foundational and redefine human nature instead of reflecting on how we can comprehend the relationship between man and technology and how we can regulate it for the benefit of humankind.

We can still open up ourselves to the last suggestion that Heidegger himself makes in the concluding lines of the *Question Concerning Technology*: the reflection on and the dispute with technology might take place in that realm both related to and fundamentally different from the essence of technology, but so proper to man and the highest expression of life. Heinrich Heine bears witness to this: "Music is the last word of art just as art is the last word of life".

We can also remember that, in search of a new objectivity that includes technology and artificial intelligence, perhaps the only form of objectivity is the gift of finding yourself in the other.

And we can still wonder, for in wonder there is no fear. But we need to do so while being aware that the world of the future will challenge the limits of human intelligence and will not be, as Weiner puts it, "a comfortable hammock in which we can lie down to be waited upon by our robot slaves" (1966, 69).[1]

---

[1] Translated from Romanian by Oana Celia Gheorghiu

References

Alexander, L. & Besnier J-M. 2018. Do Robots Make Love? From AI to Immortality – Understanding Transhumanism in 12 Questions. London: Hachette.

Fukuyama, F. 2003. Our Posthuman Future: Consequences of the Biotechnology Revolution. New York: Picador.

Harari, Y. N. 2016. Homo Deus. A Brief History of Tomorrow. London: Harper Collins.

Heidegger, M. 1977. The Question Concerning Technology and Other Essays. Translated and with an Introduction by W. Lovitt. New York and London: Garland Publishing.

Levin, S. B. 2021. Posthuman Bliss? The Failed Promise of Transhumanism. New York: Oxford University Press.

Philbeck, T. 2014. Ontology. In: R. Ranisch and S. L. Sorgner (eds.), Post- and Transhumanism. An Introduction. Frankfurt am Main: Peter Lang GmbH, pp. 173–183.

Popović, U. 2016. Heidegger's Transformation of Traditional Concept of the Human Being. In: I. Deretić and S. L. Sorgner (eds.), From Humanism to Met-, Post- and Transhumanism? Frankfurt am Main: Peter Lang GmbH, pp. 115–129.

Rughiniş, R. 2022. Societateadigitală. Stăpâni, cetăţeni sau sclavi? Bucureşti: Humanitas.

Wiener, N. 1966. God and Golem, Inc. A Comment on Certain Points where Cybernetics Impinges on Religion. Cambridge MA: MIT Press.

Wolfe, T. 1997. Sorry, but your soul just died. https://www.independent.co.uk/arts-entertainment/sorry-but-your-soul-just-died-1276509.html, (accessed December 15, 2022).

TRANSHUMANISM, POWER, AND ANARCHY: EMBRACING COLLECTIVE EMPOWERMENT THROUGH TECHNOLOGIES

Jozef Jenčík

MOTTO: *Indeed these are the mere edges of His ways, and how small a whisper we hear of Him! But the thunder of His power who can understand?*
(Job 26:14, English Standard Version)

1. Introduction

The intersection of transhumanism, power, and anarchy presents a captivating field of study, exploring the transformative potential of emerging technologies and the socio-political implications they carry. In this paper, we delve into the intricate relationship between transhumanism, power, and anarchy, with a particular emphasis on collective empowerment and the restructuring of societal norms.

Drawing inspiration from ancient wisdom, we turn to the Book of Job, where we encounter profound reflections on the limitations of human comprehension and the awe-inspiring power of the divine. "Indeed these are the mere edges of His ways, and how small a whisper we hear of Him! But the thunder of His power who can understand?" (Job 26:14, English Standard Version). These words encapsulate the humbling recognition that our understanding of the world is limited, mere fragments in the vast tapestry of existence. The thunderous power that reverberates through the cosmos is a force beyond our comprehension, reminding us of the boundless mysteries that surround us.

Within the context of our exploration, we juxtapose the cautious reservations often expressed regarding transhumanism with a resolute affirmation of the potential for technological progress to empower individuals and foster collective liberation. As we navigate this discourse, we eschew idealistic notions and embrace a pragmatic understanding of liberty. Liberty is not merely the absence of obstacles but an active manifestation of individual and collective agency. Embracing the transformative potential of technological advancements, including transhumanism, we seek to dismantle traditional barriers, expand the horizons of human potential, and foster a society where collective rights are prioritized.

In this journey of exploration, the concept of sovereignty emerges as a critical focal point. Once a symbol of power and control, sovereignty now reveals its limitations and reinforces existing inequities. By reimagining sovereignty through a lens that embraces collective rights and inclusivity, we can strive for a society where power is shared, and decisions are made through collective consensus. It is through the harmonious integration of individual freedoms and shared responsibilities that we lay the foundation for a more egalitarian and just society.

In considering the relationship between democracy and power, it is essential to heed the insights of philosopher John Dewey, who emphasized the dynamic and adaptive nature of democracy. Dewey contended that democracy is not limited to a particular form of government but is a way of life that can be embodied in various social arrangements. Building upon this perspective, we can argue that democracy can coexist with both archy and anarchy.

However, it is essential to remain vigilant, as history has shown that even democratic systems can exhibit totalitarian tendencies. The concentration of power, erosion of civil liberties, and manipulation of democratic processes can undermine the very essence of democracy. By acknowledging these risks, we can strive to create democratic systems that are resilient, transparent, and accountable.

2. Liberty

Individual liberty stands as the defining characteristic of Western civilization, guiding its remarkable trajectory of exponential growth. This distinction, as noted by scholars like Huntington (Huntington 1996, 71) sets Western civilization apart from others by its unwavering emphasis on individual freedoms in contrast to duties. A shining example of this profound commitment to liberty can be found in Shakespeare's timeless masterpiece, *Romeo, and Juliet*, which encapsulates the essence of Western literary heritage. The tragic tale of star-crossed lovers serves as a testament to the enduring power of individual agency and the pursuit of personal desires against societal constraints. Through such cultural touchstones, Western civilization reaffirms its deep-rooted belief in the value and sanctity of individual liberty, fostering an environment conducive to progress, innovation, and the flourishing of human potential.

While individual liberty is a cornerstone of Western civilization, it does not advocate for the atomization and fragmentation of collective units, as suggested by some postmodern critiques. On the contrary, the artificiality of such fragmented units becomes evident, as they rely on coercive measures to maintain cohesion. Shakespeare's Romeo and Juliet serves as a poignant illustration of this dynamic. Individual liberty, as portrayed in the play, is not a license for isolation, but rather an opportunity for individuals to meaningfully engage in societal relations. The tragedy unfolds as societal expectations and duties hinder the lovers' pursuit of their personal desires and authentic connections. Thus, individual liberty encompasses the freedom to forge meaningful bonds and participate actively in society, underscoring the importance of a harmonious balance between individual agency and collective responsibility. By embracing this nuanced understanding of individual liberty, Western civilization can foster a society that upholds both personal freedoms and the essential fabric of social connections.

However, the growth of Western technology in the 19th century empowered many individuals to challenge oppressive societal relations. Unfortunately, this period also witnessed the emergence of various "idealistic" notions of liberty, with Immanuel Kant's concept of liberty as the categorical imperative gaining significant influence. These notions of "liberty" placed excessive emphasis on awareness of duties, thereby obscuring the fundamental notion of liberty as the absence of external obstacles, as argued by Hannah Arendt. (Arendt 2006,134)

Regrettably, these distorted notions of liberty ultimately facilitated the rise of the methods of ideology and terror as the novel form of governance in the 20th century, as Arendt astutely predicted (Arendt 1951, 460). This transformation was evident not only in the brutal regimes of Nazism and Bolshevism but also in the contemporary democratic and legal states, as acknowledged by scholars like Jack Balkin from Yale University. (Balkin 2009, 5) The repudiation of individual liberty, which had long been the hallmark of Western civilization, can thus be seen as an epochal decline – a phenomenon keenly recognized by Spengler at the turn of the 20th century.

By critically examining this trajectory, we can gain a deeper understanding of the challenges and implications involved in the erosion of individual liberty. It prompts us to reflect on the importance of preserving and redefining the concept of liberty in the face of evolving social and political landscapes, ensuring that the essence of liberty as the absence of external obstacles remains central in our collective consciousness.

In a parallel to the Renaissance of the 15th century, where the concept of human dignity emerged as a response to oppressive social structures that had strayed from the foundations of ancient Greek traditions, a similar transformative shift can be envisaged in the 21st century through the lens of transhumanism. This movement can serve as a counterforce to the methods of ideology and terror as the novel form of governance. Transhumanism offers a path to challenge these methods by re-establishing a connection to empirical certainty and embracing the possibilities of technological advancement. By doing so, it aims to redefine societal relations and restore a sense of human agency and dignity in the face of evolving power dynamics.

The renaissance concept of human dignity, which initially emerged as a response to oppressive societal structures, underwent a transformation with the introduction of "idealistic" notions, notably exemplified by Immanuel Kant. This transformation led to the artificialization of human dignity, resulting in absurd consequences when applied in legal contexts. In contrast, the idea of transhuman dignity represents a return to the realist tradition of political philosophy, which emerged as a direct result of the impetus provided by the 15th-century Renaissance. By emphasizing the realist tradition of political philosophy, transhuman dignity offers a more grounded and meaningful approach to human worth and agency. It seeks to navigate the pitfalls of idealistic abstractions, offering a more robust foundation for ethical and political discourse.

Drawing inspiration from the Book of Job, Thomas Hobbes introduced the mythical Leviathan as a powerful symbol to advocate for the unbridled authority of the modern state, challenging prevailing historical biases that often portrayed it as an evil or malevolent entity. In a parallel vein, we can invoke the mythical Behemoth as a metaphorical tool, inspired by the same source, to advocate for the unhampered potential of modern technologies. This perspective seeks to transcend contemporary prejudices that perceive technology as inherently nefarious or diabolical (Spengler 2006, 410)

Thomas Hobbes consistently emphasized the importance of engaging in meaningful discourse, recognizing that such discourse can only be achieved by refraining from the indulgence in "idealistic" or scholastic concepts that obscure their true essence through the rejection of sensory perception. (Hobbes 1994, 25–41) Within the realm of political philosophy, this underscores the significance of reiterating the notion of liberty as the absence of external obstacles, contrasting it with the "idealistic" or scholastic interpretations that obfuscate its authentic meaning. Failure to do so has contributed to the rise of methods of ideology and terror as the novel form of governance in the 20th century. By highlighting the need to reclaim the genuine essence of liberty, we can confront the distortions that have emerged and reclaim the foundational principles necessary for a just and thriving society.

However, in response to the proliferation of contemporary "idealistic" interpretations of liberty that stem from valid critiques of purely negative conceptions, such as Hobbes' notion of liberty as the absence of external obstacles (Hobbes, 1994, 136–138), transhumanism presents an antidote in the form of a pragmatic understanding of liberty. Drawing inspiration from the exponential growth of Western technologies in the 20th century, transhumanism rearticulates the concept within the framework of realist political philosophy. Here, liberty is reconceptualized as more than the mere absence of obstacles; it becomes an active expression of both individual and collective agency. By emphasizing the proactive nature of liberty, transhumanism seeks to bridge the gap between abstract theories and lived experiences, fostering a more robust and inclusive understanding of freedom in the modern era.

That is why liberty and power are inherently intertwined, for liberty without power is rendered meaningless. The various "idealistic" conceptions of liberty that emphasize its positive manifestations, such as acting in accordance with the law, are likewise rendered absurd. True liberty encompasses not only the absence of external constraints but also the capacity to exercise one's agency and exert influence over one's own circumstances. It is through the recognition of this intrinsic link between liberty and power that a more comprehensive understanding of freedom can be attained. By embracing the dynamic interplay between liberty and power, we can move beyond simplistic dichotomies and appreciate the nuanced complexities of individual autonomy within the broader social and political context.

Furthermore, these "idealistic" notions inadvertently foster a sense of *powerlessness*, which aligns with the inherent traits of authoritarian or totalitarian tendencies. Recognizing liberty as an active expression of individual and collective agency entails acknowledging that no single voice should suppress the multitude of diverse perspectives. By embracing the transformative power of technological advancements, including transhumanism, we strive to dismantle conventional barriers, push the boundaries of human capabilities, and cultivate a society that values collective rights. This stands in stark contrast to authoritarian or totalitarian societies, which prioritize collective duties deemed necessary by their respective members. Through this paradigm shift, we aspire to create a more inclusive and empowering social order, where individual liberties and collective aspirations harmoniously coexist.

3. Critical Focal Point: Sovereignty

For that objective it is necessary to realize that modern technologies come to settle the conflict between what the will *might* and what it *wants*; from this discrepancy within the will itself, – which in our Western political tradition began St. Augustine who thematized it on the ontic level as the impotence of the will, (Arendt, 2006, 168) – it is possible to understand the modern contradiction between the individual and society in a more ontologically-fundamental way.

The sovereign will, originally driven by the maximization of *wanting* (as the technology of that time did not provide the means for maximization of *might*), has historically culminated in the concept of the sovereignty of the people. The sovereignty of the people is thus not an ideal, but a reminder of the limited power of the individual. A free individual was forced by external circumstances to enter a social contract, through which he would see himself as a member of a social body, which allegedly concentrates the *might* of all.[1] (Jean Jacques Rousseau 1994, 54)

---

1 But it is rather the common fallacy to which Jean Jacques Rousseau befallen because

Simultaneously, technologies emerge as an ally to sovereignty, amplifying the potency of the human will. Yet, the introspective nature of sovereignty often overlooks this transformative potential. In the technological era, it becomes increasingly plausible to argue that human rights would no longer need to be seen as inherently opposed to the public interest. After all, why impose penalties for various transgressions if modern technologies can effectively eliminate the threats they pose? Similarly, why curtail social rights due to lack of public funding when these very technologies can provide abundant resources seemingly out of thin air? By rendering these dialectical contradictions within the will redundant, technologies have the capacity to resolve them in a decisive manner.

However, for the first time in history, we are facing the threat that the sovereignty of will prevail over power. For the first time in history, it may happen that the will *might*, but no longer *want*, which is the logical completion of the sovereignty of wanting *par excellence* and not recognizing the help of technologies. Thus, the concept of sovereignty has emerged as a critical focal point, particularly in its insistence on exclusivity, revealing that the mere sum of individual wills does not constitute the general will. This notion of sovereignty poses a threat to individual liberty, as exemplified by Hannah Arendt's insightful analysis (Arendt 2006, 150), which highlights Jean Jacques Rousseau's advocacy for coercion in the pursuit of "liberty" within a sovereign state governed by the social contract. (Rousseau 1994, 58).

The concept of sovereignty has undeniably yielded various positive outcomes in its historical context, including the emergence of individual human rights and freedoms, the division of power, and the establishment of free market economies. However, in the technological era of the 21st century, the limitations of sovereignty become apparent, as it tends to reinforce existing inequities and perpetuate systemic imbalances. Spengler therefore imploringly fought against what he called "provincial" thinking; he recommended devoting himself to the improvement of technology (Spengler 2006, XIII). Therefore, Spengler's work, *The Decline of the West*, can be seen as a harbinger of hope amidst the looming specter of a dystopian future. In essence, it reveals the inherent hollowness that underlies the un-

---

if the individual parts of the social body are not powerful, neither can be the social body as the whole.

folding events of the technological epoch, thus offering a glimpse into the true nature of our reality.

Some scholars have put forth the notion of shared sovereignty as a potential alternative, one that does not turn a blind eye to the natural power dynamics at play – an idea that has been deemed logically absurd by certain scholars. Nonetheless, our task is crystal clear: we must embark on a journey to reimagine sovereignty through a lens that embraces collective rights and inclusivity. It is through the seamless integration of individual freedoms and shared responsibilities that we can establish the groundwork for a more egalitarian and just society. Embracing the transformative potential of transhumanism and the progress of technology, we have the opportunity to challenge the oppressive chains of totalitarianism and powerlessness. We recognize that by empowering the collective and enhancing our physical capacities, we can foster a society where individual agency thrives and the coercive dominance of majority rule gives way to consensus-driven decision-making.

4. Democracy and Anarchy

In considering the relationship between democracy and power, it is essential to heed the insights of philosopher John Dewey, who emphasized the dynamic and adaptive nature of democracy. In the John Dewey's essay titled *Creative Democracy – The Task Before Us* (Dewey 1988, 209–239), Dewey explores the vision of democracy as an ongoing, dynamic process that requires active participation and engagement from citizens. Dewey emphasizes the importance of democratic values in shaping society and advocates for a more inclusive and participatory form of democracy that empowers individuals to actively contribute to social and political change. He argues for the need to align democracy with the changing needs of society, fostering creative and innovative approaches to problem-solving. Dewey's essay continues to be influential in the fields of political philosophy, education, and social theory, and it highlights his belief in the potential of democracy as means to achieve social progress and human flourishing.

Acknowledging this versatility allows us to recognize that democracy is not solely reliant on a particular system or institution but is rooted in the active engagement and empowerment of individuals. It is the spirit of democracy that matters most – a commitment to fostering open dialogue, respecting individual rights, and promoting the common good.

Expanding upon this perspective, it becomes evident that democracy transcends rigid power structures or predetermined governing frameworks. Rather, democracy has the potential to flourish in diverse contexts, embracing both hierarchical elements (archy) and the absence of a central authority (anarchy). Anarchy champions horizontal relationships, mutual support, and voluntary associations, emphasizing autonomy and voluntary cooperation. In contrast, archy relies on vertical relationships and hierarchical power dynamics, often concentrating power in the hands of a few, which can result in abuses and inequalities. Embracing anarchy fosters a more widespread distribution of power among individuals or decentralized groups, prioritizing self-governance, and nurturing an environment conducive to autonomy and voluntary cooperation.

Emphasizing Individual Empowerment: Dewey highlights the need for individuals to actively participate in shaping democracy. In the context of transhumanism and anarchy, this can be interpreted as encouraging individuals to embrace their autonomy and agency in enhancing their own capabilities and determining the course of societal organization. It advocates for self-directed human enhancement and the empowerment of individuals to activelycontribute to the creation of a society that aligns with their values.

Valuing Innovation and Adaptability: Dewey argues for a democratic process that is flexible and adaptive to societal changes. In relation to transhumanism and anarchy, this can be seen as endorsing the exploration of new technologies, ideas, and social structures that promote human enhancement, individual freedom, and decentralized decision-making. It encourages a dynamic and evolving approach to governance and societal organization, driven by innovation and experimentation.

Promoting Inclusivity and Equality: Dewey emphasizes the importance of inclusivity and equal participation in democracy. In the context of transhumanism and anarchy, this can be reinterpreted as advocating for the elimination of hierarchical structures and power differentials that limit individual freedom and access to enhancement technologies. It supports a vision of society where all individuals have equal opportunities to enhance themselves and actively participate in decision-making processes.

However, anarchy has often been burdened with negative connotations, as it is commonly believed that the absence of a central authority would lead to a state of the war of all against all (*bellum omnium contra omnes*). This prejudice was further reinforced by Thomas Hobbes, (Hobbes 1994, 84) whose firsthand experience of civil war during the tumultuous 17th century deeply influenced his conceptualization of the modern state. Despite these prevalent biases against anarchy, the trajectory of democratic and legal systems in the 21st century has become increasingly clear: a reduced reliance on hierarchical systems of representation and a growing recognition of alternative democratic models. Prominent among these emerging models are forms of participatory democracy (Pateman 1970) and discursive democracy (Habermas 1996) which emphasize active citizen engagement and deliberative decision-making processes.

The development in the theory of democracy throughout the 20th century, despite prevailing prejudices against anarchy even among esteemed scholars, is indicative of an underlying objective cause.

According to Spengler, (Spengler 2006, 371) the decline of representative democracy, similar to the decline of privileges held by the nobility and clergy in the late 18th century, was a natural progression in the development of Western civilization. However, if we seek to understand the reasons behind this decline in the system of representation, we must look to the exponential growth of powerful modern technologies.

Through meticulous examination of the narrative of Job, striking parallels are unveiled that illuminate the intricate ramifications of technological advancement. Analogous to the profound insights and blessings that emerged from Job's profound suffering, the challenges, and potential perils inherent in technology expose a transformative capacity. Following this intellectual trajectory, it becomes increasingly discernible that within the realms of contemporary democratic and legal praxis, the emergence of anarchical facets can be attributed to responsive reactions necessitated by a plethora of crises encountered during the 20th and 21st centuries, encompassing environmental, financial, health, and security predicaments, wherein modern technologies have played a pivotal role. The quintessential embodiment of this phenomenon lies within the advent of the atomic bomb, a weapon of mass destruction that engendered a profound change of heart, thereby directly contributing to the emergence of a novel international order characterized by legalistic norms rather than arbitrary expressions of power, while its anarchic power dynamics remained steadfast. This evolution is epitomized by the emergence of the third generation of human rights and liberties, which has recently engendered environmental claims, exemplified by the case against the Czech Republic. (Municipal Court Ruling in Prague, č. ř. 4A 101/2021 – 248)

Our exploration of the intricate interplay between technology, human potential, and societal frameworks necessitates the adoption of a nuanced vantage point. While technology has frequently instilled apprehension and caution, it is imperative that we acknowledge its inherent duality. Drawing insights from the profound narrative of Job, we come to comprehend that technology harbours the capacity for both devastation and empowerment. Embracing this nuanced understanding, anarcho-transhumanism emerges as a paradigm congruent with the divine blueprint for humanity – a pathway that enables individuals to attain elevated levels of knowledge, capabilities, and liberation. It presents a transformative avenue to liberate oneself from oppressive systems and hierarchical constructs, empowering individuals to exercise their autonomy and contribute to the progressive advancement of society.

The metaphor of "mere edges" and "small whisper"(Job 26:14, English Standard Version) illuminates the limitations of human comprehension in the face of technological advancements, akin to a faint sound in comparison to the thunderous power of God. It acknowledges our incomplete understanding and highlights the vast realms yet to be explored and comprehended.

Recognizing the pervasive limitations inherent in our current mode of being, which often elude our notice, necessitates an almost childlike naiveté to question and transcend them (Bostrom 2005, 5). At the core of transhumanism lies the belief in overcoming our biological limitations. However, it is essential to acknowledge that certain limitations may be insurmountable, not solely due to technological obstacles but also on metaphysical grounds.

To realize the transhumanist dream, it is imperative that the necessary technological means for venturing into the posthuman realm be made available to those desiring to explore it. Furthermore, society must be organized in a manner that allows for such explorations without causing irreparable harm to the social fabric and without imposing unacceptable existential risks.

Given the limitations of our current wisdom, a measured epistemic tentativeness is warranted – an openness to continuously reevaluate our assumptions as new insights unfurl. We cannot presume that our preexisting habits and beliefs will prove adequate in navigating the intricacies of our ever-evolving circumstances.

5. Possibility: Empowerment

The exponential proliferation of contemporary technologies in the 21st century engenders the prospect of collective empowerment. Our discerning analysis of sovereignty reveals its function as a compensatory mechanism for the constrained power of the individual – a paradigm profoundly disrupted by the transformative potential of technological advancements, notably transhumanism. Given that sovereignty shepherds individual human rights, power distribution, and the principles of free market economics, the transformative trajectory of technological progress, including transhumanism, necessitates a reconfiguration of their respective connotations. It remains paramount, however, to safeguard the invaluable legacy of Western civilization's paramount value – individual liberty. One salient manifestation of this imperative lies in the escalating need to fortify privacy, for the precipitous advancements in surveillance technologies call for intensified protection. The scientific discourse resonates with proclamations of privacy's death, "the end" or "destruction" (Solove 2011, 20, 22). Hence, the contention arises that preserving privacy in the modern epoch mandates a recalibration of its antiquated understanding as a mere clandestine realm, and instead, pivots towards a legalistic paradigm rooted in safeguarding trust, confidentiality, and the prerogative to govern the dissemination and utilization of information. The exigency of this undertaking chiefly emanates from the peril that democratic societies encountered during the tempestuous years of the 1980s and 1990s – a peril arising from the enticements faced by public authorities.

However, while the attainment of this task may be within the realm of *possibility*, it by no means assumes the status of inevitability. In truth, there exist more grounds to harborskepticism regarding the realization of the desired outcome than not. As previously expounded upon, the myopia of sovereignty towards the transformative potential of modern technologies renders it prone to willingly overlook the opportunity for radical human transformation, instead acquiescing to the prevailing impotence of the individual, inadvertently perpetuating it. An exemplar of such circumstances can be found in the Chinese civilization, currently positioned as a prominent rival to Western civilization. Considerably, Xi Jinping bases his visionary blueprint for China on developmental trends already prevalent within Western countries. Consequently, in recent years, we have witnessed Western political representatives expressing admiration for the Chinese model, given its remarkable economic accomplishments. This affinity for the Chinese model has further burgeoned in Western nations with the advent of the COVID-19 pandemic, as Chinese policy of zero tolerance for the virus – albeit entailing substantial violations of human rights and liberties – was presented as a paradigm to be emulated, following its initial successes in 2020. Among other implications, this underscores the waning influence of Western states, which presently regard their most esteemed cultural achievements – such as market economy, power distribution, and individual human rights and freedoms, which once fostered the prosperity of the West – as impediments to enhancing efficiency in the governance of public affairs. Thus, unless Western countries tenaciously uphold the legacy of individual freedom as their distinguished value and devise means to perpetuate the inheritance of their cultural achievements amidst the inevitable structural transformations arising from the decline of Western culture, Xi Jinping's China model will inevitably assert its dominance on a global scale.

Therefore, the successful realization of this transformative endeavor necessitates an embrace of the anarchic and collective implications inherent in the notion of transhuman liberty, thereby amplifying both individual and collective agency. In alignment with the renaissance tradition, wherein the essence of humanity resides in its sentience, human enhancement holds the potential to augment our sensory capacities, which serve as the portals through which we engage with others. This augmentation may even extend to realms reminiscent of Pentecost, as described in the New Testament (Acts 2:1–13), wherein the disciples of Jesus were imbued with the Holy Spirit and miraculously spoke in diverse languages previously unknown to them. This extraordinary event facilitated effective communication of the

Gospel to a diverse audience, each hearing the disciples in their own native tongue. Thus, human enhancement opens avenues for more spontaneous and consensus-driven interactions, akin to the formation of communities and networks based on shared values and aspirations.

This proposition draws upon a confluence of sociological and psychological factors, underpinned by the assumption that individuals endowed with heightened physical agency are more inclined to seek out others who align with their interests and aspirations. *In this dynamic, the transformation from individual human rights and freedoms, division of power, and free market economy becomes an invitation to embrace collective human rights and freedom, distribution of power, and a shared economy.*

Self-Determination Theory: Self-Determination Theory posits that individuals have innate psychological needs for autonomy, competence, and relatedness. When individuals have increased physical agency, they have a greater sense of autonomy and control over their lives, which can lead to a stronger motivation to seek out like-minded individuals and form connections based on shared values and interests. (Deci 2002, Ryan 2017)

Social Identity Theory: Social Identity Theory suggests that individuals derive a part of their self-concept and self-esteem from the groups they belong to. When individuals have increased physical agency, they may seek out others who share their experiences and values, as this can provide a sense of belonging and validation. Forming communities and networks based on shared values can enhance social identity and promote a sense of solidarity. (Tajfel 1986, Worchel 1998)

Homophily: Homophily is a sociological concept that refers to the tendency of individuals to associate with others who are similar to themselves in various aspects, such as attitudes, beliefs, and interests. When individuals have increased physical agency, they may actively seek out others who share their experiences and perspectives, creating communities and networks where they feel understood and supported. (Mena 2017)

Common Goals and Interests: Increased physical agency often allows individuals to pursue specific goals or engage in activities that align with their personal interests and aspirations. When people have the freedom and capability to pursue their passions, they are more likely to gravitate towards others who share those goals and interests. This can lead to the formation of communities and networks centered around common objectives. (Duckworth 2016)

6. Necessity: Powerlessness

However, it is imperative to maintain a state of unwavering vigilance, for historical evidence reveals that even within democratic systems, latent totalitarian tendencies can emerge. They are the *necessity* if proactive political measures are not undertaken to safeguard the preeminent value of Western civilization: human liberty. The seductive allure of Xi Jinping's vision for Western countries serves as a stark reminder of this peril. The consolidation of power, erosion of civil liberties, and subversion of democratic processes intrinsic to such a vision have the potential to undermine the very fabric of liberal democracy. By recognizing these lurking dangers, we are compelled to endeavor towards the creation of democratic systems that embody resilience, transparency, and accountability.

Furthermore, we must concede that in times of crisis, incipient participatory frameworks may be susceptible to the machinations of centralized authorities who wield power. This vulnerability has become starkly apparent in recent times, notably during the global COVID-19 pandemic.

When confronted with a crisis, governments and institutions often adopt expeditious measures and make consequential decisions that profoundly impact the lives of individuals and communities. While certain actions may indeed be imperative for the preservation of public health and safety, it is of utmost importance to remain ever watchful for any encroachment upon the sanctity of individual rights and liberties.

In certain scenarios, the exigency of the situation can precipitate the centralization of decision-making and the suppression of participatory processes. *This summons forth the necessity to recalibrate individual human rights and freedoms, division of power, and the free market economy towards collective duties, the concentration of power, and a state-regulated economy*. Emergency powers may be invoked, circumventing democratic checks and balances in the name of expeditious action. While these measures may be deemed indispensable in the immediate term, their enduring ramifications for democratic principles and citizen empowerment should not be disregarded. This underscores the significance of our unwavering commitment to active citizenship and the continual assessment of democratic mechanisms, even in the face of crises. It serves as a poignant reminder that democracy is not a static state but an ongoing process that necessitates collective engagement and vigilant protection against the encroachment of power. Let us consider following example in this regard; in the case of Vavřička and Others v. the Czech Republic (application n. 7621/13, 3867/14, 73094/14, 19306/15, 19298/15, and 43883/15) before the European Court of Human Rights (ECtHR), which pertained to the mandatory vaccination scheme in the Czech Republic, the principle of social solidarity towards the most vulnerable was underscored. The ECtHR emphasized that social solidarity towards the most vulnerable requires the rest of the population to take minimal risk in the form of vaccinations. This decision carries a significant message that alongside fundamental rights, there exist fundamental obligations and responsibilities. This position aligns with the viewpoint expressed by Lemmens in his "supplementary" opinion, emphasizing the importance of *duties* (see resolution 1845(2011) of the Parliamentary Assembly of 25 November 2011 on fundamental rights and responsibilities cited in point 143 of the judgment). However, there is a stark divergence between collective duties and collective rights which ECtHR failed to thematize in the case of Vavřička and Others v. the Czech Republic (application n. 7621/13, 3867/14, 73094/14, 19306/15, 19298/15, and 43883/15):

Conflicting Priorities: Collective rights and collective duties can sometimes have conflicting priorities. Collective rights focus on protecting and promoting the interests and well-being of a group or community, while collective duties emphasize the responsibilities and obligations that individuals have towards the collective. In certain situations, fulfilling collective duties may require sacrificing or limiting certain collective rights, creating a tension between the two.

Individual Autonomy: Collective duties often involve imposing obligations and responsibilities on individuals for the benefit of the collective. This can be seen as limiting individual autonomy and freedom, as individuals may be compelled to act in ways that go against their own preferences or interests. The emphasis on collective duties may undermine the ability of individuals to exercise their individual rights and freedoms fully.

Limited Individual Agency: When collective duties take precedence, individuals may have limited agency and decision-making power. The focus on fulfilling collective obligations may restrict individual choices and limit opportunities for self-expression and personal development. This can hinder the realization of individual rights and autonomy.

Potential for Abuse: In some cases, the imposition of collective duties in the name of collective rights can lead to the abuse of power. Those in positions of authority may exploit the concept of collective duties to suppress dissent or control individuals, eroding individual rights and freedoms.

Therefore, it is imperative for the European Court of Human Rights (ECtHR) to consider not only the quality but also the quantity of infringements that may occur as a result of the decision. This includes examining the structural consequences and potential impact on individual liberties. By scrutinizing the use of dystopic constitutionalism (Crocker 2015, 649) as an interpretive framework for the European Convention on Human Rights, the ECtHR can ensure that the essence of Western civilization – individual liberty – is preserved. It is crucial to recognize that halting the implementation of "necessary" measures can initiate the transformation of what is merely possible, thereby preventing the erosion of fundamental rights and freedoms. By upholding the principle of preserving individual liberty, the ECtHR plays a pivotal role in safeguarding democratic values and ensuring the protection of human rights in Europe.

To elucidate the method of dystopian constitutionalism, accentuating the objectives of anarcho-transhumanism, let us contemplate the following scenario. The economic situation of the wealthiest oligarchs bears resemblances to the late 18th century, a time when royal dynasties lost their legitimacy. Piketty argues that the revenue generated from capital now resembles annuities. (Piketty, 2013, 131 – 134) While the *necessary* in the absence of proactive political approach involve taxing the wealthy and redistributing wealth among citizens, such measures could potentially undermine the foundational principles of the free market that form the bedrock of our civilization's heritage.

In this context, the ζῷον πολιτικό recognizes the potential for establishing a new power order and fostering a fresh political tradition that deviates from the "normal" capitalist relations of the 19th and the 20th centuries.

Here, the involvement of institutions such as the ECtHR or CJEU becomes crucial in preventing excessive taxation in the name of the free market, thereby provoking a restructuring of the system. Capitalism is currently experiencing a rapid transformation towards socialism, albeit not in the traditional sense of merely redistributing wealth for the sake of fairness. Rather, this shift seeks to transcend the deteriorating economic relations that typify the decline of Western civilization.

The envisioned concept of real socialism does not rely on external assistance or exclusively provide social benefits. It is a system that empowers every individual within its realm, enabling them to enhance their autonomy and agency. Rather than reducing individuals to mere vassals of the state, real socialism equips them with the means to elevate their own capabilities and exercise greater control over their lives.

In the midst of the aforementioned deliberations on the purported "necessary" measures, an unsettling undercurrent emerges: the implicit inquiry of how to exert the most efficacious control or subjugation. This particular paradigm manifests a deep-seated departure from the principles of anarcho-transhumanism, as it affords primacy to a notion of stagnant humanity defined by fixed values and desires, subsequently subjecting non-human intellects to serve these predetermined objectives. Such an approach stands in stark contradiction to the very essence of transhumanism, which strives to embrace the fluidity and transient essence of the "human" experience, rather than clinging rigidly to the present state of humankind.

The outcome hangs in the balance, swaying on the path we willingly tread towards transhumanism, where individual liberation and empowerment await, or on the adherence we are compelled into, where the preservation of a fixed human paradigm threatens to intensify oppressive tendencies, leaving us with a diminished sense of agency and control.

7. Mass for the Dead

The exponential advancement of modern technologies throughout the 20th and 21st centuries has unveiled remarkable possibilities for shaping our socio-political relationships through the augmentation of individual and collective agency. However, intertwined with this potential lies a somber inevitability: the exponential growth of modern technologies may also lead to the preservation of artificial socio-political arrangements through the exertion of brute force.

The precondition for a radical transformation of individual human rights and freedoms, the division of power, and the free market economy into collective human rights and freedom, the distribution of power, and a shared economy necessitates acknowledging the stark reality that these existing structures are no longer vibrant; they are deceased, and a proper burial is requisite if we are to forge a meaningful future. Let us delve into the following considerations.

Featherston asserts that the collapse of the nation-state and the subsequent global dominance of neoliberalism have contributed to the prevailing sentiment that state regimes have lost their prospective vitality. (Featherstone, 2017, 3, 15) The rational state model, inspired by Plato's ideal state regime in his *Republic*, (Plato 1997, II. – XI) raises pertinent questions about the authenticity of the future it embodies. Has the notion of "future" been vulgarized and flattened into a mere mode of presence, subject to our rational disposability?

Fukuyama famously posits that liberal democracy concluded history following the events of 1989. While his thesis may have empirical implications, it stems from Kojév's (mis)interpretation of G. W. F. Hegel's philosophy of history, as elucidated in Fukuyama's renowned work, *The End of History, and the Last Man*. (Fukuyama, 1992, 42) Hegel's philosophy suggests that at the end of history, spirit does not stagnate but rather becomes temporal. (Matějčková 2018, 334) Paradoxically, this temporal spirit is precisely what Fukuyama's liberal democracy denies, as it endeavors to invent multifarious substitutes for *thymos* at any cost to achieve immobilization.

In this context, we must ask ourselves: can the constant invention of substitutes for *thymos* in democratic and legal states sustainably persist? Do the lingering specters of Lenin and Mao Tse Tung, whose embalmed bodies have not found peaceful repose, demand significance from us? (Featherstone, 2017, 221) Does the veil merely engender more authentic forms of ideology and state-regime terror, ultimately leading to their inevitable eruption?

Drawing upon Friedrich Nietzsche's words, "*Man is something that shall be overcome*", (Nietzsche 1961, 7) we are confronted with a crucial question from the ghosts of our past: What have we done to surpass this limitation? By examining Job's journey from suffering to redemption, we uncover insights into the transformative potential of technology. Just as Job's challenges led to a deeper understanding of God's wisdom, the challenges and opportunities presented by technology can redefine our understanding of power, authority, and the boundaries of sovereign control. Let us dare to transcend the constraints of our present selves and embark on a collective journey towards empowerment, where the convergence of technology and human potential paves the way for a world that cherishes beauty and embraces diversity.

References

Arendt, H. 2006. *Between Past and Future*. London: Penguin books.

Arendt, H. 1951. *The Origins of Totalitarianism*. New York: Harcourt Brace Jovanovich.

Balkin, M. J. 2009, The Constitution in the National Surveillance State. *Minnesota Law Review*, 98(4): 1–25.

Bostrom, N. 2005. Transhumanist Values. *Journal of Philosophical Research*, 30: 3–14.

Crocker, T. 2015. Dystopian Constitutionalism. *Journal of Constitutional Law*, 18(2): 593–655.

Derrida, J. 1994. *Specters of Marx*. London: Routledge.

Dewey, J. 1988. Creative Democracy. In: J.A.Boydston (ed.), *The Later Works, 1925–1953*, Volume 14: 1939–1941: Essays, Reviews, Miscellany, and the Public and Its Problems. Carbondale: Southern Illinois University Press, 209–239.

Deci, E. L., & R. M. Ryan (Eds.). 2002. *Handbook of Self-Determination Research*. Rochester, NY: The University of Rochester Press.

Duckworth, A. 2016. *Grit: The Power of Passion and Perseverance*. New York: Scribner.

Featherstone, M. 2017. *Planet Utopia (Utopia, Dystopia and Globalisation)*. New York: Routledge.

Fukuyama, F. 1992. *The End of History and the Last Man*. London: Penguin.

Gillis, W. Anarchy and Transhumanism. In:G. Chartier and C. V. Schoelandt (eds.), *The Routledge Handbook of Anarchy and Anarchist Thought*. London: Routledge, 416–428.

Habermas, J. 1996. *Between Facts and Norms: Contributions to a Discourse Theory of Law and Democracy*. Translated by William Rehg. Cambridge, MA: The MIT Press.

Hobbes, Thomas. 1994. Leviathan. Indianapolis/Cambridge: Hackett Publishing Company, Inc.

Hobbes, T. 2010. *Behemoth: The History of the Causes of the Civil Wars of England*. New York: Cambridge University Press.

Huntington, S. 1996. *The Clash of Civilizations and the Remaking of World Order*. NY: SIMON &SCHUSTER.

Kojève, A. 1980. *Introduction to the Reading of Hegel (Lectures on the Phenomenology of Spirit)*. New York: Cornell University Press.

Matějčková, T. 2018. *Hegelovafenomenologiesvěta*. Praha: OIKOYMENH.

Mena, S. R., & J. K. Maner (Eds.). 2017. *Homophily in Social Networks*. New York: Oxford University Press.

Miller, D. 1999. Principles of Social Justice. Cambridge, MA: Harvard University Press.

Nietzsche, F. 1961. *Thus Spoke Zarathustra: A Book for Everyone and No One*. New York: Penguin Books.

Pateman, C. 1970. Participation and Democratic Theory. Cambridge: Cambridge University Press.

Plato. 1997. *Complete Works*. Indianapolis/Cambridge: Hackett Publishing Company.

Piketty, T. *Kapitál v 21. storočí*. Bratislava: Ikar, 2013.

Pink, D. H. 2011. *Drive: The Surprising Truth About What Motivates Us*. New York: Riverhead Books.

Rousseau, J.-J. 1994. *The Social Contract*. New York: Oxford University Press.

Ryan, R. M., & E. L. Deci. 2017. *Self-Determination Theory: Basic Psychological Needs in Motivation, Development, and Wellness*. Rochester, NY: The University of Rochester Press.

Solove, D. 2011. Speech, Privacy and Reputation on the Internet. In: S. Levmoreand M. Nussbaum(eds.), *The Offensive Internet: Speech, Privacy, and Reputation*. Cambridge, Mass.: Harvard University Press, 312.

Spengler, O. 2006. *The Decline of the West*. New York: Vintage Books Inc.

Tajfel, H.& J. C. Turner. 1986. *Social Identity and Intergroup Relations*. Cambridge, UK: Cambridge University Press.

Worchel, S., J. Morales, & D. Paez (Eds.). 1998. *Social Identity: International Perspectives*. London: Sage Publications.

Pink, D. H. 2011. *Drive: The Surprising Truth About What Motivates Us*. New York: Riverhead Books.

A Note on Anarcho-Transhumanism

Martin Turčan

1. Introduction

Among the latest forms of anarchism, one can also find the so-called "anarcho-transhumanism". This approach combines the political ideas of anarchism with the transhumanist vision of the future "man" (or rather "trans-human"). Anarcho-transhumanists even claim anarchism is the only thinkable political model compatible with transhumanism and they believe it will work. This paper aims to evaluate such an idea from a theological perspective. I will focus namely on the theological evaluation of (1) human perfection and (2) human freedom, which are essential to the concept of anarcho-transhumanism (plus (3) the value of human education, which is also relevant in this context). I will show some parallels between the idea of anarcho-transhumanism and one story from the Bible – namely from Genesis 6 – which contains these values. In this brief paper, I will thus take a narrative type of approach[1] that could serve as a theological voice in the discussion about transhumanism.[2]

2. Transhumanism and anarchy

According to a well-known anarcho-transhumanist philosopher William Gillis transhumanism implies anarchism. Gillis' reasoning is quite simple in this regard. It is based on the notion of risks implied by the technological advancement culminating in the very idea of transhumanism:

---

1 And my approach will also be "canonical" in nature – i.e., I will deal with the biblical text as we have it.

2 I am not aware of any published comparison of the story with the idea of anarcho-transhumanism so far. Thus, the contribution of my paper is to sketch the value parallels (and perhaps stir a further theological discussion in this respect).

> "The more means by which people can act the easier attack becomes and the harder defense becomes. It's a simple matter of complexity. The attacker only needs to choose one line of attack, the defender needs to secure against all of them. This isn't just true of small thermal exhaust ports, it's true in our software ecosystems today and any other system with many dimensions of movement. Complexity – more degrees of freedom within a system – allows for greater attack surface. [...] Freedom-to is disruptive and complex. It expands options. And when truly decentralized – spread to individuals – it makes it impossible for power to function. For any actor, individual or institution, to control the vast unfathomable diversity and complexity of the world. Impossible to impose edicts, even 'democratic' ones. When liberal or social democrat transhumanists declare that what we need is technology 'under the control of The People', what is never included in that is how exactly that kind of control is supposed to work. [...] We cannot control advanced technology without an authoritarianism so complete it would make Hitler and Stalin salivate in their graves. So what can we do?" (Gillis 2015).

Gillis answers the question by pointing to the long-standing tradition of anarchism which can, in his view, help us reach what we need – "an ethical awakening, a singularity of empathy that clarifies and refines our values". (Gillis 2015). Thus, according to Gillis, it is possible to have a world functioning without structural power relations (i.e. to have a world of anarchy) where human (or rather trans-human) beings flourish on their way to their highest potential.

However, as Paweł Malendowicz points out, in order for anarcho-transhumanism to count as a genuine form of anarchism it is relevant whether human perfection is seen as the highest goal or whether human freedom is the goal – i.e. whether freedom is just a means by which human perfection can be reached, or whether human perfection is a means of reaching freedom.[3] Because the appeal to the value of freedom is the basic

[3] "Freedom is a postulate of anarchism, but the values in transhumanism are improvement and perfection. Their combination constitutes the essence of anarcho-transhumanism. Anarcho-transhumanism is the recognition that social freedom is inseparable from material freedom, and that freedom is ultimately a matter of extending human possibilities and opportunities to engage with the world around human beings. This means not only freeing oneself from the arbitrary constraints that bodies can impose on humans, but also being free to shape the world around us. It is transcending the limitations of gender, genetics and all human experience. It is questioning limitations and seeking to change the conditions that govern human beings. Anarchotranshumanism is the claim that if the tools exist to improve the quality of life, they should be used, for no one should experience hunger or other scarcity if they can be eliminated (Gillis, n.d.). In the above view, anarcho-transhumanism is a consequence of tran-

tenet of anarchism in general, having human perfection as the highest goal is not enough for any approach to count as truly anarchist. If we agree with Gillis about the anarchistic implications of transhumanism (with which we may not, and some – like democratic transhumanists – certainly do not), from the anarchist perspective it is substantial to have human freedom as the goal to which enhancement of our capabilities (our perfection) is only instrumental. So the question should not be: *Does transhumanism imply anarchism?* Rather: *Does anarchism imply transhumanism?*

But be that as it may, let us suppose that transhumanism and anarchism go hand in hand,[4] and within this, that transhumanism implies either anarchism or tyranny. What can be said about the relationship or interaction of the two fundamental values at play which constitute the whole issue – human perfection and human freedom – from the theological perspective and what light does it shed on the very concept of transhumanism?

3. Perfection and freedom through a biblical lens

It is quite clear that the Bible values both human perfection and freedom in some sense. The notion of human perfection, including bodily perfection, is there. The man was originally created perfect ("very good") according to the narrative of Genesis and his physical condition began to go down only after the Fall. Even the length of human life before the flood and its rapid decrease after the flood shows that the human condition was originally perfect in some sense. In the New Testament, the idea of human bodily perfection has an eschatological charge. Apostle Paul speaks of the glorious bodies given to believers at Christ's *parousia* (1 Corinthians 15). Humans are going to return to their original state of flourishing (bodily and

---

shumanist thinking. For it means freedom from the limitations of human nature and freedom to improve and perfect the human being. Anarcho-transhumanism is a current of anarchist thought when it treats the idea of freedom as a primary value and as a condition for other values, and the improvement and perfecting of man as methods for achieving the goal of freedom. Anarcho-transhumanism is not a current of anarchist thought when its primary value is the perfection of man and his transformation into a posthuman, and a state without power and hierarchy is the result of posthumans achieving perfection". (Malendowicz 2022, 80).

4 Anarcho-transhumanism stands in direct opposition to another extreme called "anarcho-primitivism", which views technology primarily as a danger and wants people to live without it.

mental perfection) in the era of eternal life. The idea of human beings with enhanced physical and mental capacities (compared to our contemporary state, at the least) both originally and in the future kingdom of God is thus certainly not unbiblical. The Bible also speaks of God's interest in human flourishing during the age after the Fall and before the Second Coming. We find both explicit mentions and implicit allusions to the idea of human flourishing throughout the Bible (Psalm 35:27 might be an example).

The value of freedom is, in a certain sense, illustrated by the story of the Fall. God values human freedom and lets people choose. Even the meta-narrative of Lucifer's fall which has traditionally been seen in the parables of the king of Tyre (Ezekiel 28) and the king of Babylon (Isaiah 14) presupposes the eminence of freedom (freedom to choose either to love God or reject Him). It is true that in the normative texts of the Law of Moses and also in various biblical stories human freedom is not seen as the absolute value in human relations. At least not in the sense of negative freedom (i.e. freedom *from*). Sometimes people are required to do something for someone else in these texts (for instance Deuteronomy 22:1–4). But this would, at its best, exclude anarcho-capitalism which is based purely upon the idea of negative freedom. Most anarcho-transhumanists, however, are not anarcho-capitalists. They are rather left-wing anarchists, which means they believe also in the idea of positive freedom (as, after all, can been seen in the above-mentioned quotation of Gillis who explicitly speaks of "*freedom-to*"). The notion of human perfection culminating in the reality of transhumanism is typically linked to the concept of positive freedom (i.e. freedom *to*) which, if valued highly, means we all ought to do something for each other in order to be all free.[5]

What is the biblical view of the relation or interaction of these two values – human perfection and freedom? Will they work for good and does

---

5 This may be tied to Kropotkin's reversal of *ought implies can* to *can implies ought* (Kropotkin 2000, 40–41). Even though Kropotkin is just trying to explain the idea of moral duty when talking about *can implies ought* (following Jean-Marie Guyau he bases it on our natural – biologically determined – capacities and inclinations), I think, in the wider context of his anarchist thought we can see a deeper sense of this principle: If you can develop your potential (say, in order to be truly free and help others to be free), you should (ought to) do it. If we all should (ought to) be something more, we must cooperate (applied in the transhumanist context: we ought to do something for each other in order to reach our liberated trans-human condition as the highest achievement of what we can be).

anarcho-transhumanism appear as an acceptable view, theologically speaking? Of course, it may be asked whether transhumanism is really unavoidably linked to (left-wing) anarchism. Several years ago, Elizabeth Kolovou and Stavros Karageorgikas pointed out that according to a survey done in 2007, only two percent of the members of the World Transhumanist Association identified as left-wing anarchists. (Kolovou andKarageorgikas 2010, 315).[6] The mentioned authors themselves are trying to separate anarchism from transhumanism as two not really compatible ideas.[7] But let us suppose that it is impossible to have transhumanism without either (left-wing) anarchism or dystopia. Can theology give us some advice in the evaluation of the very idea of transhumanism then?

There are several biblical passages that might be used as a theological argument against anarchism (e.g. Romans 13:1–7, 1 Peter 2:13–17, Judges 21, etc.). But there is, I think, one particular passage that is of a special interest now because it has the potential to be theologically instructive concerning the key values behind anarcho-transhumanism as this passage seems to presuppose a non-negligible degree of human perfection and also a non-negligible degree of human freedom (plus knowledge). Genesis 6 describes the state of humankind in the time before the flood. To set the wider context briefly: In Genesis 3 we encounter the human Fall, Genesis 4 illustrates the impact of expanding sin and describes the first murders, Genesis 5 records genealogy from Adam to Noah, and Genesis 6 speaks of human wickedness as the reason for God's punishment (the flood).

3.1 Human perfection

One of the two key parts of Genesis 6 concerning our issue is found in the verses 1–8 (NIV):

> "When human beings began to increase in number on the earth and daughters were born to them, the sons of God saw that the daughters of humans were beautiful, and they married any of them they chose. Then the LORD said, 'My Spirit will not contend with humans forever, for they are mortal; their days will be a hundred and twenty years.'The Nephilim were on the earth in those days – and also afterward—when the sons of God went to the daughters of humans and had children by them. They were the heroes of old, men of renown. The LORD saw how great the wickedness of the human race had become on the earth, and that every inclination of the thoughts of the

[6] Maybe the data has changed meanwhile in favor of left-wing anarchism; I don't know.
[7] Their views have been criticized by John Danaher (see Danaher 2014).

human heart was only evil all the time. The LORD regretted that he had made human beings on the earth, and his heart was deeply troubled. So the LORD said, 'I will wipe from the face of the earth the human race I have created – and with them the animals, the birds and the creatures that move along the ground – for I regret that I have made them.' But Noah found favor in the eyes of the LORD".

This text is famous for the mention of the mysterious *Nephilim* (traditionally translated as *giants*)[8] – *"the heroes of old, men of renown"*, whoare children of the *"sons of God"* and the *"daughters of humans"*.[9] Whether they are what they appear to be at first glance – half human and half angelic – or whether they are merely human – namely descendants of Sethites mingled with Cainites – is not really decisive for our purposes.[10] In any case, these are "superhumans" in some sense (either metaphysically, or at least as to their particular physical and perhaps also mental capacities). We could thus say they are some sort of enhanced human beings (at least compared to what we have today and also compared to other men of those times). And yet they seem to use their capabilities for evil rather than for good. It is true that the text does not explicitly evaluate them in the moral sense. It only states that they were *heroes* or *men of might*, which is basically a neutral designation denoting their strength and success. But the fact that only Noah and his family were saved when the flood came implies that these Nephilim were not good men. Liberated individuals with great abilities, but not good ones.[11]

---

8 "The only other OT reference to the Nephilim is Num. 13:33, where they form part of the pre-Israelite population of Palestine. This passage indicates strongly that the Nephilim (here associated with the sons of Anak) were individuals of imposing stature beside whom the Hebrew spies appeared as grasshoppers. Probably for this reason the LXX (and see AV) translated Nephilim as 'giants' (hoi gígantes)". (Hamilton 1990, 270).

9 However, not everyone identifies the Nephilim with the heroes. As Hamilton states: "The translation we have offered understands the Nephilim to be distinct from the mighty men, who alone are the offspring of the union of the sons of God and the daughters of men. Thus we have set off the first part of the verse in parentheses". (Hamilton 1990, 270). Peter Gentry also doesn't think the Nephilim are offspring of the sons of God and the daughters of men. But, unlike Hamilton, he seems to identify them with the mighty heroes. (Gentry 2019).

10 On possible interpretations see for instance Westermann 1984, 371–372; Hartley 2000, 96.

11 Perhaps fighting warriors, as might be suggested by the very term gibborim which is translated as heroes or mighty men. "The LXX translated nephilim by gigantes,

When we look at verse 3 we read: "*Then the Lordsaid, 'My Spirit will not contend with humans forever, for they are mortal; their days will be a hundred and twenty years.'*" This phrase may also be translated: "*Then the Lordsaid, 'My Spirit will not remain in humans forever, for they are corrupt* [...]" We may even combine the versions to also say: "*My Spirit will not contend with humans forever, for they are corrupt*", or: "*My Spirit will not remain in humans forever, for they are mortal*". Either translation is theologically instructive when deliberating about the idea of anarcho-transhumanism.

The expression that God's Spirit will *not contend* with humans forever suggests that God is trying to appeal to human conscience for quite a long time, but humans are not responding accordingly. They are *corrupt*, following their own ways. The expression that God's Spirit will *not remain*[12] in humans forever refers to the judgment tied to the fact that they are *mortal*, as another possible translation puts it. The first translation implicitly collides with anarcho-transhumanist optimism – with the idea of a good man, who can be learned and follow the right paths. The Socratic idea that humans only need to be well-informed and they will choose the good rather than the bad. Plus the anarchist idea of the need for a complete empowerment of individuals in order to self-actualize and enjoy full freedom. We have Nephilim in Genesis 6 and God trying to speak to their hearts, and yet they do not listen. They, together with other people, remain *corrupt* (as

---

from which the English 'giant' is derived. In Num. 13:33 the Israelites reported that they felt like mere grasshoppers in the sight of the nephilim, which the KJV translates 'giants'. There is reason to believe that this Hebrew word may come from the root naphal, and that the nephilim were 'violent' ones, or terrorists, rather than physical 'giants'. Since in those days the entire human race was of great stature, it must be that character rather than height is designated. The antediluvians generally possessed great physical and mental strength. These individuals, renowned for wisdom and skill, persistently devoted their intellectual and physical powers to the gratification of their own pride and passions and to the oppression of their fellow man [...]". (Nichol et al. 1978, 251).

12 This reading is supported by LXX and Vulgate's translation of the Hebrew word *yadon*. If it is a form of *din*, it should be translated *to judge* (hence the meaning *to strive* or *to contend*), as in many other places of the Old Testament including other parts of the book of Genesis. However, many exegetes seem to favor the translation *to remain* (Wenham 1987, 142). The problem is that *"if the form in question is to be connected with the verb dîn, 'to judge'* [...] *one would expect yādîn, not yādôn".* (Hamilton 1990, 266).

it is possible to translate the Hebrew phrase *bešaggam hu basar* – i.e. *for indeed he is flesh*). The second translation – i.e. *"My Spirit will not remain in humans forever"*, together with another possible translation of the Hebrew word *basar (flesh)* as *mortal*, collides with a well-known idea behind some extreme versions of (anarcho-)transhumanism which expect humans to be able to live forever. The way of securing this should be via uploading human consciousness into a technological facility. But the idea of fallen humans living forever is rejected (in the normative sense) by the very narrative of the Fall in Genesis 3:22 (NIV): *"The man has now become like one of us, knowing good and evil. He must not be allowed to reach out his hand and take also from the tree of life and eat, and live forever"*. Eternal existence in the fallen state would only amplify the problem of evil.[13]

Thus Genesis 6:1–8 shows human wickedness (which is not reduced but rather enhanced by super-human might, fully revealed during a hundreds-of-years-long life span) as the grounds for God's judgment. After the flood, human age decreases significantly and the wickedness of men may be viewed as the reason. Genesis 6:3b says that "*their days will be a hundred and twenty years*", which is basically the maximum age of humans since some time after the flood according to subsequent biblical stories (only a few people live longer in these stories). But the phrase may also be understood as delineating the time of grace while Noah is building the ark (Clines 1998, 14). In this sense, he is preparing the means of rescue for a hundred and twenty years, while God's Spirit is still trying to appeal to human hearts (c.f. 1 Peter 3:20).

This story shows us that people in super-human conditions (either those extraordinary Nephilim or other "ordinary" men who are able to live for a very long time with well-functioning bodies and minds)are prone, or at least capable, to aggregate evil drastically. This is, at the minimum, a raised finger against a human pursuit of super-human perfection in the fallen state where people are unrestrained from using their super-human capacities, as they please. I say *unrestrained* because, in my view, the original civilization resembles anarchy in some sense.

---

[13] This is not to say we should not try to prolong human life. The problem arises, at the minimum, when such an effort springs from the human desire (whether conscious or unconscious) to be independent of God.

3.2 Human freedom (and knowledge)

Saying this I move to the second important anarcho-transhumanist value which is also implicitly present in our story – *human freedom*. In Genesis 6 in verses 5, 11, and 13, representing the second key part of that chapter in the given context, it is said:

> "The LORD saw how great the wickedness of the human race had become on the earth, and that every inclination of the thoughts of the human heart was only evil all the time. [...] Now the earth was corrupt in God's sight and was full of violence. [...] So God said to Noah, 'I am going to put an end to all people, for the earth is filled with violence because of them. I am surely going to destroy both them and the earth [...].'"

If the earth is filled with violence, because everyone is corrupt, and because every inclination of the thoughts of the human heart is only evil all the time, then it looks much like the Hobbesian *bellum omnium contra omnes*, where *homo homini lupus est*.[14]

I do not deny that some systemic power structures might be presupposed by the story, but the mention of the widespread violence gives the impression of much freedom of individuals in dealing with their neigh-

---

14 Hamilton points out that *lawlessness* (a wider term than *violence*) is perhaps a better translation of the Hebrew term *hamas* or *chamas* (but he seems to agree that violence was definitely present in the situation of Genesis 6): "In a sense vv. 11–12 are a condensation of the narratives extending from Gen. 3:1 to 6:4. This is most apparent in the report in v. 11 the earth was full of lawlessness (ḥāmās, LXX adikía). Such lawlessness, which may lead to violence, permeates both the Cain story (ch. 4) and the Lamech scenario (4:23–24)". (Hamilton 1990, 278). Wenham states: "'Chamas is cold-blooded and unscrupulous infringement of the personal rights of others, motivated by greed and hate and often making use of physical violence and brutality' (TDOT, 4:482). In this context Gen 4 well illustrates the meaning of 'violence', although the word itself is not used here. The post-flood decrees in 9:4–6 attempt to limit human and animal violence". (Wenham 1987, 171). Robert Alter notes: "Humankind had been enjoined to multiply and fill the earth, but the proliferation of human population leads to a proliferation of lawless behavior. This is one of several verbal echoes of the Creation story, suggesting, first, a perversion of creation and, then, a reversal of creation by God". (Alter 2004, 40). Derek Kidner notes that "the words corrupt(ed) and violence give new inside into the prevailing anarchy (and into the ugly side of the might and fame noted in verse 4). The Hebrew for corrupt(ed) (or 'destroyed') also makes it plain that what God decided to 'destroy' (13) had been virtually self-destroyed already". (Kidner 1967, 87).

bors (it seems like there is no centralized power to restrain them).[15] Just like Lamech in Genesis 4 (who kills a boy for a mere insult), whose story seems to sketch out human relations of those times.[16]James G. Murphy,

[15] Of course, the question is who could hold such centralized power if everyone is corrupt. Perhaps only the righteous Noah and his family, but probably not for long. The problem of people of those times (except Noah and his family) is their distance from God and we see that even the super-condition of humanity does not help in this respect. From the theological point of view, in any society, there will always be some people (even though not all) as evil as those in the time of the flood. Therefore the idea of either dystopian or anarchistic implications of transhumanism sounds troubling.

[16] Sidney Greidanus notes: "Lamech is a brutal killer. God's law for Israel demanded that punishment must fit the crime [. . .]. But Lamech moves far beyond this principle of justice: He kills a man for wounding him, a young man for striking him. And then he brags, 'If Cain is avenged sevenfold, truly Lamech seventy-sevenfold.' He takes God's words to Cain of complete vengeance and goes them seventy times better. He vows unending vengeance. No one, but no one, will touch the violent Lamech. He does not need God's protection. He can fend for himself. The story is almost finished. The narrator has sketched the awful development of sin in human history. Only seven generations from Adam, a complete number of generations, and sin has come to full fruition: human beings boast about their power to defend themselves; they don't need God; they don't need his law; they themselves will decide what is good and what is evil (3:4); they can be gods for themselves. This is the sin of Adam and Eve, only far more defiant. With their cultural developments they can fend for themselves. Only seven generations, and humanity has disintegrated from a world where God was worshiped and adored to a world where humans think they can live without God". (Greidanus 2007, 98). Similarly, John E. Hartley states: "In contrast to Cain, who sought protection from Yahweh, Lamech shamelessly boasted as he threatened with vengeance anybody who would hold him accountable, up to seventy-seven times. This number symbolizes the utmost extent. J. Gabriel [. . .] posits that Lamech made such an outrageous boast because he had available new weapons forged by Tubal-Cain. [. . .] He claimed to be his own law. This song reveals that with the rise of the human thirst for violence increases dramatically. The threat to human existence then becomes the abuse of human inventiveness". (Hartley 2000, 85–86). John Skinner even thought that "Lamech habitually avenges the slightest personal injury by death of a man or child of the tribe to which the assailant belongs", – i.e. "not a fighting 'youth,' – a sense it rarely bears [. . .] – but an innocent man-child [. . .]". (Skinner 1910, 121). Craig Bartholomew and Michael Gohen point out that Lamech is not misusing just material things (like iron), but also immaterial things like poetry when bragging: "Poetry is a wonderful gift from God, and the Bible contains many songs and poems that develop the beauty and power of language in obedience to God's order. Lamech is the first poet in the Bible. But in his poem God's wonderful gift has already been distorted, twisted into an instrument to threaten with revenge and violence [. . .]". (Bartholomew, Goheen 2006, 32).

who wrote a commentary on the book of Genesis as part of a commentary series edited by the famous 19th-century biblical scholar Albert Barnes, once noticed:

> "It is remarkable that we have no hint of any kind of government in the antediluvian world. It is open to us to suppose that the patriarchal polity would make its appearance, as it is an order based upon natural relations. But it is possible that God himself, being still present and manifest, was recognized as the governor. To him offerings were brought, and he deals with Cain on his first and second transgression. In that case the lawless violence of the strong and willful is to be regarded as rebellion, not only against the patriarchal rule, but the divine supremacy". (Murphy 1867, 181).

It seems to me, just like to Murphy, that there is rather a lack of power needed to hold back the widespread aggression in Genesis 6.[17] The first mention of a human ruler appears four chapters later – in Genesis 10:10 (i.e. after the flood), where the kingdom of Nimrod is mentioned. Before that, no kings or rulers are mentioned.[18] This is, of course, an argument from silence.[19] But a relevant one, in my opinion.

A Christian anarchist needs an optimistic anthropology which does not seem present in our story either. This optimism is typically linked to the value of education (the third important value of anarcho-transhumanism). As I have already noted, anarchists sympathize with the Socratic idea of a well-informed individual who is able to live in harmony with other well-informed individuals. But there is, I think, a presupposition of well-informed individuals (or at least something of that sort) in our story too. In Genesis 4 God and Cain are talking together which, say, suggests God

---

17 Which is not to say, as Murphy correctly mentions, there would not be any strong versus weak people; there are definitely differences among people concerning their power. This is, after all, suggested by the very mention of the heroes of might, and it is also quite natural for the fallen world (Genesis 3:16b).

18 "Nimrod appears in the register of nations as the author of imperialism. Under him society passed from the patriarchal form to the monarchical. He is the first man mentioned in the Bible as the head of a kingdom". (Nichol et. al. 1978, 275). I am aware that some think the Nephilim are "dynastic rulers, an early royal aristocracy". (Hamilton 1990, 263). This is the third traditional explanation besides the "human-angelic" and "Setho-Cainitic" explanations. And it places the appearance of a monarchy even before the flood. But it seems somehow less persuasive to me.

19 Jewish tradition seems to support it, however. For instance, Slovak Catholic Biblicists point in their commentary on the book of Genesis to Jewish rabbis Radak and Ramban who view Nimrod as a warrior who became the first ruler. (Dubovský et al. 2008, 88).

is still communicating in some empirically perceivable way with humanity after the fall until the flood, even though people have been removed from paradise. There is also this implicit idea of the Garden of Eden being still present on Earth before the flood (it is the flood that destroys it), even though nobody can come in. This means people do (or at least can) have information about God and his will. Methuselah is the former contemporary of Adam and he dies in the very year of the flood. So he is able to testify about the story of the Fall almost until the very end of the first civilization. And God is trying to plead with human hearts, as has been said. So it is not impossible for humans to turn away from evil (unless one accepts the Calvinistic paradigm, which I do not) if only they were willing. But they are not. Thus the story reminds us that we cannot rely on human reasonableness – on the good choices of (actually or at least potentially) well-informed individuals.

My point is simple: The story of Genesis 6 speaks of (1) free (2) superhumans who (3) do, or at least can, have the right information, and yet, they create a brutal world. Human perfection does not work with human freedom and knowledge for good here. Biblical anthropology is just not that optimistic. And because of this, the idea of an anarcho-transhumanist society seems somewhat illusory.[20]

---

[20] Gillis speaks of social singularity and apparently believes in the idea of deep social unity. But the Bible sketches a different picture of the fallen humanity. As Denis Farkasfalvy notes: "The Book of Genesis begins with the narration of humans' multiple fall(s) and God's corresponding judgment. This judgment initially exiles the humans from the garden, yet they continue to fall away from God, who sees 'that the wickedness was great in the earth, and that every inclination of the thoughts of their hearts was only evil continually. And the LORD was sorry that he had made humankind on the earth and it grieved him to his heart' (Gen. 6:5–6). Although through the flood God terminates all human existence except that of Noah and his family, he makes a covenant with them and promises never to repeat this act of universal punishment. Nonetheless, as Genesis continues its narrative, humanity's conceit and wickedness continue to grow, knowing no limit, so that God, in reply to their repeated attempted rivalries with him, deprives humanity of their ability to establish universal community as he confuses their languages and scatters 'them abroad over the face of all the earth' (Gen. 11:8). In the Bible, the preamble to human salvation is described not by a narrowly individualized concept of original sin, but by humankind's ongoing advancement toward subjugating the earth as an expression of their conceit, while failing to establish lasting communion with other human beings through culture. In this way, humanity allows their Creator and their own creaturely status to fall into oblivion. At the same time, the Bible presents humankind as the one project God wants to save [. . .]. [. . .] The morality of each Testament establishes unbreakable links between the love

4. Conclusion

It is not necessary *toprove* that politically liberated and technologically perfected people *will* fill the Earth with violence (lawlessness), similar to what we see in the story of Genesis 6. The mere threat is, I think, enough for a critical approach to the idea of anarcho-transhumanism. It is good to note that the first chapters of the book of Genesis are paradigmatic for the whole Bible in some sense. Thus they have an important bearing on the formation of all of our theology, including anthropology and (social) ethics. If it is true that transhumanism implies either dystopia or anarchism then, I think, an implicit theological warning can be deduced from our story against such risky pursuit of human enhancement.

---

of God and the love of the neighbor. Consequently, restoring one's union with God cannot happen without re-creating also communion with fellow human beings, nor can one's commitment to the one God validly exist without the search to promote humanity's unity, in both senses of restoring wholeness and integrity in the individual as well as binding ties of understanding and love with other human beings". (Farkasfalvy 2016, 227). In light of the New Testament, this is undoubtedly one of the roles of the Church. However, applying it to a wider social context, including the political realm, is another thing. Of course, there are values relevant to our political life in the Bible, that might have a-kind-of-utopian flavor – like equality of all, justice and peace, hope as the most practical political emotion, reverence for the earth, etc. (Maguire 2005, 37–38) – but these do not imply anarchy. Not even in the Church are people able to function without any authority structures, let alone in civil life. The need for some restrictions on human freedom in the fallen state is the basis of *usus politicus legis* in traditional protestant ethics (Ebeling 1982; Westberg 2015, 130). Christian anarchists, like Tolstoy for instance (to whom Kropotkin points (Kropotkin 2000, 73–87) while rejecting his faith-based approach), would surely disagree. Unlike Luther, "Tolstoy believed in the ideal and possibility of human moral perfection […]. This ideal of perfection will become the basis of human social life. […] Tolstoy identifies coercive human institutions as the major constraint upon the bursting forth of the new consciousness of love and its capacity to govern human life. The state, with its coercive instruments of armies, police, and prisons is the basic impediment. If the state and the instruments of coercion can be abolished, the new reality of love in the kingdom of God will be free to burst forth". (Wogaman 2011, 186–187). The Bible, however, does not seem to count on harmonious moral and political unity of humanity until the very end. To say otherwise requires some form of post-millennial eschatology, which I do not endorse (whereas I don't believe the problem of eschatology is the institution of the state as such, although it is true the apocalyptical books of Daniel and Revelation depict a misuse of the state power).

References

Alter, R. 2004. *The Five Books of Moses: A Translation with Commentary*. New York: W. W. Norton & Company.

Bartholomew, C., & Goheen, M. 2006. *The Drama of Scripture: Finding our place in the biblical story*. London: Society for Promoting Christian Knowledge.

Clines, D. 1998. The Significance of the "Sons of God" Episode (Genesis 6:1–4) in the Context of the "Primeval History" (Genesis 1–11), online: https://www.academia.edu/5570561/The_Significance_of_the_Sons_of_God_Episode_Genesis_6_1_4_in_the_Context_of_the_Primeval_History_Genesis_1_11_ (accessed April 28, 2023).

Danaher, J. Is Transhumanism Compatible with Anarchism? 2014. *Philosophical Disquisitions*, online: https://philosophicaldisquisitions.blogspot.com/2014/05/is-transhumanism-compatible-with.html (accessed April 28, 2023).

Dubovský, P. (ed.) 2008. *Komentáre k Starémuzákonu. I. zväzok. Genezis*. Trnava: Dobrá kniha.

Ebeling, G. 1982. Usus politicuslegi – ususpoliticusevangelii. *Zeitschrift für Theologie und Kirche*, 79(3): 323–348, online: https://www.jstor.org/stable/23584857 (accessed May 11, 2023).

Farkasfalvy, D. 2016. A Framework for Theological Interpretation. In:C. G. Bartholomew and H. A. Thomas (eds.), *A Manifesto for Theological Interpretation*. Grand Rapids: Baker Academic, 218–236.

Gentry, P. 2019. Were the sons of God in Genesis 6 fallen angels? Who were the Nephilim? online: https://www.youtube.com/watch?v=qKtHwc3mMY8 (accessed April 28, 2023).

Gillis, W. 2015. Transhumanism Implies Anarchism, online: https://c4ss.org/content/44993 [April-13–2023].

Greidanus, S. 2007. *Preaching Christ from Genesis: Foundations for Expository Sermons*. Grand Rapids: Eerdmans.

Hamilton, V. P. 1990. *The New International Commentary on the Old Testament: The Book of Genesis. Chapters 1–17*. Grand Rapid: Eerdmans.

Hartley, J. E. 2000. *New International Biblical Commentary: Genesis*. Peabody: Hendrickson Publishers.

Kidner, D. 1967. *Genesis: An Introduction & Commentary*. Leicester: Inter-Varsity Press.

Kropotkin, P. 2000. *Anarchistickáetika*. Olomouc: Votobia.

Kolovou, E. & Karageorgikas, S. 2010. Free from Nature or Free Nature? An Anarchist Critique of Transhumanism, 315–332, online: https://www.academia.edu/2183083/Free_Nature_or_Free_From_Nature_An_Anarchist_Critique_of_Transhumanism_in_New_perspectives_on_anarchism (accessed April 13, 2023).

Maguire, D. C. 2005. *A Moral Creed for All Christians*. Minneapolis: Fortress Press.

Malendowicz, P. 2020 Non-anarchist anarchisms and anarchisms of the non-anarchist origin in contemporary political thought. *Athenaeum*, 75(3): 67–86., online: https://bibliotekanauki.pl/articles/2163345.pdf (accessed April 13, 2023).

Murphy, J. C. 1867. *Critical and Exegetical Commentary on the Book of Genesis with A New Translation*. Boston: Draper and Halliday, online: https://archive.org/details/criticalexegetic00murp/page/n1/mode/2up (accessed May 22, 2023).

Nichol, F. D. (ed.) 1978. *The Seventh-day Adventist Bible Commentary. Volume 1*. Hagerstown: Review and Herald.

Skinner, J. 1910. *Critical and Exegetical Commentary on Genesis*. Edinburgh: T. & T. Clark.

Wenham, G. J. 1987. *Word Biblical Commentary: Genesis 1–15*. Grand Rapids: Zondervan.

Westberg, D. A. 2015. *Renewing Moral Theology: Christian Ethics as Action, Character and Grace*. Downers Grove: InterVarsity Press.

Westermann, C. 1984. *Genesis 1–11: A Commentary*. Minneapolis: Augsburg Publishing House.

Wogaman, J. P. 2011. *Christian Ethics: A Historical Introduction*. 2nd ed. Louisville: Westminster John Knox Press.

Transhumanism as a New Topic in Education

Noemi Bravená and Helena Hejlová

1. Introduction

Primary school education, a foundational component of academic development, is structured and regulated by the national curriculum, which is a mandatory framework adopted by all schools. This curriculum undergoes periodic revisions conducted by specialized teams of pedagogical experts with the intent of reflecting and accommodating the prevailing needs of society, advancements in scientific disciplines, and significant societal shifts. Through a specific case study from the Czech Republic, this study seeks to identify potential sectors within the state curriculum where topics concerning transhumanism could be incorporated. It posits that the sensitization of children to these emerging concepts is no longer a prospective idea but rather an immediate necessity.

In 2021, the Czech Basic Education Curriculum witnessed the incorporation of digital competence, emblematic of technological literacy, a change expedited by the global COVID-19 pandemic. However, its current interpretation within the curriculum is largely reduced to pragmatic and quotidian utilization of technology, overlooking its broader social and ethical implications. This issue extends beyond the realm of cyberbullying or the dependency of students on media associated with emerging technologies. Transhumanism, a rapidly burgeoning field, poses a multitude of ethical and technological conundrums that warrant consideration (Žalec 2021; Huberman 2021). This study contemplates these emergent educational challenges and is guided by the following research questions:

1. Where can room be accommodated within the state syllabus to familiarize children with issues pertaining to transhumanism?

2. What overarching objective can such an education cater to and what are the fundamental challenges inherent to this task?

This study also proposes the implementation of a systematic methodology that integrates a comprehensive literature review and critical analysis of the current state syllabus, with the objective of identifying potential areas of inclusion for the subject matter. Additionally, this research aims to elucidate the fundamental learning outcomes and challenges associated with introducing transhumanist topics into primary school education. By employing a multidisciplinary approach, this study attempts to bridge the gap between the technological and ethical implications of transhumanism and the necessary adaptability of our educational structures.[1]

2. Transhumanism as Part of the Main Goals of Education

With the growing discourse on the significance of technologies for humans and the possibility of enhancing the physical aspects of human beings, a corresponding question must be how to introduce this topic as a subject in primary schools. Children's education must respond to new ways of thinking about technology and its significance to humans. While we do not yet need to ask ourselves whether an "imperfect" human being will one day have significance for "perfect" technologies, it is indeed a question whether artificial intelligence might one day pose this question to us. While AI is not yet at this stage of development, inaction may be robbing humans of the time in which future boundaries between humans and technologies are defined and future forms of cohabitation of the "imperfect" human, his variously enhanced forms, and entities of artificial intelligence are delineated. It may sound like science fiction, but so did the books of Jules Verne for many people. Our text aims to open a discussion about transhumanist ideas as a subject that equips students with an aspect of competence that connects the technological, ethical, and transcendent dimensions of being human.

A new aim in the curricular document titled "Framework Education Programme for Basic Education" (hereafter referred to as the Framework or RVP and cited as 'RVP') is: "to help students navigate the digital envi-

---

[1] This paper was supported by the "Cooperatio project research area Pedagogy" of the Faculty of Education, Charles University in Prague.

ronment and guide them to the safe, confident, critical, and creative use of digital technologies at work, in learning, in leisure time, and in participating in society and civic life" (RVP 2021, 9). We believe that the term "utilization of technology" does not reflect all needs of the present. It would be beneficial to open a discussion on how to guide students to reflect on current topics concerning the human-technology relationship. Here, we see an opportunity to motivate teachers and the professional public to engage with other current topics besides the basic utilitarian use or the misuse of technologies.

It is essential to view transhumanism not as a separate entity, but as a significant component within the broader scope of education goals. The incorporation of transhumanist ideals within educational objectives could pave the way for fostering a more technologically inclusive and forward-thinking mindset among students. This will enable learners to better understand and adapt to rapidly evolving technologies and their potential impact on human life. In essence, integrating transhumanism into education will equip students with a future-oriented vision, encouraging them to participate proactively in shaping our technologically augmented future.

3. Transhumanism and Media Education

In recent years, pedagogy has placed growing emphasis on *interdisciplinary and inter-thematic connections*, as it is likely that key employees in the future will be those who can work at the intersection of multiple fields. This correlates with the trend of integrating fields with new technologies (such as vertical farming, telemedicine, teaching in virtual environments, etc.). For this reason, the Czech curriculum includes so-called cross-sectional themes (RVP 2021, 132–146). These are not separate educational areas due to their smaller content but contain significant contemporary issues and an intentional requirement to guide children towards a more comprehensive reflection on topics. For example, *Media Education* primarily aims to analyze and improve communication strategies, but there is also a certain space for topics of transhumanism. The concept of "media literacy" includes its connection with digital literacy, aimed at "acquiring some basic knowledge about the operation and societal role of current media (their history, structure, and function)". We believe that under the terms "role" and "function", we can subsume both the consequences of using technologies and the future role of media in society.

Here, we see the opportunity for discussing these topics:

1. "The societal role of current media" (RVP 2021, 144) and their *connection to ethical-transcendent themes*.
2. Media literacy in the RVP includes guiding students towards the "ability to choose the appropriate media as a means to fulfill various needs – from acquiring information through education to fulfilling leisure time" (RVP 2021, 144). Here, a discussion is offered on the *connection between media and leading a meaningful life*. We refer to the broader definition of media as an intermediary of information (Middendorf 2017, 13; Herzig 2017, 41–42) and the growing connection, or even dependency, of students on new technologies. Therefore, the relationship to technology must be discussed from the perspective of values and meaning of life.
3. Another topic missing from this cross-sectional theme is understanding the ethics of media and would therefore be a suitable addition to the thematic circle Functioning and influence of media in society (RVP 2021, 146).

The intersection of transhumanism and media education provides a unique platform for exploring the impact of digital media and technologies on the human condition. Given the omnipresence of digital media in today's world, it is imperative to develop media literacy in a transhumanist context. By doing so, pupils would gain the skills to critically analyze the media's influence and foresight to anticipate and evaluate the potential outcomes of transhumanist tendencies reflected within media narratives. This awareness would be crucial in navigating the complexities of our increasingly digital and technologically intertwined existence.

4. Transhumanism and Ethical Education

Ethical education serves as an additional subject in the RVP, which schools are not obliged to incorporate into their educational programs (RVP 2021, 121–125). In the Czech curriculum, religious education is not included as a mandatory (Germany) or optional subject (Slovakia) (Hanesová 2006), for which ethical education is offered in parallel for interested parties. This disrupts the cross-curricular dimension among IT, media, ethics, and comprehensive (interdisciplinary) literacy. Consequently, there is insufficient integration of digital and media themes with ethical, worldview, value conceptions, and reflections on the meaningfulness of human existence. In this sense, RVP is inflexible and deficient, and does not meet the requirement of connecting themes, as is the case in educational areas.

The themes of transhumanism are complex issues, similar to global development and multicultural topics, and cannot be isolated into a few separate lesson scenarios. The authors believe it is necessary to:

- Initiate a discussion about *complex and cross-curricular themes* regarding their significance in education and their practical realization in schools.
- Question whether to redefine the significance of ethical education as such and introduce a NEW cross-sectional theme titled "*Current Ethical Topics*" (such as transhumanism, euthanasia, immoral and illegal activities on the internet, new technologies as a current form of a new religion, etc.).

We are compelled to think this way based on the following consideration: *Ethical Education* in the Czech Republic focuses on the development of pro-sociality (Pachelová 2022), and thus overlaps with the cross-sectional theme of *Personal and Social Education* in some topics. Therefore, it is understandable that many educators do not see the practical significance for students in *Ethical Education*. The inclusion of "Current Ethical Topics" does not disrupt the importance of *Ethical Education* as currently conceived in RVP but extends the opportunity for schools to respond to significant ethical issues of today. It reflects on the essence of ethics and non-ethics, including criminal liability for specific actions. At the same time, it involves a closer connection between ethical education and current ethical-philosophical theories (e.g., situational ethics, utilitarianism, hedonism, moral dilemmas) on one side and theories of other fields (IT, media, communication, medicine, human rights, minorities, etc.) on the other. Drawing conclusions from ethical reflection for technological literacy is a different methodological and didactic approach than what is now presupposed by RVP, i.e., that the student reflects on technological, digital, and media issues and estimates the ethical and non-ethical nature of actions within them.

To conclude, in the scope of ethical education, transhumanism implies fundamental questions about human nature and identity, as well as the aspect of morality complicated by extensive technological advancements. Therefore, the topic requires consideration in the scope of ethical education. Incorporating these topics into Ethical Education would encourage students to discuss transhumanist ideas and critically assess their moral aspects. Thus, students would be equipped with an understanding of the complex ethical issuesconcerning technological enhancement and a basis for a moral approach to the age of transhumanism.

5. Transhumanism and Key Competence

The majority of European countries define general educational goals with a cross-curricular character as key competencies. These are defined in the Czech document as a "set of knowledge, skills, abilities, attitudes, and values ... " (RVP 2021, 9). Topics of transhumanism can currently best be categorized within digital competence under the key competencies framework. This competence is linked to the limits of technology in this way: the student "critically evaluates the contributions (of IT technologies) and reflects on the risks of their use". This definition contains two areas that cannot be properly reflected without ethical reflection.

1. In what ways and for whom are IT technologies beneficial? How is the benefit for individuals, society, specific fields, or specific cultures defined?
2. Who determines the risks and is it possible to know all the risks? We assume that the one who determines the risks has good intentions toward us or has all the information necessary to determine these risks. Some technologies have been in use for too short a time for all health, ethical, and criminal risks to be established. Another question arises about the requirements for those who monitor risk determination.

The RVP states that the student learns to "prevent situations that threaten the security of equipment and data, situations with *a negative impact* on his physical and mental health and the health of others". It is further stated that the student: "acts ethically in collaboration, communication, and sharing information in a digital environment". The consequences for humans are broadly defined in terms of physical and mental health, but when considering this issue from the perspective of transhumanism, other questions arise. If technology improves someone's health, is it therefore guaranteed to be good? This involves resolving dilemmatic situations: my physical health is helped; my mental health is burdened – is this then good (positive impact) or bad (negative impact) technology?

The quotation suggests that the student should be guided to ethical behavior in the technological environment, but it is clear that each environment is specific and has its own community of users, vocabulary, rules, and thus ethical requirements based on different theories and worldviews. This essentially refers to *applied situational ethics*. This topic could be covered in the optional subject of *Ethical Education* (see the quote: "The student analyzes the ethical aspects of various life situations", RVP 2021, 124). However, there are two problems here: *Ethical Education* is not part of every school curriculum, and there is again a deficit in connection with new technologies.

Another question needs to be asked: What if the environment itself does not fulfill ethical values?; what if the defined scope of the technology is debatable, if not unethical? How is a student supposed to question this type when they do not look at technology from a higher perspective and are led to believe that danger is primarily hiding in overuse, cyberbullying, and misuse of technology for criminal activity? Ethical questions are often posed from the perspective of the IT industry in the school environment, not from the perspective of ethical concepts, and we see this as a fundamental deficiency. Is it possible to reflect on ethical topics without knowledge of ethical concepts? These theories become meaningful for teachers when they respond to specific phenomena in society, which are clarified by philosophizing thought. Without a more thoughtful development of ethical competence in children, any guidance to ethical behavior is a one-sided fast product, which partly fulfills its purpose but is unable to withstand the more serious pressures of today.

The digital competence in the RVP currently does not open the question of human enhancement through technologies with all subtopics. The focus is on data security and minimizing misuse risk. For example, the student "describes how a computer works in terms of hardware and operating system; discusses the functioning of digital technologies defining trends in the world, … can direct his activity to minimize the risk of data loss or misuse; describes the functioning and discusses the limitations of security solutions" (RVP 2021, 43).

To pave the way for topics related to transhumanism in the educational process, it is important to discuss expanding Digital and Technological Competence through an anthropological-ethical dimension. Emphasis should be placed on the student recognizing the uniqueness of a human being living in a world of technology, and the benefits and limits of improving the quality of life through technology. The student should be guided to technologically independent thinking about the meaning of human life.

Our main argument in this section is as follows: Therefore, since key competencies in education are some kind of synthesis of knowledge, skills, attitudes, and values, it is especially relevant and wise to embed the concept of transhumanism in one of the existing key competencies. The competence approach to education cultivates the readiness for change and the ability to adapt to them, technological literacy, and critical thinking. The involvement of learners in the educational process as a competence in the context of transhumanism will also ensure their readiness and ability to respond quickly and adequately to the changes that will inevitably happen in a future society more influenced by technology.

6. Transhumanism and the Purpose of Human Education

Themes relating to new technologies pose serious ethical questions, particularly in the context of human enhancement (Strahovnik 2021, 37–38). In pedagogical discussions, these are emerging as practical requirements for the inclusion of specific topics into the national curriculum. Examples include topics related to transhumanism and artificial intelligence, which are still relatively unexplored by educators, or the currently debated issue of "the relationship between digital wellbeing and overall wellbeing of children and young people" (Konference 2022). According to the authors, the essence of these new topics extends beyond the topics themselves.

Czech pedagogical psychologist ZdeněkHelus was ahead of his time when he advocated for a pedagogy that addresses all qualities of personality (the so-called "education of the turn"). The depth of his reflections rested on his ability to skillfully link personal thinking about the child to question the essence of education. In his text "Is education what it is supposed to be?", he defined *six purposes of education*, which do not fully capture its essence, but resonate with both the lay and expert public. Education, he posits, should:

1. "Shape human resources" and ensure "economic growth" and career possibilities;
2. Serve "individualistic hedonism" (enjoying life);
3. Develop various competencies;
4. Enhance the quality of life;
5. Lead to "the correction of human matters", i.e., by demonstrating the leading role of a specific idea in times of crisis;
6. Guide creative "concern for humans, so that they find their calling, fulfill the meaning of their own life, personal and generally human" (Helus 2012, 1–2).

Helus does not state that we cannot strive for such goals, but rather that the essence of education lies outside these definitions in the *education of the turn*. This approach "asks about the qualities of personality that enable a person to meet the demands of their time: in other words, the qualities that allow one to resist the pressure of deforming crisis phenomena – including pressures causing reductionism and individualistic hedonism". The reduction of human personality and personal happiness are important concepts in discussions about the benefits of connecting humans with technology. Helus's new concept of education is also linked to a new definition of man as the "*man of the turn*". Such an individual can only be educated when education evenly considers four dimensions:

- "Anthropological" – a genuine interest in humans is emphasized;
- "Ethical" – education evenly connects knowledge and morality;
- "Contextual" – education leads to the recognition of causes and consequences in all phenomena and promotes responsible action;
- "Transcending" – education guides the student towards a supra-personal (non-egocentric) sense of action, and simultaneously leads them towards a "cosmic" orientation of life, which "raises questions about the meaning of humanity and its history" (Helus 2012, 4; Bravená 2019).

The personality that can adequately reflect the issues of transhumanism is Helus's "man of the turn". This figure is the goal of education, which, in a certain sense, can be seen as a profane form of Imago Dei. The "man of the turn" not only targets all the potentialities of the human personality that can be developed through education but also re-evaluates the meaning of all his actions and knowledge, i.e., undergoes a constant inner turn (*metanoia*) with the goal of serving the whole and the non-egocentric dimension of human existence (Helus 2012). The education of the turn strives for a child's development that is both personally and cosmologically (i.e., transcendentally) oriented while also based on a clear anthropological appeal to children's rights. According to H. Hejlová, everyone has the right "to be guided towards good" and "protection from discernable evil, which goes against good, beauty, and love, thus against values that are believed to be understood by all, shared by all, and for which there is a common will to share, as they make human beings human and enable them to live with human dignity" (Hejlová2010, 99). Z. Helus defined a transcendental yet anthropologically and contextually firmly anchored paradigm of pedagogy (Bravená 2019, 144–145), thereby paving the way for responsible discussions about the relationship between humans and technologies.

The committing of transhumanism into the essence of human education challenges us to question what humanity entails in a world characterized by rapid technological revolution. It requires educators and educational departments to embrace a whole-system approach to education: one that does not only prepare students for the present but also instills in them skills necessary for a future world in which the distinction between human and technological integration becomes less defined. Embedding Transhumanism in the purpose of education might motivate responsible learners who will influence, engage and guide a future planet in which the evolution of humans and technology seems inseparable.

7. Conclusion

The incorporation of transhumanism into the educational system necessitates a broad-based dialogue on pedagogical objectives, academic domains, and the nature of the topics themselves, as well as the preparedness of educators to engage in such discourse. It also necessitates a future orientation, preparing students for a universe where the line between fragile beings and breakthroughs is often blurred. Despite the significant limitations of integrating transhumanism into the curriculum, this responsibility can create a generation of fully educated learners prepared to be multiliterate and agile in technology, grounded in ethics, and dexterous enough to be future makers, not merely victims.

Like any research endeavor, the present study is not without its limitations. One key constraint lies in its largely theoretical nature. While it draws on existing literature, especially from the *Framework* and Czech theories to explore the integration of transhumanism within various aspects of education, there remains a lack of empirical evidence to substantiate these discussions. Consequently, the applicability of the suggestions provided may be dependent on context and subject to the variability of practical realities. Further, given the vast and multidimensional nature of transhumanism, the study might not encompass all potential implications of transhumanism in education, focusing only on its integration within main education goals, media education, ethical education, competence, and the overall purpose of human education.

We considered in our work how to start conversations about transhumanism in the classroom. Implementing empirical research in the future could provide concrete proof of the effects of transhumanism integration in education. This might be action research of experimental implementation in classrooms, case studies, or surveys to find out how teachers and students see and feel about things. Future study might also look at other areas of educational practice, such pedagogy, curriculum design, evaluation, and educational policy, where transhumanism might have a significant impact. " With the variety of socio-cultural norms and technological accessibility across areas, studies could also look into the difficulties and possible solutions in introducing transhumanist ideas into various educational contexts.

References

Bravená, N. 2019. *"Do Not Be Concerned Only About Yourself… " Transcendence and Its Importance for the Socialization and Formation of a Child's Personality*. Kassel: Kassel University Press.

Hanesová, D. 2006. *Náboženskávýchova v Európskejúnii*. Banská Bystrica: PedF UMB.

Hejlová, H. 2010. *Práva dětí ve vzdělávání – výzva pro učitele*. Praha: PedF UK.

Helus, Z. 2012. *Je vzdělávání tím, čím má být? A ne-li, v čem je problém?*https://skav.cz/wp-content/uploads/2012/06/skav_konf12_prof_helus.pdf (accessed April 15, 2023).

Huberman, J. 2021. *Transhumanism. From Ancestors to Avatar*. Cambridge: Cambridge University Press.

Konference: Digitální wellbeing dětí. 2022. https://digitalniwellbeing.skav.cz/ (accessed April 15, 2023).

Middendorf, W. 2017. Pädagogischer Mehrwert?: Digitale Medien in Schule und Unterricht – eine Einführung. In: Ch. Fischer (ed.), *Pädagogischer Mehrwert?: Digitale Medien in Schule und Unterricht*. Münster: Waxmann Verlag, pp. 11–24.

Herzig, B. 2017. Digitalisierung und Mediatisierung – didaktische und pädagogische Herausforderungen. In:Ch. Fischer (ed.), *Pädagogischer Mehrwert?: Digitale Medien in Schule und Unterricht*. Münster: Waxmann Verlag, pp. 25–58.

Pachelová, M. 2022. *ImplementacedoplňujícíhovzdělávacíhoboruEtickávýchova na prvnímstupnizákladniškoly*. Praha: PedF UK (Ph.D. thesses).

Petkovšek, R. & Žalec, B. (eds). 2021. *Transhumanism as a Challenge for Ethics and Religion*. Zürich: LIT Verlag.

Rámcovývzdělávací program pro předškolnívzdělávání[RVP]. (2021). Praha: VÚP. https://www.msmt.cz/vzdelavani/predskolni-vzdelavani/opatreni-ministra-zmena-rvppv-2021 (accessed April 15, 2023).

Strahovnik, V. 2021. Virtues and transhumnist human enhancement. In: R. Petkovšek and B. Žalec (eds.), *Transhumanism as a Challenge for Ethics and Religion*. Münster: LIT Verlag, pp. 37–44.

THE EFFECTS OF TECHNOLOGY ON HAPPINESS: A VIETNAMESE PERSPECTIVE

Hang Thi Thu Vu

1. Introduction and Overview

Technology is the realization and reflection of human desires. To reach the potential in their bodies and minds that are becoming more and more demanding better fulfillment, people use technological ways. Technology thus strives to meet every need, feeling, and want of people.

Technology comes in numerous forms to satisfy the wide range of interests and demands of people, simplifying and improving their quality of life. Artificial intelligence is one of these intelligent tools that enables humans to use scientific knowledge to carry out different tasks fast and efficiently; Information and communication technology that enables people to connect from anywhere in the world using amazing technologies like social networking platforms, virtual assistants, Wi-Fi, and Bluetooth; Entertainment technology applied to simulation, automation, augmented reality, and virtual reality; Medical Technology facilitates more precise and efficient health evaluation, diagnosis, and treatment. For those with impairments, assistive technology can greatly enhance their quality of life by facilitating their ability to hear, see, and move more easily. Technology also exists in agriculture, business, industrial robotics, education, food, manufacturing, architectural, construction, environmental, chain, and industry sectors; it also includes biotechnology, electronics, military, and science.

A major turning point in the Fourth Industrial Revolution was the introduction of big data, artificial intelligence, the Internet of Things and digitization. At a rate of growth never seen before, these technologies are dramatically changing the global production and economic landscapes by promoting higher efficiency and brilliance. Simultaneously, they improve connection, supporting strong and varied partnerships arising from the most basic human drives, regardless of distance or cultural background. Such developments include improving spiritual life, fostering democratic and communal values, and fostering conditions that are favorable to cultural evolution.

For the most part, technological advancements have significantly impacted people's lives in all aspects, both physically and mentally, including happiness. There are many different views on the concept of happiness; happiness is each person's desire in life. Humans are born with the pursuit of happiness, as declared by the United Nations Resolution (2012) to be a fundamental human goal. Epicurus argues that happiness is pleasure; all things are to be done for the sake of the pleasant feelings associated with them; when people are satisfied with life, they are happy. Happiness is an abstract issue; to measure and count it, one needs to be based on various criteria because it reflects aspects of human life. Some are personal, and others are related to physical environmental conditions and social relationships close to family, friends, and colleagues. Frey and Stutzer (2002, 6) mentioned, "Individual well-being is not an isolated feeling, but strongly depends on the conditions in which the persons concerned live". There is a lot involved with the work environment; job benefits, relationships between colleagues, leadership, inspiration at work, recognition, and promotion all govern a person's level of happiness.

Happiness is also the goal and value of society, and happiness is associated with the people's interests (Communist Party of Vietnam 2021). Happiness plays an essential role in assessing each country's good governance level. The happiness index shows changes in people's emotions and needs, accurately grasping the direction and requirements of social development, thereby formulating scientific policies to develop society materially and spiritually. According to research by authors Mai N.T.N. and Linh N.P.D (2022), the assessment is reflected in the level of satisfaction in each person's life. It pertains emotional well-being, physical well-being, social well-being, professional happiness, intellectual happiness, environmental well-being, and spiritual well-being.

In a research paper on some of the factors that impact employee happiness, the author Phi N.Q. (2022) focuses on a study that aimed to understand the factors that impact the happiness of workers. The study found that workers who are happy in their jobs contribute more effort to the company's growth. The study also found that happy workers are more productive, stay with their company longer, and have higher energy levels than unhappy workers. The study used the JD-R model, which is a leading workplace stress model, to define job demands and resources as factors that impact worker happiness.

The research used a combination of qualitative and quantitative research methods. The qualitative research was conducted through group discussions and in-depth interviews to improve the measurement scale and survey form. The quantitative research was conducted by collecting data from 50 workers in Ho Chi Minh City to analyze the reliability of the measurement scale. The survey form officially included one dependent variable, seven independent variables, and one control variable, with the dependent variable "Happiness" having seven observation variables and the seven independent variables being "Job Satisfaction" (5 variables), "Relationship with Leaders" (4 variables), "Relationship with Colleagues" (4 variables), "Recognition" (4 variables), "Career Opportunities" (4 variables), "Salary and Benefits" (4 variables), and "Work-Life Balance" (4 variables), and the control variable being "Covid-19 Impact" (4 variables). The quantitative research was conducted with a survey of 350 workers through Google Drive due to the Covid-19 pandemic. The author filtered and checked the responses and kept only 303 valid responses for the study. The author used data analysis methods such as the reliability of the measurement scale with the Cronbach Alpha coefficient, exploratory factor analysis (EFA), and linear regression analysis. The research results show that the majority of the 303 respondents were between 20–25 years old, female, and had a college or higher education level. Most were single and had a monthly income of 10–20 million VND. The average scores of the different variables were calculated, with "Job Satisfaction" having the highest average score of 3.76 and "Happiness" having an average score of 3.98. The results of the reliability analysis of the measurement scale and the exploratory factor analysis are also presented in the thesis.

The author of the text conducted a study to analyze the impact of 33 variables on the happiness of workers. The Bartlett test was used to test the hypothesis that the variables were not related to each other. In contrast, the KMO test was used to check the appropriateness of the sample size for the exploratory factor analysis. The results of the simple linear regression showed that the variables impacting worker happiness were an inspiration in work, relationship with superiors, relationship with colleagues, recognition, opportunities for advancement, salary and benefits, and work-life balance. The outbreak of COVID-19 in Ho Chi Minh City harmed worker happiness, particularly in work-life balance, salary and benefits, and opportunities for advancement. The discussion emphasized the importance of worker happiness for companies and the need for companies to create a positive work environment to ensure workers are motivated and contribute to the company's success.

The text further describes the factors contributing to employees' workplace happiness. It discusses the relationship between employees and their leaders, the importance of interaction with coworkers, recognition, opportunities for personal growth, and the need for a fair and transparent promotion system. The text also emphasizes the importance of creating a supportive work environment that encourages employees to improve themselves and contribute to the company. These are the main takeaways that we can learn from the author:

The relationship with leadership: The concern and involvement of leadership is just a part of creating happiness for workers, but their management skills, direction of employees, and implementation of company policies will bring good results for the team and the business.

The relationship with coworkers: Positive relationships and learning from coworkers are positive factors that contribute to job satisfaction. The company should encourage these relationships through team building and sharing experiences between departments.

Recognition: Workers' recognition is a highly valued factor but needs to be given more fairly in many businesses. Recognition can motivate and improve the learning and development of employees.

Opportunities for advancement: In today's changing and developing society, workers value personal growth and development highly. Companies should provide opportunities for advancement and support for continuing education.

Clear and fair advancement system: A clear and transparent advancement system is necessary to give workers confidence in their future within the company. Providing benefits such as retirement support and education assistance can help retain and motivate employees.

Let us examine another happiness research report, namely "Lessons learned from countries around the world" – by Hông(2020). The text discusses the World Happiness Report of 2019 (Helliwell et al. 2019), which evaluated 156 countries based on six key criteria. These criteria include average GDP per capita, social support, healthy life expectancy, freedom to choose, generosity, and perception of corruption. The report found that these factors did not always correspond with the overall happiness of a country. For example, Costa Rica ranked high in happiness despite having a lower GDP than other countries. Meanwhile, China and the United States ranked 19th and 18th in terms of GDP, but their rankings in the World Happiness Report were lower, at 95th and 19th, respectively. The author also mentions that social support, as determined by the Gallup World Poll, is an important factor in determining happiness, with countries with higher social support generally ranking higher in happiness.

The text further discusses the results of a Gallup World Poll on various aspects of well-being, including Generosity, Healthy Life Expectancy, Freedom, and Corruption. Generosity is measured based on the average response to a question about giving money to help others. Healthy Life Expectancy is based on the average life span of a person from birth to death, as determined by the World Health Organization. Freedom is measured by the results of a Gallup World Poll on the freedom to choose one's own life and make decisions. Corruption is also considered an essential aspect of well-being and is determined by two questions about corruption in the government and businesses. The poll's results may vary depending on the methods and accuracy of the survey.

The text further compares the well-being of citizens in four countries, namely Denmark, New Zealand, Spain, and Bhutan, based on the 2019 World Happiness Report. Denmark ranks second and has a high standard of living. New Zealand ranks eighth and is highly ranked in well-being due to its national happiness budget and strong community spirit. Spain ranks 30th and values social relationships but faces a high unemployment rate and increasing political instability. Bhutan ranks 95th and uses Gross National Happiness as a well-being metric, emphasizing spiritual and emotional well-being over wealth and material development. The text concludes that happiness is a subjective concept that varies greatly depending on a person's individual experiences and circumstances.

The following key takeaways can be drawn from the text:

1. Denmark ranks 2nd in the 2019 Global Happiness Report by the World Happiness Council (WHC). The country's high ranking is due to its strong economy, efficient public services, and emphasis on work-life balance.
2. New Zealand ranks 8th in the same report, with a focus on social support and strong community spirit as factors contributing to its high ranking.
3. Spain ranks 30th in the 2019 Global Happiness Report, with strengths in social relationships, work-life balance, and personal freedom.
4. Bhutan ranks 95th in the same report, but the country prioritizes Gross National Happiness (GNH) over economic growth. Bhutan believes happiness is more important than wealth and focuses on maintaining a balanced and sustainable way of life for its citizens.
5. Happiness is a subjective concept and can mean different things to different people. It is influenced by factors such as the natural environment, social relationships, and personal values.
6. Vietnam ranks 94th in the 2019 Global Happiness Report, with a high ranking considering its average income. The country values family, work, and a sense of community, and its citizens are content with their current way of life.

Further, we have analyzed the content of the Proceedings of the first Southeast Asia regions psychology conference "Human well-being and sustainable development" held by the University of Social Sciences and Humanities, Hanoi National University: Institute of Psychology (Vietnam Academy of Social Sciences), International Association of Applied Psychology, International Board of Surveying, International Society for Transcultural Psychology, Australian Psychological Association and Chinese Psychological Society (VNU USSH 2017). The conference obtained 454 abstracts by individuals and research groups from 35 countries and regions, with 13 symposia held with 24 sub-committees presenting various topics related to human well-being, physical and spiritual health, and sustainable development in different contexts, sectors, and environments in the diversity and constant transformation of global culture and society. The authors focused on the following topics: happiness in life, marriage, emotions, emotional capacity, personality, mental health, education and learning, culture, and nation.

In relation to happiness and technology, Section 10 of the Proceedings contains studies on the impact of the Internet and social media on well-being. In this part, the authors focus on evaluating the following: Social Media and Youth Risk Behaviors: A Mini-Review and Social Media and Human Relationships (Mai 2017, 303); Cyberbullying and Its Effects on Vietnamese Youth (Linh 2017, 313); Effectiveness of Online Peer Support Group and Its Interventions, A Case Study of Beautiful Mind Vietnam (Kha, Thanh, & Linh 2017, 324); Considering Innovativeness and Engagement to Overcome Online Disinhibition Effect on Facebook (Sadida, Fitria, &Caninsti 2017, 333); Self-Assessment and Internet Addiction Among Adolescents in Dong Nai, Vietnam (Cong & Chi 2017); The Impact of Information and Communication Technology on the Ethics and Lifestyle of Today's Youth (Ha 2017); The Situation of Cyberbullying Among High School Students in Da Nang City (Hanh & Cong 2017).

The above studies indicate that, in terms of happiness, technology contributes to increased happiness through emotional technology devices, media, online services, and social networks. However, technology can also lead to feelings of loneliness, reduced engagement, and negative sentiments, which diminish happiness. More practical studies are needed in specific countries to better understand this relationship. Additionally, it is necessary to study the impact of technology on the well-being of Vietnamese people in the current context.

2. Status of Technology in Vietnam

In fact, Vietnam has now emerged as a dynamic development hub in the region, the new digital powerhouse in Southeast Asia. Vietnam is also known as one of the countries with the most modern Internet technology infrastructure in the world and a high level of Internet access. In particular, mobile broadband infrastructure has covered 99.73% of villages nationwide. Fiber optic cable system has been deployed to 100% of communes, wards, and townships, 91% of villages, 100% of schools and 19.79 million households have fiber optic cable, reaching 72.4% (Communist Party of Vietnam 2022).

With modern technology infrastructure and nationwide coverage, the Internet has brought the opportunity to access the achievements of technology to people from urban to rural, from the delta areas to the mountain areas, and from North to South. It is easily used in daily life.

Vietnam officially joined the global Internet network on 19/11/1997; at that time, the number of Internet users in Vietnam was just over 200,000 people, and by 2002 there were about 3 million Internet users (about 4% of the country's population at that time), in 2007 it was nearly 20 million people. The number of social network users in Vietnam now is nearly 76 million, an increase of nearly 10 million people within 1 year (equivalent to 73.7% of the population) (Datareportal 2023). Vietnam has the 12th highest number of Internet users worldwide and ranks 6th out of 35 countries/territories in Asia (People Army Newspaper 2022).

In addition to equipping synchronous and developed technological infrastructure, with living standards and incomes increasing, Vietnamese people have now equipped themselves with various modern and high-tech means of communication to quickly access the Internet and make the most of the technological utilities offered. According to the statistics from the White Book on Vietnamese E-business 2022, the devices used by people to access the Internet in 2021 included desktops and laptops at 78%; mobile phones at 88%; and other devices such as tablets and iPads at 14% (Ministry of Industry and Trade 2022).

More specifically, the number of mobile phone subscribers using smartphones is 94.2 million; the number of mobile broadband subscribers is 82.2 million, accounting for 74.3% of the population. Vietnam has more than 564 thousand domain names, with ".vn" ranked 2nd in ASEAN and in the top 10 in the Asia-Pacific region. Vietnam is among the top 30 leading countries in information technology (Long 2022). Statistics from "We Are Social" indicate that 70% of the population in Vietnam currently uses mobile phones, and 64% of subscribers are equipped with 3G, 4G, and 5G connections. With a high rate of smartphone and Internet usage and gradually changing daily habits, Vietnam is becoming a potential land for developing digital economic models (VNN 2021a).

Not only is the number of internet subscribers growing, but Vietnam's digital businesses are also expanding rapidly. According to data from the Ministry of Information and Communications, Vietnam currently has about 64,000 digital technology enterprises. In 2021, 5,600 new digital technology enterprises were established (VNN 2021b). Vietnam is also recognized as a country with a fast pace of innovation compared to other lower-middle-income economies. According to the 2022 Global Innovation Index, Vietnam ranks in the top 50 countries for innovation achievements. The rate of scientific and technological development in Vietnam is high compared to regional and global standards; Vietnam ranks 48th out of 132 ranked countries (WIPO 2022). Vietnamese technology enterprises such as FPT, VNPT, and Viettel are continuing to invest in AI, the metaverse, 6G, NFTs, blockchain, smart devices, vaccine production, and healthcare technologies, considering these as ongoing breakthrough trends in technology infrastructure development in Vietnam. Viettel Group has proposed the pilot deployment of satellite Internet services. FPT announced it will spend VND 300 billion on AI research and development over the next five years. VNPT is promoting the development of AI technology for smart cities and e-government (Nham 2022).

In particular, in the coming years, Vietnam will prioritize science and technology as central to the country's development goals, aiming to use science and technology to enhance happiness. Resolution No. 23-NQ/TW, dated March 22, 2018, from the Politburo outlines the national industrial development policy up to 2030 with a vision to 2045. The overall targets are for Vietnam to achieve its industrialization and modernization goals by 2030, positioning itself as a modernity-oriented industrialized country among the top three in ASEAN in terms of industry, with some industries achieving global competitiveness and deep integration into the global value chain. By 2045, Vietnam aims to become a modern and industrialized country. To implement these goals, the National Digital Transformation Program up to 2025, with an orientation towards 2030, and the Prime Minister's Decision to issue the National Strategy on Research, Development, and Application of Artificial Intelligence (AI) until 2030 have been launched.

With the current robust technological development, coupled with the identification of technology development strategies in national goals for the upcoming period, Vietnam is poised to become a technologically advanced country. This demonstrates that the impact of technology on the lives and emotions of the Vietnamese people is inevitable. Whether technology makes people happier or leads them to feel lonelier, more alienated, and more negative are issues we will study in the next section.

3. Effectiveness of Technology on happiness in Vietnam

3.1 Positive effects of technology on happiness in Vietnam today

This part addresses how different technologies may promote social connection, improve social life conditions, and enhance mental health for Vietnamese people.

First, Social Connection

In growing up, each person is associated with close relationships with family, community, village, school, and office, to new social relationships while interacting with new conditions. This process helps people expand their circle of connection, promote various development capacities, and find meaning and happiness in life.

The integration hypothesis proposes that when individuals and groups associate with and identify with both the heritage of their own culture and that of other groups in the larger society, they are more successful in achieving higher levels of perceived well-being (both psychologically and socially) than if they were associated with just one or a few others in the same cultural group (Berry 2020). Communication and Information Technology are tools to connect, share knowledge, and empower people more substantially. Indeed, social media, especially Facebook, has been providing an ideal place with many different features for people to express themselves, share information, join groups, and connect with people around the world.

In Vietnam, technology has transformed the living habits and interactions of the Vietnamese people, both within the country and with the region and the world. With the development of the Internet, 4G, and 5G networks, smart cellphones and computers have turned residents from rural areas to cities, and from remote islands to high mountains, into technologically savvy individuals. They use social networking platforms for communication, business, shopping, studying, entertainment, and work.

In 2021, according to the Mobile Application Report published by Appota, among the popular applications in Vietnam, social networks are the most downloaded apps by Vietnamese people, with 28%. The report also shows that Facebook and YouTube are the two applications that users spend the most time on when using smartphones.

Specifically, Vietnamese spend 25% of their time using Faccbook and 12% watching YouTube. The number of Facebook users in Vietnam in 2023 is more than 75.6 million, ranking in the top 10 countries with the most significant number of users in the world are Indonesia and Brazil (more than 114.2 million people); Mexico (more than 93.3 million); the Philippines (more than 91.9 million), and more than Bangladesh (more than 54.2 million); Thailand (more than 51.6 million); Egypt (more than 47 million people) according to Data report statistics.

According to a Q&Me report, of the 97% who use Facebook, 94% are active daily. Research has also shown that the fact that users have many friends on social networking sites helps to present they are friendly, sociable, and easier to share their feelings (Q&Me 2022)

Besides Facebook, Zalo, a social network created by Vietnamese developers, is also leading with a usage rate of 87%, while Messenger and Instagram account for 58% and 15%, respectively (Nhandan online 2023). TikTok has also become the fourth most popular social network in Vietnam. DataReportal estimates that there are about 49.9 million TikTok users in Vietnam, ranking it sixth among the top ten countries globally for TikTok usage as of February 2023 (VET 2023). These platforms are among the most popular social networks worldwide; participating in these networks has created opportunities for contact, cultural exchange, and mutual understanding between individuals and social groups, from which each individual can build good relationships or cooperate in many aspects, promoting cultural exchange between Vietnam and the world. Research conducted by Vero and Insight Asia in 2019 with 300 people aged 15–45 also confirmed this: 85% of respondents said that technology opens many new opportunities, and the influence of technology is quite positive on people's lives.

The group of social network users is significant and often young. The Ministry of Education and Training statistics (2019)show that more than 22 million students use social networks. The results of a sociological survey in 2014 by authors Tran T.M.D. and Bui T.H.T.(Hanoi National University) on 4,247 students in 6 big cities of Hanoi, Hai Phong, Vinh, Hue, Da Nang, and Ho Chi Minh City on the current situation of using social networks of students showed that 99% students participating in the survey use social networks – Facebook and YouTube is 86.6%, Google is 56.2%.

Regularly being on social media and sharing positive emotions on online platforms has been shown to generate more social interactions and lead to favorable communication responses (Linh 2022). Research by Huong (VNU USSH 2017, 302–311) on social media and human relationships also highlights these benefits. Her article collected data from 150 high school and university students from Ho Chi Minh City and Hanoi, exploring the reasons for the excessive use of social media among Vietnamese youths. It then discussed the evening effects of social media, such as Facebook and Instagram, on human relationships among Vietnamese youths. The results of the research presented that 108 people, accounting for 72%, use the social network for keeping in touch; 138 people, or 92%, use it for making new friends; and 54 people, or 36%, use it for self-expression. Many respondents, 79.3%, said they use social media to make friends because it is difficult to speak directly, and 80% stated that they did not have time to meet face-to-face, so they used social media to communicate quickly (VNU USSH 2017, 302–311). However, it can also be said that these data in Vietnam are not comprehensive in capturing the effects of social media on the development of young people, especially in their relationships with family, friends, and others. Thus, the assessment remains incomplete. The impact of technology on social connections is exceptionally positive in emergency situations and epidemics. Notably, during the COVID-19 pandemic, when countries implemented social distancing and most people stayed at home, digital technology enabled teachers and students to continue with their lessons; employees could still maintain their work using computers connected to the Internet. People easily expressed their emotions through touching and loving personal status updates to encourage relatives, friends, nurses, and doctors to overcome the challenging times. Thanks to technology, social connections were only somewhat interrupted, and people were less anxious about being apart because they could still see each other on video calls, update each other's situations, and feel relieved to know their loved ones were still healthy and continuing their work and lives.

Thus, it is evident that the convenience and efficiency of technological utilities in work and life have made people's lives more fulfilling. People are more satisfied with life, which leads to increased happiness.

Second, improve living, working, and leisure conditions

Another benefit of technology to happiness is the improvement of people's living, working, and entertainment conditions. Science has shown that people with comfortable living conditions, high income, and easier access to meet their physical, spiritual, and entertainment needs have a higher quality of life and feel happier. Workers' working conditions and environments are increasingly invested in, improved in quality, and bring a sense of happiness to employees at the workplace due to the impact of technology. In Vietnam today, some businesses have adopted virtual office technology and Chatbots working 24/7 to help increase labor productivity, free employees from tedious tasks, and promote creativity to build a happy office. FPT is a typical technology company with a happy office model and is ranked among the best workplaces in the Information Technology industry in 2022. It is not only with large companies like FPT, but, under the philosophy of "happy boss, happy business" (Vnexpress.net 2022a), many digital businesses in Vietnam (about 70,000 enterprises) are now committed to creating thousands of happy workers in their working environments (Vnexpress.net 2022a).

The application of technology at work also helps tasks to be handled faster, and revenues to increase. As commented by Luong Dang Khoa, General Director of Boston Pharmaceutical Vietnam, the company achieved a threefold increase in revenue in three years thanks to FPT's digital products. "I myself am happy after using the Base ecosystem, which helps everything to be solved on the system, quickly processing", he said (Vnexpress.net 2022b).

In addition, thanks to technology, we have become globalized, transforming into borderless individuals who transcend the limitations of place and space. Some people work in offices, while others work from their homes or cafés. This flexibility meets the varied requirements of people's lives, making it easier for them to organize their lives, balance work and life, and thereby increasing their happiness. Especially after the COVID-19 pandemic, with the support of technology, various companies in Vietnam, particularly those related to technology, have allowed employees to work 60% at home and 40% at the workplace to enhance labor productivity and reduce many costs, while also improving well-being for office workers. According to the latest survey by PwC Vietnam, as of 2019, 33% of respondents favored a hybrid model combining office work with remote work. It is predicted that by 2025, Generation Z (born between 1996–2012) will comprise one-third of Vietnam's working age population. Moreover, up to 80% of this group believes they can work remotely effectively. However, this model is more suitable for several fields such as technology, communication, advertising, design, tourism, fashion, cosmetics, and home appliances. For industries requiring strict information and process security, such as banking and securities, this model will be challenging to implement (Vnexpress.net 2023).

Furthermore, science and technology, especially new, modern, and intelligent technologies along with the digital transformation process, have been utilized in daily life, providing state-of-the-art educational links and spreading content to people as quickly as possible, helping people enjoy high-quality services, reducing labor load, creating more jobs with high incomes, and improving the quality of life. For example, FPT Company has integrated AI into online education services, focusing not only on the transmission of learning content but also on personalizing user experiences, stimulating excitement, and promoting self-discipline.

Additionally, the development of information technology has also led to more positive and democratic changes in social life. This is true not only in centers and cities but also in most localities across the country, from rural to mountainous and island areas. Thanks to the multidimensional, fast, and unlimited information sources across regions and national territories, people have access to diverse cultural values and global information, thereby gaining a rich and extensive understanding of all fields of social life. Technology facilitates easier access to services and information, especially in public affairs, connecting people and authorities. With the policy of "strengthening information and propaganda work, promoting the strength of mass media agencies, expanding traditional information channels, and direct dialogue with people, contributing to relieving skepticism in society" (Resolution No. 25-NQ/TW of the Central Committee of the Party (XI term)), the Vietnamese Government has built a digital database from the central to the local level and created conditions for people to update necessary information about the operation of the state apparatus. People also actively propose aspirations and suggestions and participate in supervising the government's activities. At the same time, thanks to the application of technology in administrative management, the collection, synthesis, management, and analysis of people's aspirations are accurate, fast, and timely, aiding leaders in directing, coordinating, handling, and reconciling conflicts in society. Vietnam currently has 1,952 general websites and 935 social networks that have been licensed to operate. These are all online forums where people can freely share and express information and personal views (Communist Party of Vietnam 2022).

Regarding access to information for personal purposes, thanks to technological support, the spiritual life of people is enhanced. Statistics from the Ministry of Information and Communications indicate that Vietnamese people lead Southeast Asia in online video viewing at 92%, with 70% of Vietnamese watching videos on mobile devices. Readers now spend 75% of their time watching videos instead of reading articles. Another study reveals that Internet usage is mainly for research and study (69%), watching movies and listening to music (61%), shopping online (59%), searching for purchasing information (56%), reading newspapers (55%), gaming (30%), and other activities (31%) (Ministry of Industry and Trade 2022). Additionally, according to the statistics from the White Book on Vietnamese E-Business 2022, the types of goods and services people buy online through technological means primarily include clothes and shoes (69%), household appliances (64%); technology and electronics (51%); books, stationery, flowers, and gifts (50%); food (44%); train, air, and car tickets (27%); hotel and tour bookings (25%); movie tickets (22%); watching movies online (20%); online consulting and training services (17%); music/video/DVD/Games (14%); service incentives on platforms (12%); beauty and spa services (10%); and other goods and services (20%).

Furthermore, as internet communication technology develops, establishing online peer support groups can be an effective way to help reduce the burden of disease, anxiety, and stress disorders for different social audiences. Online support services are also expanding, including school counseling, reproductive health counseling, and mental health support, which contribute to healthy mental development among Vietnamese people. For example, the Beautiful Mind Vietnam group's online peer support service offers online peer counseling, psychological first aid, and offline help for people with acute stress and mental disorders in Vietnam. This support has helped individuals with mental health problems alleviate acute stress, reduce symptoms of psychosis, and foster a sense of community belonging (VNU USSH 2017, 325–331).

3.2 The adverse effects of technology on happiness

In addition to studies on the positive impact of technology on happiness, it is also true that technological advancements can equally be a source of stress and frustration for people. This section will examine the potential adverse effects of technology on happiness, such as technology addiction, social isolation, cyberbullying, and information overload.

First, dependence on technology, the virtual world, virtual interaction

Dependence on Information and Communication Technology (ICT) is one of the most common adverse effects of technology on people's lives. It represents a state of personal incontinence, loss of initiative, and disbelief in one's ability to solve problems without external help. This condition often results from the excessive use of ICT, leading to a loss of self-control and a distorted sense of time spent aimlessly online, searching for information without purpose, and immersing oneself in entertainment to escape reality. A study conducted by the Ho Chi Minh Communist Youth Union during 2014–2015 on "the impact of ICT on the ethics and lifestyle of adolescents in the current period" with 1,000 young people living in Hanoi and Danang found that 14.5% of adolescents show signs of ICT dependence. Additionally, teenagers who are active members of virtual friend groups on social networks and forums are more susceptible to adopting negative habits due to group pressure mechanisms (VNU USSH 2017, 347–354).

Furthermore, with technology, and more specifically the Internet, spending excessive time online can lead individuals to isolate themselves almost completely from the real world. The results of a sociological survey conducted in 2014 by Tran Thi Minh Duc and Bui Thi Hong Thai on 4,247 students in six major cities –Hanoi, Hai Phong, Vinh, Hue, Da Nang, and Ho Chi Minh City – revealed that students spend considerable time on social media: 43.5% of them between 1 and 3 hours per day, 31.5% from 3 to 5 hours per day, and about 7.2% go online for up to 8 hours per day (Tran & Bui 2014). Therefore, some Vietnamese youth today spend excessive time on and frequently use social networks. Despite the benefits of social networks, technology also adversely affects students and young people mentally, and in terms of health, learning, and work efficiency. Spending substantial time on social networks can distract them from their studies and lead them to chase virtual emotions and victories. Notably, children addicted to social networks may experience brain damage, causing cognitive decline, depression, and negativity.

Second, information overload affects the quality of relationships and makes people lonelier.

According to several studies, some people's reduced ability to communicate with family members, a shrinking social circle, and increased levels of depression and loneliness are associated with their time spent online (Linh 2022). Susan Pinker argues, "Without face-to-face contact, the socially poor also get poorer" (Pinker, 2014, p. 265). Regular face-to-face social connections can enhance physical and mental health by producing the hormone dopamine, which makes people happier, improves their study habits, and extends their lifespan. However, with the rapid advancement of technology today, people often feel lonelier because their interactions occur online rather than face-to-face and can sometimes be superficial. Technology can make us lazy, sometimes selfish, distant, and less interactive, reducing direct meetings and exchanges between individuals. Excessive use of social media also affects the quality of face-to-face relationships.

Dr. Elias Aboujaoude, a psychologist at Stanford University, commenting on the intersection between human psychology and technology, emphasizes: "The Internet confers new qualities like anonymity, virtual connectedness, omnipotence, and the possibility of personal reinvention" (Aboujaoude 2011, 220). However, spending a lot of time and energy on a multitude of 'virtual connections' can make real-life relationships less of a concern. He notes, "become excessively daring or less diplomatic in our day-to-day interactions and relationships, even when there is no open browser or iPhone in sight ... or felt away from the screen, in the form of tension at home, as when new Facebook friends start taking too much time away from family" (Aboujaoude 2011, 23). Similarly, the results of author Nguyen Mai Huong's research on the relationship between social media and human relationships show that the majority of respondents admitted that excessive social media use affected their relationships with parents and siblings at home. They also reported feeling isolated from relatives and friends. Furthermore, a high percentage of respondents said they had become quieter after using social media; specifically, as many as 54.7% of 150 respondents said they did not talk to their parents despite being at home because they were busy using social media; 80% think social media has taken away much time spent together; and 20.7% became more introverted(VNU USSH 2017, 302–311).

Due to easy access to the Internet, users spend considerable time and energy on virtual relationships and often feel insecure when they are not engaged in online activities. People frequently find themselves spending time on platforms like YouTube, Netflix, and Facebook because the data available is overwhelmingly vast; thus, they spend all day and night surfing social networks and tackling many tasks online, leading to overload and causing their brains to fall into a state of fatigue. Additionally, with a vast array of apps and network connections, users often do not feel the need to engage with others physically. As a result, they become ensnared in virtual realities and, when existing in real life, often feel isolated and lonely.

Moreover, people are easily manipulated by media discourses, such as companies publishing false advertising or exaggerating product effects. Nevertheless, people often believe these claims because they are broadcast publicly on television, leading them to spend money on advertised products. Furthermore, the rapid spread of media can also disseminate the inappropriate behavior of some individuals without verification, causing many to believe and emulate such behaviors, only to end up disappointed and, in some cases, financially depleted or falling into depression and negativity. According to a recent report by the Global Anti-Scam Alliance (GASA), Vietnam is currently a country with a high rate of online fraud. The report noted that there were 87,000 recorded cases of fraud in Vietnam, with Vietnamese network users losing 374 million USD in 2021 (Global Anti-Scam Alliance 2021). The situation continues to worsen as the number of network users increases; the Authority of Information Security reports that in the first six months of 2023, instances of online fraud in Vietnam increased by 64.78% over the same period last year and 37.82% compared to the last six months of 2022 (Microsoft 2023).

Besides, the constant novelty of technology also negatively affects individual happiness because people can hardly be satisfied with what they have when they are aware that others possess more or better things. Technological changes now occur so rapidly that when we purchase any technological product (like a mobile phone, computer, or television), we know there will be a better and faster version of that product in a few months. Consequently, we are left with outdated products while others acquire newer and more advanced technologies, which negatively affects our mental health.

Moreover, there are growing concerns about artificial intelligence replacing humans in many jobs, a trend likely to intensify as interactions between robots and humans increase. A Microsoft study from the 2023 Work Trends Index, which surveyed 31,000 people representing various occupations across 31 countries, including Vietnam, posed the question, "Will AI Fix work?". A report published on May 16 revealed that 54% of Vietnamese workers are worried that AI might replace their job positions, while up to 90% expressed a desire to delegate as much work as possible to AI to reduce their workload (49% and 70% globally, respectively) (Microsoft 2023). This data indicates that while there is optimism about the emergence of AI and a desire to utilize it to enhance work productivity and alleviate pressure on employees, the technology also leads to concerns about future job security for workers. Consequently, there may also be an underlying mentality of needing to compete more strenuously with AI.

Third, cyberbullying

In Vietnam, in recent years, cyberbullyinghas become a serious topic. With the rapid rise of digital tools, social media, messaging platforms, gaming, and mobile phones, more and more people, especially children and teenagers, are being bullied online. Cyberbullying is bullying with the use of digital technologies. It can occur on social media, messaging, gaming, and mobile phones. It is repeated behavior aimed at scaring, angering, or shaming those who are targeted (UNICEF 2023)

Some acts of cyberbullying are mainly detected in online communities such as fandoms, fan groups, and pages, where individuals bully the targeted person by isolating, alienating, and badmouthing them. Other forms of bullying include arbitrarily editing photos to provoke and mock, and using sexual symbols in online conversations to bully social media users.

A study of 500 high school students in Da Nang City, Vietnam, conducted in both a public and a private school, showed that 19.3% of students were perpetrators of cyberbullying and 16.7% had been victims. Specifically, 11.7% of students regularly engage in cyberbullying, and 7.6% do so very often, while 29% of students occasionally engage in cyberbullying. On the victims' side, 21.1% of students were bullied, 28.4% occasionally, and 7.7% were frequently bullied, with 9% very often. The report also found that the more time people spend on the Internet, the more likely they are to bully others online; students who bully others are more likely to be bullied in return. Many individuals who are bullied experience panic, irritability, and depression, which can even lead to suicide(VNU USSH 2017, 355–362).

A more in-depth study by a non-profit organization that provides peer counseling and mental health services to Vietnamese youth has yielded clearer results on the effects of cyberbullying on young people's psychophysiology. The study, which analyzed 1,345 responses from individuals affected by cyberbullying, utilized stratified sampling to focus on 550 samples. Among these, there were 473 respondents, including 45 males and 32 individuals who did not declare their gender, aged between 10 and 30, from both urban and rural areas. Notably, 45 men and 473 women reported being affected by cyberbullying, either as attackers or victims. A significant finding from the study is that 83%, or 460 respondents, experienced emotional and psychological changes after being bullied. Respondents reported feelings of panic, irritability, and depression, some even contemplating suicide.

Prominent acts of cyberbullying included negative comments on a 22-year-old female victim's profile and severe harassment, including rape threats through ask.fm accounts after a girl posted photos showing her breasts online. This resulted in numerous derogatory comments about her body and unwelcome sexual demands, leading her to carry knives and scissors to school for self-defense. Another case involved a 16-year-old girl who fell into severe depression, experienced a mental breakdown, and contemplated suicide due to cyberbullying. An 18-year-old and a 21-year-old expressed suicidal thoughts, the latter feeling compelled to stay online for a sense of care and attention. A 25-year-old woman, haunted by the bully's words and actions, attempted suicide but was ultimately rescued. Despite these severe consequences, many victims prefer to keep their experiences private and try to cope alone, with 19.8% of respondents expressing fear of judgment and believing that no one cares about their problems; 20.7% felt they could handle it themselves.

The research suggests that living in rural areas might be less prone to cyberbullying, possibly due to limited access to network devices like smartphones and computers. The study indicates that with more technological utility, the risk of cyber violence from anonymous users increases. As technology advances, the consequence is that cyberbullying escalates, significantly affecting individuals' emotions and psychology, both now and in the future. For those who have been victims, happiness in their future remains uncertain. For example, one male respondent from the study reported feeling consistently confused and scared whenever he saw any emoji from social media, as it brought back memories of being bullied with words like "stupid" or menacing greetings(VNU USSH 2017,313–323). This raises deep societal concerns and requires further multidimensional research to find suitable solutions.

4. Conclusion

The development of science and technology in Vietnam today has substantially impacted people's perceptions and emotions. People now have many tools to express themselves, create, and spread happiness; they also have numerous information channels to acquire knowledge, raise awareness, and express opinions both directly and indirectly to social management and development actors. Technology contributes to improving aesthetic qualifications and tastes, diversifying the aesthetic needs of the Vietnamese people, bringing confidence and joy to their lives. It helps individuals experience a range of emotions more profoundly, reduces the burden of hard work, and allows more time to enjoy life.

Nevertheless, technology also brings negative consequences for the happiness of individuals and society. These include the reduction in the quality of natural, emotional, and psychological relationships, especially as more young people experience bullying and isolation online; or even the spread of virtual values, which can delude many about their capabilities, potentially harming their development. Therefore, for society to achieve greater happiness, the process of technological development needs to be carried out comprehensively. This includes combining technological policies with social development policies, cultural development strategies, and enhancing the spiritual lives of people. Integrating technology projects to optimize the happy experiences for the masses, and aligning smart gadgets with human needs appropriately, are crucial. Above all, the development of technology must prioritize the interests of people and not just focus on economic growth.

References

Aboujaoude, E. 2011. *Virtually You: The Dangerous Powers of the E-Personality*. New York, NY: W.W. Norton.

Berry, J. W. 2020. How shall we all live together? In: S. Safdar, C. Kwantes, & W. Friedlmeier (Eds.), *Wiser world with multiculturalism: Proceedings from the 24th Congress of the International Association for Cross-Cultural Psychology*. https://scholarworks.gvsu.edu/iaccp_papers/284

Communist Party of Vietnam. 2021. The Internet is an essential infrastructure, an important component of digital transformation [online]. https://dangcongsan.vn/khoa-hoc/internet-la-ha-tang-thiet-yeu-thanh-to-quan-trong-cua-chuyen-doi-so-626820.html, (Accessed May 16, 2023).

Communist Party of Vietnam. 2022. Internet freedom in Vietnam is an undeniable fact [online]. https://dangcongsan.vn/bao-ve-nen-tang-tu-tuong-cua-dang/tu-do-internet-o-viet-nam-la-mot-thuc-te-khong-the-phu-nhan-626055.html, (Accessed July 22, 2023).

Datareportal. 2023. Digital 2023: Vietnam [online]. https://datareportal.com/reports/digital-2023-vietnam. (Access May 21, 2023).

Frey, B. S. & Stutzer, A. 2002. *Happiness and Economics, How the Economy and Institutions Affect Well-Being*, Princeton University Press.

Global Anti-Scam Alliance (GASA). 2021. Online Scams in Vietnam increased by 64.78% in the first 6 months of the year [online]. https://vneconomy.vn/lua-dao-truc-tuyen-tai-viet-nam-tang-64--78-trong-6-thang-dau-nam.htm, (Accessed July 23, 2023).

Helliwell, J., Layard, R., & Sachs, J. 2019. World Happiness Report 2019. New York: Sustainable Development Solutions Network.

Hong, D. N. 2020. A Study on The World Happiness Report – Lessons from Successful Countries. *Industry and Trade Magazine*, 7, 189–195.

Linh, N.T. 2022. Share happy feelings and express yourself on social networks [online]. https://lyluanchinhtrivatruyenthong.vn/chia-se-cam-xuc-hanh-phuc-va-the-hien-ban-than-tren-mang-xa-hoi-p26450.html, (Accessed July 21, 2023).

Long. P. 2022. Internet Day 2022: Vietnamese Internet users reach more than 70% of the population after 25 years [online]. https://vtv.vn/cong-nghe/internet-day-2022-nguoi-dung-internet-viet-nam-dat-hon-70-dan-so-sau-25-nam-20221204111428 02.htm, (Accessed May 21, 2023).

Mai, N. N & Linh, N.P.D. 2022. National happiness index – a new assessment indicator in "good governance". *State Management Magazine*, 1, 73–77.

Ministry of Education and Training (MET). 2019. 22 million Vietnamese students use social media [online]. https://giaoduc.net.vn/22-trieu-hoc-sinh-sinh-vien-viet-nam-su-dung-mang-xa-hoi-post203870.gd, (Accessed July 25, 2023).

Ministry of Industry and Trade (MIT). 2022. Vietnam E-Commerce and Digital Economy Agency, Ministry of Industry and Trade. The White Book on Vietnamese E-Business [online]. https://trungtamwto.vn/file/21930/bctmdt2022-final-pdf_08c88.pdf, pp 36–39 (Accessed July 18, 2023).

Microsoft. 2023. Work Trend Index: Annual Report [online]. https://assets.ctfassets.net/y8fb0rhks3b3/5eyZc6gDu1bzftdY6w3ZVV/93190f5a8c7241ecf2d6861bdc7fe3ca/WTI_Will_AI_Fix_Work_060723.pdf, pp. 25, (Accessed August 2, 2023).

Nhandan online. 2023. Zalo continues to be the most popular messaging app in Vietnam [online]. https://nhandan.vn/zalo-tiep-tuc-la-ung-dung-nhan-tin-pho-bien-nhat-viet-nam-post741283.html, (Accessed May 24, 2023).

Nham, N. 2022. Digital technology for human life [online]. https://dangcongsan.vn/khoa-hoc/cong-nghe-so-phuc-vu-cuoc-song-con-nguoi-602930.html, (Accessed May 23, 2023).

Phi, N.Q. 2022. Factors Affecting the Happiness of Workers. *Industry and Trade Magazine*, 13, 199–206.

People Army Newspaper (PAN). 2022. Vietnam's internet development is safe and sustainable [online]. https://www.qdnd.vn/kinh-te/cac-van-de/phat-trien-internet-viet-nam-an-toan-ben-vung-714298, (Accessed May 21, 2023).

PwC Vietnam. 2019. What's in the pioneering self-service restaurant chain in Vietnam? [online]. https://kenh14.vn/co-gi-trong-chuoi-hang-an-tu-phuc-vu-tien-phong-tai-viet-nam-2019032219 1434074.chn.

Q & Me. 2022. The popularity of social networks in Vietnam [online]. https://qandme.net/vi/baibaocao/muc-do-pho-bien-cua-mang-xa-hoi-tai-vietnam-2022.html, (Accessed May 24, 2023).

Pinker, S. 2014. *The Village Effect: How Face-to-Face Contact Can Make Us Healthier and Happier*. New York: Spiegel & Grau.

Tran, T.M.D & Bui, T.H.T. 2014. Use Of Social Networks Among University Students In Vietnam. *Vietnam Social Sciences*, 8(81): 50–60.

UNICEF. 2023. Cyberbullying: What is it and how to stop it [online]. https://www.unicef.org/end-violence/how-to-stop-cyberbullying, (Accessed May 21, 2023).

VET. 2023. Comprehensive inspection of TikTok's operations in Vietnam from May 15 [online]. https://vneconomy.vn/kiem-tra-toan-dien-hoat-dong-cua-tiktok-tai-viet-nam-tu-ngay-15--5.htm. (Accessed July 28, 2023).

Vnexpress.net. 2022a. Vietnam has 70,000 digital technology enterprises, https://vnexpress.net/viet-nam-co-70--000-doanh-nghiep-cong-nghe-so-4544939.html, (Accessed July 21, 2023).

Vnexpress.net. 2022b. Technology make people happy [online]. https://vnexpress.net/ong-truong-gia-binh-cong-nghe-phai-lam-con-nguoi-hanh-phuc-4544881-tong-thuat.html, (Accessed May 26, 2023).

Vnexpress.net. 2023. Businesses prefer the working model of 'now at home, tomorrow at work' [online]. https://vnexpress.net/doanh-nghiep-chuong-mo-hinh-lam-viec-nay-o-nha-mai-len-cong-so -4382873.html, (Accessed July 22, 2023).

Vietnam E-Commerce and Digital Economy Agency, Ministry of Industry and Trade (MIT). 2022. The White Book on Vietnamese E-Business [online]. https://trungtamwto.vn/file/21930/bctmdt2022-final-pdf_08c88.pdf, (Accessed July 18, 2023).

VNN. 2021a. Vietnamese people "burn time" on smartphones the most for Facebook [online]. https://vietnamnet.vn/nguoi-viet-dot-thoi-gian-tren-smartphone-nhieu-nhat-cho-facebook-734893.html, (Accessed May 21, 2023)

VNN. 2021b. Vietnam has 5,600 more Make in Vietnam technology enterprises [online]. https://vietnamnet.vn/viet-nam-co-them-5600-doanh-nghiep-cong-nghe-make-in-viet-nam -i399722.html, (Accessed May 22, 2023).

VNU-University of Social Sciences and Humanities. 2017. Human Well-being and Sustainable Development: Proceedings of International Conference the First Southeast Asia Regional Conference of Psychology. Hanoi: VNU Publishing House.

VTV. 2022. 87,000 online scams cases recorded in Vietnam [online]. https://vtv.vn/cong-nghe/87000-vu-lua-dao-qua-mang-duoc-ghi-nhan-tai-viet-nam-20221020170555126.htm. Accessed July 22, 2023.

WIPO. 2022. Global Innovation Index [online]. https://www.wipo.int/edocs/pubdocs/en/wipo-pub-2000--2022-section1-en-gii-2022-at-a-glance-global-innovation-index-2022--15th-edition.pdf, (Accessed May 21, 2023).

Contingency, Relationality, and Narrativity: Three Constitutive Aspects of Human Identity

Michal Valčo and Radoslav Hanus

1. Introduction

While we live in some of the most uncertain and decisive times for the human experience, our mutual effort to describe the nature of what it means to be human has never been so vital. Contingency, relationality and narrativity are key features of human existence, and like the famed labyrinth, they imperfectly co-exist, at times becoming entangled and at times disentangling themselves. This paper seeks to explore the interplay between contingency, relationality and narrativity as they are vital features of human experience and together form an integral framework to understand the human condition in modern times. Human contingency reminds us that we are vulnerable and interdependent beings, for it destroys the dream of self-sufficiency and situates us in a profoundly interconnected reality. In so doing, it changes how we view the world, and we are compelled to see the human in more vivid and existentially frail terms. The second component of our reflection on human contingency, relationality, highlights the fundamental ways in which we are interconnected. Relationality extends beyond human interactions, and our interconnection is not exclusively limited to a social nature, but extends to a divine connection that enriches our understanding of our dependence on the Other and situates our communal nature. The third part of our reflections on the nature and foundation of the human experience is narrativity. Narrativity highlights the power of stories for narrating selves and lives. The human is understood as a storyteller, a subject who dwells in historic human communities and narrates her or his existence.

Fundamental to this investigation is the understanding of the enormous effects of our inability to fully express ourselves as relational and real people because of innate corruption or sin. History has repeatedly demonstrated that this failure causes a chain reaction of depersonalization that finally dehumanizes and destroys the core of our humanity (Wojtyla 2013). Reevaluation is desperately needed, as seen by the emergence of personalism in philosophical debate from the ashes of catastrophic global events and the collapse of once-cherished ideologies. But personalism has its own conundrums; it swings between an inward concentration on oneself and a wider concern for all of mankind (Williams and Bengtsson 2022).

We combine theological analysis, historical context, and comparative narrative analysis in a mixed-methods approach. With each of them contributing a special perspective to our comprehension of the human story, Tillich (1965), Taylor (1989; 1991; 2003; 2007), MacIntyre (2007), Luther, Wojtyla (2013), Zizioulas (1985), and Pöhlmann (2002) are all consulted in this approach. A key component of our research is a theological study on imago Dei, a notion that Luther, Wojtyla, Pöhlmann, and Zizioulas, among others, have thoroughly examined to connect human relationality with divine relationality. This theological anthropology holds that because humans are made in God's image, they reflect the relational aspect of the divine. This viewpoint gives a helpful understanding of the relationship between human and divine nature that goes beyond simple individuality and includes our communal and spiritual aspects.

In exploring these ideas, we also participate in the critical conversation about transhumanism. With its emphasis on technology-enhanced human potential, this contemporary movement raises important theological, philosophical, and ethical issues. In light of possible technical change, it forces us to reevaluate the essence of human identity and dignity. In a society on the verge of significant transformation, our article is therefore a theological/anthropological investigation into the essence of what it is to be human. Through the prisms of contingency, relationality, and narrativity, the complexity of human identity is attempted to be untangled, therefore adding to the current discussion of what makes us human in the face of social change and technical breakthrough.

2. Contingency: The Existential Fabric of Human Existence

In the investigation of the human essence, the idea of contingency becomes essential and provides deep understanding of our existence, identity, and purpose. When used broadly, contingency describes the innate ambiguity and reliance that define human existence. Humans are contingent beings, entwined into a wider, interrelated reality that itself depends on a transcendent source, rather than being self-constituted individuals. Examining its ontological, ethical, and spiritual aspects as well as its significant ramifications for our comprehension of human identity, dignity, and the general story of creation, redemption, and fulfillment, this section seeks to peel back the layers of human contingency. This section will include Lutheran anthropology, which provides deep knowledge of this idea, especially in its conception of human nature as essentially sinful yet bearing the image of God (imago Dei).

2.1 The Ontological Dimension of Contingency

According to Tillich (1965), humans are not necessary entities but rather live in a position of "thrownness", which is a reflection of our temporal, constrained, and conditioned character. We are "tossed into existence" by forces that are beyond our comprehension or immediate control; this reality starts with our parents' biological act of conception of us. Deeply embedded in the human mind and experience, this ontological contingency evokes ontic, spiritual, and moral uneasiness. It is not just a philosophical concept. It molds how we see the world and ourselves, giving us awe and humility in the face of the enormous and enigmatic cosmos we live in.

2.2 The Ethical and Theological Aspects

According to phenomenology and ethics, human contingency shows up as our desire for purpose, fulfillment, and a moral life. Being dependent, we are not self-referential; our existence is intrinsically linked to a larger story that goes beyond each of our personal lives (Valčo and Šturák 2018). Themes of creation, atonement, and fulfillment are all included in this story, and each deepens our grasp of what it means to be human (Colorado 2014).

We are reminded, for example, of our interdependence with the world and its Creator by the story of creation. We are part of a deliberate and planned act of creation, not the outcome of random accident. This insight infuses a deep sense of obligation and thankfulness into our lives. We are required to meaningfully add to the world's story as it is being written, not just to exist. Redeeming also emphasizes how dependent we are on divine favor to reach our ultimate goal. It redefines what it is to be human, based as it does on our intrinsic value as God's created rather than our accomplishments or talents. This viewpoint recognizes our common vulnerability and contingency, therefore promoting a more inclusive and compassionate understanding of human dignity.

According to Lutheran doctrine, people are both sinners and saints living in a condition of "simul justus et peccator" (WA 56,272). This perspective emphasizes our innate limits, vulnerabilities, and dependence and is consistent with the idea of human contingency. Living thereby under the forgiving eye of a redemptive God is one of the conditions of being a contingent being from a Lutheran perspective. Within this Lutheran perspective, original sin emphasizes the element of human contingency. It explains, as Luther clarified, the intrinsic sinfulness of human nature (WA 39,1,174–180; WA 56,277,12). But our being inherently sinful does not make us less like God. "Even after the fall, this nature still is and remains a creature of God" (Pöhlmann 2002, 195), says the author. This contradiction in human nature, which combines fallen nature with divine image, captures the intricacy of human contingency.

The fulfillment story also asks us to consider our ultimate goal and fate in the larger scheme of the history of the globe. The quest of justice, love, and peace is part of the Creator's goal for the world, which we as contingent creations help to realize (Wojtyla 2013). This knowledge gives our life direction and purpose and motivates us to reach our greatest potential as individuals and as members of a community.

A more encompassing, sympathetic, and meaningful understanding of what it is to be human results from accepting our sensitivity and contingency. It serves as a reminder of our basic relationality – our need for and reliance on people, both divine and human. This relational component of contingency provides a counter-narrative to the isolated, independent self frequently praised in contemporary culture. It is not a weakness but rather a source of strength and solidarity. We thus argue that realizing the transience of human existence and our position in the larger stories of creation, atonement, and fulfillment enhances our comprehension of human identity, dignity, and potential. It emphasizes how interrelated, dependent, and wonderful life is, and it motivates us to live a life that accepts and values these basic realities.

Relationality: The Interconnected Self

Relationality becomes a key idea in the attempt to understand the core of the human being since it provides a deep insight of our existence as intrinsically linked entities. Foundational to human existence, identity development, and community cohesiveness is relationship.

To get beyond the bounds of phenomenological personalism is necessary on the path to a relational knowledge of the human person. Even if phenomenological personalism offers insightful knowledge about human experience, it frequently falls short in establishing a thorough basis for human rights and dignity. For example, the whole of human personality is not sufficiently explained by concentrating only on the individual's intrinsic abilities, such reason, emotion, or will. This kind of thinking misses the point of relationality, which is a fundamental aspect of who we are rather than merely an extra (Grenz 2001; 2002; Zizioulas 1985).

3.1 Taylor's Dichotomy: Buffered vs. Porous Self

Understanding relationality in the contemporary setting is made crucial by Charles Taylor's 2008 contrast of the "Buffered vs. Porous Self". With meanings and purposes coming only from within, the "buffered self" represents the contemporary autonomous person cut off from the outside world. By contrast, the "porous self" is by nature responsive and open to the world outside of the mind. This porousness suggests that the people and places in our lives have an impact on our deepest feelings and meanings. Taylor's distinction highlights the glaring difference between a self-contained individualism and an intrinsically connected self.

> "The dominance of instrumental rationality in our world and the ubiquity of the secular age go hand in hand. The *buffered identity of a* disciplined individual moves in a constructed social space in which instrumental rationality is a key value and time is secular through and through. This is all what I call the immanent frame. To this must be added only one idea behind it: that this framework creates a natural order, which must be seen in contrast to the supernatural order; an immanent world as opposed to a possible transcendent world". (Taylor 2007, 542)

3.2 The Constitutive Nature of Relationality

Relationality is not merely a characteristic of the human person; it is fundamental to our existence. Being a gift of relational love, we are shaped by a network of interactions that form our identity and sense of belonging from birth. As seen by the close relationship that develops between a mother and child, this relational matrix starts well before self-awareness. Known by developmental psychologists as psychological imprinting, this relationship is intricate and essential to the formation of the self. It emphasizes how relationships, both chosen and given (as with family) constantly interact to create our identity (Valčo and Šturák 2018, 293).

Deeply based on Martin Luther's theology, Lutheran anthropology stresses how human beings are inherently relational – not just to God but also to one another. Luther emphasizes the intricacy of human interactions when he describes the human state as "simul justus et peccator", or simultaneously sinner and saint. It implies that, although sin has left humans fundamentally defective, divine grace has also enabled them to have deep relationships with God and other people. This viewpoint fits very nicely with Charles Taylor's idea of the "Porous Self", which holds that our relationships with other people and our environment have an impact on our innermost feelings and meanings (Taylor 1989; 2003). Within the Lutheran framework, this porousness also has a spiritual dimension in which people are receptive to the power and mercy of God.

Relationality thus plays a critical role in the formation of individual identity and the cohesion of communities. Our interactions with others – through communication, shared experiences, and mutual understanding – forge our personal identities. As we engage with the world, our sense of self evolves, influenced by the narratives, symbols, and rituals that we share with our community (MacIntyre 2007). This communal aspect of relationality is vital in fostering a sense of belonging and solidarity, which is crucial for the health and sustainability of any society.

But in this day of growing individualism and technology breakthroughs, the idea of relationality has many difficulties. Many people now feel disconnected and alone because of the emergence of the "buffered self", which undermines the innate interconnection that is essential for human development. We think that realizing how important relationship is creates chances to rebuild relationships and strengthen communal links.

It stresses the need of empathy, interdependence, and reciprocal care and asks us to rethink how we see ourselves and society. Not just a quality, but the core of what it is to be human is relationship. Offering a more complex, interwoven picture of human existence, it questions the contemporary idea of the independent, self-contained individual. Viewing ourselves, our interactions with others, and our place in the larger fabric of life are all profoundly impacted by accepting relationality as a fundamental part of who we are. We can really understand the intricacy and beauty of the human experience only through this lens of interconnection.

3. Narrativity: Crafting the Human Story

Narrative is an essential component in the complex fabric of human existence as it shapes our conception of experience and identity. Explored in this part is the complex field of narrativity, including its function in the creation of individual and collective identities, its impact on human development, and its importance for psychological and social well-being.

As MacIntyre defined it, narrative places people essentially as "storytelling animals". Understanding human identity and experience requires this viewpoint since tales are how we make sense of our lives and the world around us. Stories have meanings and interpretations that influence how we see the world, not just being accounts of what happened.

> "A central thesis then begins to emerge: man is in his actions and practice, as well as in his fictions, essentially a story-telling animal. He is not essentially, but becomes through his history, a teller of stories that aspire to truth. But the key question for men is not about their own authorship; I can only answer the question, 'What am I to do?' if I can answer the prior question, 'Of what story or stories do I find myself a part?' We enter human society, that is, with one or more imputed characters – roles into which we have been drafted – and we have to learn what they are in order to be able to understand how others respond to us and how our responses to them are apt to be construed". (MacIntyre 2007, 216)

MacIntyre's conception invites us to view narrativity as an essential lens through which human life is understood and experienced. The concept of narrative identity plays a crucial role in how individuals perceive and construct their sense of self. It involves weaving together life experiences into a coherent story/narrative that integrates the past, present, and future. This narrative is not static but continually evolves, reflecting the fluidity and continuity of human identity. Personal and collective histories are interwoven in this narrative tapestry, each influencing and shaping the other.

> "It is because we all live out narratives in our lives and because we understand our own lives in terms of the narratives that we live out that the form of a narrative is appropriate for understanding the actions of others. Stories are lived before they are told – except in the case of fiction". (MacIntyre 2007, 211–212)

When told dynamically, stories help to shape how one sees oneself and how one grows personally. Our own and others' stories shape our perceptions of ourselves and our place in the world; they are not merely passive reflections (Jenson 1993). MacIntyre's observations show how socially embodied traditions, through personal tales, shape our perceptions of both ourselves and our community. These narratives, which revolve on important topics and life events, are essential to the development and metamorphosis of identity.

Personal and group identity development are double functions of embodied narratives. This section of the conversation combines Kierkegaardian emphasis on personal introspection and responsibility with MacIntyrean emphasis on socially embodied historical traditions. It exposes how stories, based in our social and historical backgrounds, shape our own identities and also help to define our communities as a whole.

Furthermore acting as a link between relational empathy and personal comprehension is narrative. Shared personal stories help people better understand themselves and others. The communal component of identity creation and the interdependence of human relationships are highlighted by this process, which also fosters social cooperation. Lastly, the part narrativity plays in social and psychological health is discussed. In the field of psychotherapy, rewriting one's story can result in a person's life making tremendously good improvements. Furthermore, storytelling is also important for strengthening community ties and a shared sense of identity in social and educational settings. The therapeutic and social features of narrativity emphasize its value for society building as well as for individual growth.

4. Synthesis: The Interplay of Contingency, Relationality, and Narrativity

Deeply entwined ideas, contingency, relationality, and narrativity each affect and are affected by the others. Because it emphasizes how dependent and non-self-sufficient human existence is, human contingency draws attention to our basic need for stories and relationships. Our lives are shaped and given significance by a wider network of relationships and stories than by an isolated occurrence. We are all interrelated as everyone of us has a story that is molded by their interactions and unforeseen events. Relationship, then, is not only a result of our contingency but also a primary factor in how our stories are formed. Our relationships – both divine and human – form the narratives we create about the world and ourselves. These stories are the outcome of a complicated network of relationships that determine our identity and position in the world; they are not produced in a vacuum. A basic human quality, narrative offers the relational and contingent parts of our life structure and purpose. Influenced by our connections and changing circumstances, the tales we create enable us to make sense of our lives and locate our role in the greater story of creation, atonement, and fulfillment.

Philosophically, this synthesis emphasizes the interwoven and narrative character of human experience rather than the idea of the autonomous, self-determined individual. It challenges conventional philosophical ideas of identity and agency by arguing that they are greatly impacted by our relationships and unforeseen situations rather than being the result of our own reasoning or will.

Theologically speaking, this synthesis provides a deep grasp of people as made in the image of a relational God. Understanding human relationality is profoundly facilitated by the Christian theology of the Trinity, which presents God as a communion of persons (or different centers of consciousness). Our interactions with other people and our place in the story of creation are mirror images of the divine. Based in their creation in the image of a relational God and their involvement in the divine story, this theological perspective highlights the dignity and worth of every person. Moreover, the combination of these elements provides knowledge of the Christian concept of fulfillment and atonement. Through our stories, we represent our dependent and relational existence, which is aimed toward a bigger goal than itself. The Christian story of redemption presents a fresh story of hope and change by telling of a God who enters our relational and contingent existence. Moving toward the ultimate fulfillment of all creation in God, this story urges us to engage in the divine life.

So we have come to contend that a thorough framework for comprehending human existence and identity is provided by the synthesis of contingency, relationality, and narrativity. With roots in both theological and philosophical views, this paradigm highlights how human life is narrative and interwoven. It asks for a more profound comprehension of humans as relational and legendary beings, whose lives are influenced by and find their ultimate meaning in their involvement in the divine story, challenging individualistic and autonomous notions of the self. The human person is thus understood:

> "as a personal, holistic unity of […] ontology and ethics as they were captivated by the Gospel narrative, integrating them with transcendent, spiritual realities. These provide an invaluable life orientation, inner motivational force, along with a structure of meaning and purpose. While the spiritual aspect of human existential experience can be expressed through biopsychosocial media, it should be distinguished as a unique, separate anthropological entity that overlaps into transcendent reality. Spiritual etiology, among other things, adds valuable insight into the multifaceted socio-ethical discourse in the contemporary debate between the secularists and those who point out a world-wide resurgence of religious traditions and new forms of spirituality". (Valčová and Pavlíková 2016, 100–101)

5. Philosophical and Theological Implications

Rich philosophical and theological implications are invited by the deep synthesis of contingency, relationality, and narrativity in human experience. Engaging the ideas of Zizioulas, Levinas, Buber, and others, this section investigates the depth of human relationality as a mirror of the interior relationality of the triune God as well as theological reflections on human personhood and the function of narrativity. Fundamentally, the classical, ecumenical theology tries to explain how, and to what degree, the imago Dei is maintained in humans while they are corrupted, or *status corruptionis*.

6.1 Human Relationality as a Reflection of Divine Relationality

Human relationality is, according to Christian theology, a deep mirror of the inner relationality of the triune God rather than just a social quality. In his emphasis on the communal aspect of existence, Zizioulas (2006) finds resonance with this notion. Within the Trinity, the idea of perichoresis – the mutual indwelling of the Father, Son, and Holy Spirit – offers a paradigm for human relationship. It implies that our connections are fundamental to who we are and not just outside associations. In this sense, the viewpoint of Levinas (1999) of the "Other" as an absolute, static entity finds a dynamic counterpart. Seeing the "Other" as an essential component of our relationship life rather than as a far-off, static entity is made possible by the Christian idea of God as a relational person. The dialogical principle of Buber (1970) in "I and Thou" deepens this comprehension by highlighting the reciprocal and mutual character of relationship.

6.2 Theological Reflections on Human Personhood

Understanding human personhood is made compellingly possible by the Christian notion of imago Dei, the image of God. In place of the contemporary idea of the self-sufficient, independent individual, it suggests a view of the self as essentially social and communal (International Theological Commission 2002). Advocating for a collective definition of personhood, this viewpoint is consistent with the criticism of the destabilized Nietzschean self and the "therapeutic self" of contemporary psychology.

Personhood as seen by Zizioulas (2006) is an ontological phenomenon rather than an individualized endeavor. This relational perspective is expressed by the Eastern Fathers' clarification of the difference between "image" and "likeness" in theological anthropology. Though a process firmly based in relationships and love, we are created in God's image and grow into His likeness.

Lutheran theologians like Paul Tillich and Wolfhart Pannenberg contend that the fate of Jesus, in his openness to God and the world at the same time, embodies the essence of mankind. Theologically speaking, it is unavoidably true that humans are not physiologically characterized. Still, we can characterize their destiny and some of their essence, which was the main focus of the German reformer Martin Luther's thoughts.

Typical of German Reformation theology, Pöhlmann makes a distinction between *imago generaliter* and *imago specialiter*. God is basically reflected in humans. In Christ, the imago Dei par excellence, their sin-marked imago specialiter is restored, yet their *imago generaliter* is kept even in status corruptionis. Pöhlmann discovers the *imago generaliter* in the human individuality, in their humanum, which is most expressed in connection to God and their fellow human beings. It is evident that theological discussion of humans cannot proceed without discussing their destiny and nature, most especially, *de peccato*, about sin.

Sin characterizes human behavior in connection to God, other people, and the environment. Peccatumoriginale e peccatumactuale are thus same since "sin is being and action, fate and guilt in one" (Pöhlmann 2002, 218). It violates human nature and is more than just unlike from God.

To be sure, "Even after the fall this nature still is and remains a creature of God" (BC FC I. 2000, 488). Original or inherited sin is described by the Formula of Concord as "a corruption so deep that there is nothing sound or uncorrupted left in the human body or soul, in its internal or external powers" (BC FC I. 2000, 488), adding that "the damage is such that only God alone can separate human nature and the corruption of this nature from each other". "This separation will take place completely through death, at the resurrection" (BC FC I. 2000, 489).

Disbelief in God, which comes before any impulse of human free will, is the fundamental sin according to the German Reformation. Human will is inverted because selfishness and conceit that arise from disbelief separate people from God. Humans are thus unable of upholding the law, which is the Ten Commandments. The reason is the inversion of will; they are unable to keep the First and most important commandment, which is to fear, love, and trust God above anything else.

But human predicament before God and, in the end, in their deeds toward the world is not hopelessly in a dead end. By the grace of Christ, God deems sinners to be righteous outside of the law. God forgives and accomplishes new things on people because of the merit of Christ, not because of what is in them. "We receive forgiveness of sin and become righteous before God out of grace for Christ's sake through faith when we believe that Christ has suffered for us and that for his sake our sin is forgiven and righteousness and eternal life are given to us" (BC AC IV. 2000, 38–40). By the grace of involvement in a life-giving relationship, the human agent whose inner self has been re-aligned with the transcendent Other, "recaptures" and "internalizes" our relatedness to the divine. As Maritain aptly reminds us:

> "The relatedness of human persons to the divine, Transcendent Whole, predisposes them to be related in the proper way to the common good of the Universe, that is, the created realm. … The notion of grace points us beyond the immanent frame of this world towards transcendence; this is so because the free act of the human person, considered in its pure and secret intimacy as a free act, is not of this world. By its liberty/freedom, the human person transcends the stars and all the world of nature" (Maritain, 1966: 18–20).

6.3 Role of Narrativity in Theological Reflection

The relational character of human existence is articulated and understood in this theological thought largely through narrative. Not only are the tales we create and live by personal, but they also form a part of a greater divine story. This realization helps us to realize how our stories are entwined with the stories of others and with the larger story of creation, atonement, and fulfillment.

Narrativity in the Christian tradition is a means of taking part in the divine story as well as a matter of individual or group identification. With its themes of creation, fall, redemption, and new creation, the biblical story offers a structure inside which our personal and collective stories find meaning.

It is shown that a rich area of philosophical and theological study is opened up by the synthesis of contingency, relationality, and narrativity in human existence. It forces us to reconsider how we define personhood – from individualism to a relational and group conception of the self. Inviting us into a closer contact with the divine and with one another, this synthesis also challenges us to view our lives not as separate stories but as a part of the great story of God's creation.

6. Conclusion

It is evident when we conclude this investigation that the interaction of narrativity, relationality, and contingency offers a deep and workable framework for comprehending human identity and existence.

We started by looking at human contingency, which exposed our basic reliance and weakness. With its challenge to the delusion of independence, this idea places people in a larger, more interwoven fabric of life. The second element, relationship, emphasizes how essentially interrelated people are to the divine as well as to one another. Narrativity, which emphasises the ability of stories – especially those embedded in past human communities – to shape our identities and experiences, enriches this knowledge even further. These three elements taken together provide a thorough prism through which to see human experience, dignity, and rights, promoting a comprehensive perspective that goes beyond reductionist viewpoints. This three-tiered structure has a wide range of ramifications for upcoming theological and philosophical debate. Theologically speaking, this synthesis begs a more thorough examination of the idea of imago Dei and a reworking of human identity in connection to the divine. It pushes theologians to think about how the interdependence of relationality, narrativity, and contingency might provide new perspectives on ideas like creation, redemption, and eschatology. Philosophically speaking, this framework makes one reevaluate what personality, identity, and ethics are all about. It challenges philosophers to investigate how relationality and contingency shape our ethical frameworks and self-concepts as well as to interact more fully with the story side of human existence. With its wide ground for discussion between philosophy and theology, this method encourages cooperative investigation of these essential elements of human existence.

Moreover, this strong anthropological framework provides important new perspectives on how to tackle the problems raised by transhumanism. Unlike transhumanist emphasis on technology advancement and possible modification of human nature, our tripartite framework of contingency, relationality, and narrativity highlights the intrinsic worth and interconnectedness of human beings in their inherent fragility and limitations. This viewpoint emphasizes the ethical ramifications of technical developments for human identity and society in addition to reiterating the need of human dignity and agency. It makes a strong case against the reductionist and dispersed picture of humanity put out by transhumanist ideologies for appreciating the whole and interwoven character of human existence. It therefore begs a reassessment of the interaction between technology and humans, calling for a harmony that respects the richness and complexity of the human experience. We need to rediscover the idea of agape, or unselfish love, more than a human superman. Such idea leads us to develop epistemic humility in our understanding and evaluation of our basic nature and constraints. It supports a modest approach in our conversations with people from all origins and cultures, in line with a hermeneutic inquiry of the Gadamerian kind that emphasizes sincere and honest communication. This viewpoint also fosters an attitude of unselfish, selfless service and deeds of love shown to everyone, even to those we may first think are unworthy of such compassion. We may better negotiate the complexity of the human condition and promote a more compassionate, connected, and morally sound society by incorporating this method into our life experience.

References

Buber, M. 1970. *I and thou*. W. Kaufmann (trans.). New York: Scribner

Colorado, C.D. 2014. Transcendent Sources and the Dispossession of the Self. In: Colorado C. D. and Klassen, J. D. (eds.), *Aspiring to Fullness in a Secular Age: Essays on Religion and Theology in the work of Charles Taylor*. Notre Dame, IN: University of Notre Dame Press, 2014, pp. 73–97.

Frankl, V.E. 1984. *Man's Search for Meaning: An Introduction to Logotherapy*, 3rd edition, New York, Touchstone Book.

Grenz, S.J. 2001. *The Social God and the Relational Self: A Trinitarian Theology of the Imago Dei. Vol. 1, The Matrix of Christian Theology*. Louisville: Westminster John Knox.

Grenz, S.J. 2002. The social God and the relational self: Toward a theology of the Imago Dei in the postmodern context. *Horizons in Biblical Theology*, 24(1): 33–57.

International Theological Commission. 2002. Communion and Stewardship: Human Persons Created in the Image of God. [online]. Vatican, http://www.vatican.va/roman_curia/congregations/cfaith/cti_documents/rc_con_cfaith_doc_20040723_communion-stewardship_en.html

Jenson, R.W. 1993. How the World Lost Its Story. *First Things*, 36(10): 19–24. https://www.firstthings.com/article/1993/10/how-the-world-lost-its-story

Kearney, R. 2016. Transcendent Humanism in a Secular Age: A Dialogue With Charles Taylor. In: Kearney, R. and Zimmerman, J. (eds), *Reimagining the Sacred: Richard Kearney Debates God*. New York, NY: Columbia University Press, 2016, pp. 76–92.

Kolb, R., Wengert, T.J. &Arand, C.P. (eds.). 2000. *The Book of Concord: The Confessions of the Evangelical Lutheran Church*. Minneapolis: Fortress Press [cited as: BC].

Levinas, E. 1999. *Alterity and transcendence*. Columbia: Columbia University Press.

Luther, M. 1535/1883. Disputationen 1535/38. Band I. In: *Martin Luther Werke, Vol. 39. Kritische Gesamtausgabe*. Ed. J.F.K. Knaake, et al. Weimar 1883. [citedas: WA 39].

Luther, M. 1515/18883. Römervorlesung (Hs.) 1515/16. In: *Martin Luther Werke, Vol. 56. Kritische Gesamtausgabe*. Ed. J.F.K. Knaake, et al. Weimar 1883. [cited as: WA 56].

MacIntyre, A. 2007. *After Virtue: A Study in Moral Theory*. Notre Dame, IN: University of Notre Dame Press.

Maritain, J. 1966. *The person and the common good*. New York: Charles Scribner's Sons.

Pöhlmann, H. G. 2002. *Kompendium evangelickédogmatiky*. Jihlava: Mlýn.

Pope Francis. 2015. *Encyclical Letter 'Laudatosi'*. Rome: Libreria Editrice Vaticana.

Taylor, C. 1989. *Sources of the Self: The Making of the Modern Identity*. Cambridge, MA: Harvard University Press.

Taylor, C. 1991. *The Malaise of Modernity*. Concord, ON: Anansi Press.

Taylor, C. 2003. Ethics and Ontology. *The Journal of Philosophy*, 100(6): 305–320. *JSTOR*, JSTOR, wwwjstor.org/stable/3655731.

Taylor, C. 2007. *A Secular Age*. Cambridge Massachusetts – London, UK: Harvard University Press.

Taylor, C. 2008. Buffered and porous selves. In: *The Immanent Frame: Secularism, religion, and the public sphere* [online], Social Science Research Council, 2008. Available at: https://tif.ssrc.org/2008/09/02/buffered-and-porous-selves/

Tillich, P. 1965. *Ultimate concern*. New York: Harper & Row.

Valčo, M. and P. Šturák. 2018. The "Relational Self": Philosophical-Religious Reflections in Anthropology and Personalism. *XLinguae: European Scientific Language Journal*, 11(1): 289–299.

Valčová, K., Pavlíková, M. & Roubalová, M. 2016. Religious Existentialism as a Countermeasure to Moralistic Therapeutic Deism. *Communications: Scientific Letters of the University of Zilina*, 18(3): 98–104.

Williams, T. D. & Bengtsson, J.O. 2022. "Personalism". In: *The Stanford Encyclopedia of Philosophy* (Summer 2022 Edition), Edward N. Zalta (ed.). https://plato.stanford.edu/archives/sum2022/entries/personalism/ (accessed: 20 Sep 2023).

Wojtyla, K. 2013. *Love and responsibility*. Translated by Grzegorz Ignatik. Boston: Pauline Books & Media.

Zizioulas, J.D. 1985. *Being as communion: Studies in personhood and the church* (No. 4). Crestwood, NY: RSM Press.

Zizioulas, J.D. 2006. *Communion and otherness: Further studies in personhood and the church*. London: T & T Clark.

Transhumanism as a Techno-Gnostic Challenge to Theological Antropology

Michal Valčo

1. Introduction

Fundamental concerns regarding the nature of humans and their capacity for technological change are addressed in the fascinating and complicated subject of "Transhumanism as a Techno-Gnostic Challenge to Theological Anthropology". Nevertheless, talking about this topic comes with its own set of difficulties, mostly because it is hard to define what it means to be human and since Transhumanism and Gnosticism are two very different ideologies.

Examining the relationship between religious anthropology and transhumanism, one of the main issues is the disputed conception of human nature (Roughley 2023; Hull 1986; de Sousa 2000). Any essentialist definition of a human being has been called into question by posthumanist philosophers. They contend that biological, cultural, and technological elements all influence the ongoing evolution of human identity (Chesi 2022; Braidotti 2017; Cord 2022; Haraway 2010). This viewpoint is consistent with Buddhist ideas of non-dualism, which further refutes the notion of a fixed human essence and suggests that distinctions between the self and the world are arbitrary and illusory, and impermanence, which hold that all phenomena, including human existence, are in a continuous state of change and flux (Loy 2019). Posthumanism, which frequently challenges the distinctions between natural and artificial, human and non-human, finds resonance in such reasoning. An unique and unchanging human essence/nature is further complicated by the idea of inevitable interconnectedness, which holds that all phenomena are intrinsically interconnected and mutually influencing.

Complicating things even more, generalizations regarding the objectives, beliefs, and connection to theological anthropology are challenging to make about both Transhumanism and Gnosticism because they both include a broad range of movements and concepts. As our investigation of transhumanism has shown, there are several sub-movements with different foci and goals, some of which are more directly related to Gnostic ideas than others. Gnosticism itself, too, is not a monolithic tradition but rather consists of several currents and manifestations over time (King 2003; Marjanen 2009).

Given this complexity, it is imperative to approach this subject with a sophisticated awareness of the various viewpoints and difficulties that emerge while investigating the junctions of Theological Anthropology, Gnosticism, and Transhumanism. By doing do, we may better understand the complex tapestry of concepts and opportunities that these movements offer, as well as their consequences for our knowledge of human nature and capacity for change.

Through a comparison of Transhumanism and Gnosticism, I hope to offer a critical viewpoint on the movement. I contend that transhumanism – more especially, some of its more radical manifestations – can be considered a kind of techno-Gnosticism. This is noteworthy since it shows that transhumanism is not a new invention but rather the continuation of a long-standing human ambition to get beyond our physical bounds and reach a higher degree of knowledge and applied understanding, which is supposed to have a liberating or even redemptive impact on humanity. Like Gnostics, transhumanists use knowledge and manipulation of reality to try to escape the bounds of the material world. Building on the idea of Gnosticism, which holds that the human body is to be overcome as something inherently limiting, low, and detestable and that salvation (or: liberation, elevation, fulfillment) comes through secret knowledge or gnosis, I will examine the philosophical and theological foundations of transhumanism and its implications for our understanding of human nature, ethics, and spirituality. I will also contend that transhumanism raises significant issues about the relationship between technology and human flourishing. Even as transhumanism presents exciting opportunities for human improvement, any attempt to achieve a transhumanist future must carefully weigh the substantial risks and difficulties associated with it.

2. The Concept of Gnosticism

During the first several centuries of the Common Era, a collection of theological and philosophical doctrines known as Gnosticism were common in the ancient world, particularly in the Mediterranean area. Gnostic groups were distinguished by their conviction that secret knowledge (gnosis) is essential to salvation, their dualistic conception of the universe – which holds that there is a higher, divine realm and a lower, material realm – and their conviction that the material world is intrinsically evil and defective (King 2003). Though the bulk of Gnostic doctrines hold that the human body is only a vehicle or shell for the actual, divine self, it would be false to argue that Gnostics see themselves as robots. Rather, they hold that people are entrapped in a physical form and that they can escape their material existence and re-unite with the divine by spiritual enlightenment and self-knowledge (Marjanen 2009).

The main exponents of Gnosticism in the first and third centuries and their pertinent opinions to our subject are summarized below:

Simon Magus: Simon Magus was a Samaritan who is considered to be the founder of a Gnostic sect known as Simonianism. According to Gnostic writings, Simon believed that he was the embodiment of the divine logos, and that he had come to save humanity from the ignorance of the material world. Simonianism emphasized the importance of secret knowledge for salvation and viewed the material world as a prison for the soul.

Valentinus: Valentinus was a Christian Gnostic who developed a complex system of cosmology that emphasized the existence of a divine realm and a lower, material realm. Valentinus believed that the material world was the product of a mistake made by the divine realm, and that salvation came through the acquisition of secret knowledge that allowed one to ascend to the spiritual realm.

Basilides: Basilides was a Gnostic teacher who lived in Alexandria during the second century. Basilides believed that the universe was created by a series of emanations from the divine realm, and that the material world was the product of the lowest of these emanations. Basilides believed that the soul could be liberated from the material world through the acquisition of secret knowledge.

Carpocrates: Carpocrates was a Gnostic teacher who believed that the soul could be liberated from the material world through the pursuit of personal freedom and pleasure. Carpocrates believed that the material world was the product of an evil creator, and that salvation came through the pursuit of the true self through pleasure.

Marcion: Marcion was a Gnostic teacher who believed that the God of the Old Testament was different from the God of the New Testament, and that the God of the Old Testament was an evil creator. Marcion believed that the material world was the product of this evil creator, and that salvation came through the rejection of the material world and the acceptance of the spiritual realm.

The major proponents of Gnosticism all rejected the material world as intrinsically wicked and believed that secret knowledge was essential to redemption. Each of them thought that by learning secret knowledge or rejecting the material world, one might escape the confines of the human body and reach a higher condition of existence. As it happens, a deep contempt for the physical body and the constraints of temporal life is at the heart of Gnostic philosophy. This dualistic worldview sharply divided the mind, which was thought to be spiritual and maybe immortal, from the body, which was seen to be corrupt and inferior. This contradiction was interestingly (or perhaps rather revealingly) expressed by Gnosticism in two opposing behavioral tendencies: asceticism, which rejected physical pleasures as unworthy, and libertinism, which, considering the alleged depravity of the body (Carpocrates), indulged in physical pleasures without moral restraint.

These views are pertinent to our subject since they show how Gnosticism and transhumanism, which both aim to use knowledge and manipulation of reality to overcome the constraints of the material world, are related. Gnostics frequently followed ascetic actions because they firmly believed that the material world and our bodily bodies were meaningless or even degrading. They might, for example, go on protracted fasts, follow strict diets, or give up sexual activity entirely. Most Gnostics saw physical pleasures as diversion from more important goals, and in more severe situations, as wicked diversions that took them away from their true calling.

As was already noted, Carpocrates stood in for the less prevalent libertarian branch of Gnosticism.

3. Contemporary Transhumanism

The term 'transhumanism' was first coined in the mid-20th century by evolutionary biologist Julian Huxley in the 1950s. So Julian Huxley is generally regarded as the founder of transhumanism (1957). Another one is Max More, the author of "Principles of Extropy" (1990) and founder of Extropy Institute (1992). In 1998, philosophers Nick Bostrom and David Pearce founded the World Transhumanist Association (WTA), which in 2008 became known as Humanity+. Then we have the American Sociologist and bioethicist James Hughes, former executive director of WTA (Valčo 2021, 112). Other notable names: Ray Kurzweil, Natasha Vita-More, Steven Fuller, Zoltan Istvan etc.

Over the past thirty years, transhumanism has expanded as a philosophy and field of study that uses cutting edge technology to better the lot of humanity. Its foundation is thus the developments of the Fourth Industrial Revolution (Schwab 2014). Multidisciplinary and incorporating many scientific and technological disciplines, transhumanism includes biology, neurology, engineering, computer science, and psychology. With the speed at which technology has advanced recently, it is now feasible to imagine a day when people would be able to live longer, think better, and perform better physically. Many and extensive potential advantages of transhumanism have created a significant lot of interest and excitement in the subject.

When it comes to defining what Transhumanism actually is and wishes to achieve, we turn to Max More and his early definition of the movement:

> "Transhumanism is a class of philosophies that seek to guide us towards a posthuman condition. Transhumanism shares many elements of humanism, including a respect for reason and science, a commitment to progress, and a valuing of human (or transhuman) existence in this life rather than in some supernatural "afterlife". Transhumanism differs from humanism in recognizing and anticipating the radical alterations in the nature and possibilities of our lives resulting from various sciences and technologies".(More 1996)

The World Transhumanist Association gave the following definition (originally in 2001):

> "(1) The intellectual and cultural movement that affirms the possibility and desirability of fundamentally improving the human condition through applied reason, especially by developing and making widely available technologies to eliminate aging and to greatly enhance human intellectual, physical, and psychological capacities.
>
> (2) The study of the ramifications, promises, and potential dangers of technologies that will enable us to overcome fundamental human limitations, and the related study of the ethical matters involved in developing and using such technologies. [...]
>
> We can also use technological means that will eventually enable us to move beyond what some would think of as 'human.'" (Humanity+ 2016)

Humanity is seen by some transhumanists as a stage of consciousness evolution. In this perspective, the idea that transcends conventional Transhumanism into the domain of Posthumanism is that the importance of humanity stems from its capacity to open the door for the creation of sophisticated sentient life forms. This philosophy promotes human capacities being developed beyond their inherent limits through a human-guided evolutionary process. With the ultimate goal of immortality, this includes attempts to greatly extend the healthy human lifetime.

3.1 Three New Civil Liberties

Three new civic liberties are suggested by transhumanists to guarantee that people may decide freely about their own bodies and minds, as well as their reproduction, free from coercion or undue interference. These liberties are procreative, morphological, and cognitive (Valčo 2021, 113).

Cognitive liberty is the ability of a person to manage their own mental processes, cognitive capacities, and states of awareness. This covers having the freedom to improve cognitive skills such memory, focus, intelligence, or emotional health by using different methods and technologies. As long as these decisions do not violate the rights and liberties of others, cognitive freedom also includes the freedom to decide whether or not to participate in activities that may change one's mental state, such as meditation or the use of psychotropic medications.

Morphological freedom is the ability of people to use existing technology and medical treatments to improve, enhance, or change their own bodies anyway they deem appropriate. This might include genetic changes, cosmetic procedures, cybernetic improvements, or other bodily form modifications. As long as these decisions do not hurt others or infringe their rights, morphological liberty acknowledges the value of bodily autonomy and the individual's right to establish their own identity and look as well as to achieve their preferred degree of physical performance or health.

The freedom of people to decide whether or not to have children, when and how far apart pregnancies occur, and whether or not to use reproductive technology is known as *procreative freedom*. This liberty includes everything from the availability of abortion and contraception to the application of assisted reproductive technologies including in vitro fertilization, preimplantation genetic diagnosis, and even germline gene editing. Procreative liberty stresses the value of reproductive autonomy, enabling people to choose, within moral bounds and free from discrimination or compulsion, how to design their families and the genetic characteristics of their children (Humanity+ 2016).

3.2 Examples of Currents within Transhumanism

What follows is are examples of the most common trends or currents within the diverse movement of Transhumanism:

Extropianism is a movement within transhumanism that emphasizes the use of technology to enhance the human body and mind to achieve prolonged life span, physical and mental abilities, and to transcend the limitations of the human condition. It is based on the idea of continual improvement (enhanced and expedited evolution) and the belief that technology can help humans overcome death and achieve a posthuman state (More 1990).

Immortalism is another current in transhumanism that focuses on the development of technology and medical interventions to achieve immortality and defeat death. It views death as a problem to be solved and seeks to find ways to extend human life and health span to the maximum.

Democratic transhumanism advocates for the democratization of technology and its use to enhance the lives of all people, not just the privileged few. It seeks to ensure that the benefits of technological advancements are distributed fairly and equitably, and that everyone has access to these technologies.

Postgenderism is a branch of transhumanism that explores the possibility of eliminating or transcending gender roles and differences through the use of technology. It suggests that gender is a social construct and that with advances in biotechnology, people could move beyond the binary concept of gender and create new gender identities or even do away with gender altogether.

Singularitarianism is a transhumanist movement that envisions a future in which artificial intelligence surpasses human intelligence and becomes the dominant form of intelligence on the planet. Singularitarians believe that this development will bring about a technological singularity, a point in time when technological progress accelerates so rapidly that it becomes impossible to predict the future.

Postpolitics is a transhumanist philosophy that envisions a future in which political issues and disputes are resolved through technology and science. It suggests that as technological progress continues, political and social issues will be increasingly addressed through data-driven decision-making facilitated by AI and that human nature will change as a result.

3.3 Examples of Human Enhancement Technologies

Human enhancement technologies include, among others, bioelectronics, sensory upgrades, brain interventions, bionics, exoskeletons, genetic manipulation, and drugs. To replace biological parts with artificial and/or electronic materials, for instance, is the essence of bionics. Bionic technology can be applied to enhance current human abilities, for lifting large objects or seeing a specific distance. Addition of technological gadgets or bodily substitutes, such an earthquake sensor, might improve senses. Brain interventions are medical devices and electronics used to improve memory, intelligence, or sensory experiences. To humans, exoskeletons provide resilience and strength. One can utilize genetic alteration to restore impaired abilities like hearing, vision, or mobility. Pharmaceuticals can be used to influence mood (chemical conditioning) or increase cognitive power or to relieve pain. Other technologies have already generated possible cures with great promise to enhance human health worldwide, including conjugated nanoparticles, tailored immunotherapies, and messenger therapeutics. Notable attempts in human augmentation also include wearable electronics (e.g., augmented reality glasses, smart watches, smart cloth), personal drones, and on- and in-body nanonetworks, all part of the Internet of Things (IoT).

Neil Harbisson (2019) is one of the persons whose bodies have been improved; he has an antenna inserted in his skull that enables him to hear colors. Another case in point is Jens Naumann (2012), who used a gadget called BrainPort to regain his sight after losing it when he was 20. Some people have had prosthetic limbs controlled by their brains implanted in place of severed limbs. Spanish dancer and performer Moon Ribas can feel earthquakes since she had a sensor inserted in one arm (Alcaraz 2019).

4. Similarities between the Gnostics and Transhumanists

These Gnostic inclinations are repeated in transhumanism, especially in its contempt for the constraints of the human body. The normal state of the body is not to the liking of many who support augmentation technology, who see its inherent limitations as barriers to happiness and fulfillment. They see a day when these physical constraints will be overcome by genetics, artificial intelligence, and neural interfacing technology, turning human weaknesses into assets (Pauls 2006). Like Gnosticism, transhumanism is devoted to releasing humanity from the constraints of biological existence and building new bodies that will sustain us into the future. But transhumanism brings with it a new technological assertion: the "singularity", a combination of biotechnology, nanotechnology, and artificial intelligence that will allow humans to overcome their biological bounds, is said to be imminently approaching.

As we can see, transhumanists and Gnostics have the same objective of escaping the material world since they both look for ways to free people from physical necessities. Similar attempts to divorce consciousness from the physical body are highlighted by the emphasis on mental experience over physical, embodied experiences in both Gnosticism and transhumanism. To be sure, some transhumanists appear to view the human being as a consciousness housed in a body and the body as a machine that the will may control with the aid of science and technology through reason (the intellect). Like Gnosticism, the Transhumanist movement holds that the secrets of overcoming physical limitations are knowledge and technological understanding. This theory predicts that a new, technologically advanced human race would arise, maybe dividing society between the technologically advanced and the less advanced majority. The ultimate objective is similar to the Gnostic ideal: total transcendence of the physical body, reaching a condition of existence unrestricted by time, nature, and history (Pauls 2006; Valčo, 113).

The techno-gnostic type of transhumanists (of the more extreme type) foresee a future where every aspect of human interaction, including sex, can be digitally simulated. They believe that technology will render physical touch obsolete, as digital simulation will offer the same levels of pleasure and intimacy. Furthermore, some transhumanists extend this reductionist perspective to music, envisioning a world where even music becomes a purely telepathic experience. A good example of such kind of thinking is the Hungarian transhumanist, Istvan Zoltan:

> "Mammals use sex as a means to generate offspring, to experience pleasure, and for bonding with partners… Erogenous zones and orgasms are simply the product of chemicals firing in the brain. If scientists can replicate that feeling by firing signals from an implanted chip or a brain wave headset, then it might even be the end of sex altogether". (Zoltan 2014a)

> "[T]he music concert of the future could very well be silent. Dead silent. Just like live music was replaced by vinyl record players and vinyl record players were replaced by Walkmans and Walkmans were replaced by iPods, iPods and other music-playing devices could be replaced by low-cost EEG brainwave-reading headsets. No more wires; no more earphones; [no] more play buttons. Just thoughts – and scans of those thoughts, meandering about your brain".(Zoltan 2014b)

C.S. Lewis adeptly captured the essence of transhumanism's ultimate aspirations in his 1945 novel, *That Hideous Strength.* Through a revealing conversation, one of the main characters, Professor Filostrato, shares his vision of the future:

> "A great race, further advanced than we. A pure race. They have cleaned their world, broken free (almost) from the organic… They do not need to be born and breed and die; only their common people, their canaglia do that. The Masters live on. They retain their intelligence: they can keep it artificially alive after the organic body has been dispensed with – a miracle of applied biochemistry. They do not need organic food. They are almost free of Nature, attached to her only by the thinnest, finest cord". (Lewis 2014)

5. Religious Undertones in Transhumanism

Moreover, since transcendence of the ordinary, a fundamental religious concern, motivates much of the transhumanist goal, transhumanism can be viewed in religious terms (Shalet 2019). Though using distinct methods – Gnosticism through spiritual understanding and Transhumanism through technical progress – both philosophies have as their goal transcending the material world. This similarity emphasizes a fundamental human desire for transcendence that has taken many different shapes and philosophies across generations. Traditional religious stories of salvation and this new quasi-religion of transhumanism appear to have four primary points of overlap.

First off, there is a very obvious inclination toward escape. Gnostic beliefs in leaving the earthly world to attain a higher, spiritual existence are in line with transhumanism's emphasis on surpassing human limitations. Both conceptions hold that by a process of metamorphosis, humans may transcend both intellectual and physical limitations. This common goal of transcendence emphasizes a basic human want to go above our natural constraints and live a perfect life.

Second, a fundamental idea of many religious beliefs as well as transhumanism is the quest of immortality. Christian belief in an afterlife or the bodily resurrection fits nicely with transhumanist aspirations to achieve eternal life by technological means, including mind uploading or cutting-edge medical procedures. This common endeavor emphasizes how, in the face of death, people strive for stability and permanence.

Thirdly, the transhumanist focus on scientific and technical breakthroughs is a reflection of the idea of gnosis, or knowledge, as a way to attain spiritual enlightenment. Both ideologies emphasize the need of wisdom and knowledge in determining human destiny and emphasize the path to transcendence through knowledge acquisition.

Finally, stories of both religions and transhumanism contain the idea of atonement. Whereas transhumanism sees redemption through technology's ability to end pain, disease, and death, Christianity sees redemption as accomplished by faith in Jesus Christ and his sacrifice. These comparable stories show how deeply people want to be saved and to experience an alleviation of suffering.

6. Philosophical underpinnings of Transhumanism as techno-Gnosticism

Of course, Transhumanism cannot be reduced to Gnosticism. Nevertheless, the concept of Gnosticism seems to be important for understanding the philosophical and theological underpinnings of transhumanism, which shares many of its key beliefs. To understand the source and nature of these 'underpinnings', we must go back in history and re-examine the triumph of univocity and nominalism (Milbank 2018; Haig 2015).

Univocity (Duns Scotus) and nominalism (William of Ockham) triumphing over metaphysical realism is a major change in medieval philosophy that still has ramifications for current debates of technognosticism and transhumanism. Championed by Thomas Aquinas (1225–1274), metaphysical realism is a philosophical stance that holds that there are universals, or abstract things, like "justice" or "humanity", that exist apart from particular instances. Aquinas contended that these universals were reflected in the material world and existent in God's thought, therefore anchoring everything in a divine order that was beyond human comprehension. This perspective gave great weight to each person's intrinsic worth and purpose, the boundaries of human understanding, and the need of humility before God.

But in the late Middle Ages, this philosophical realism was questioned and finally superseded by univocity and nominalism. As put out by John Duns Scotus (1266–1308), univocity is the notion that a single concept, like "being" or "existence", can be used equally to God and animals without suggesting any resemblance. This change of viewpoint made space for a more human-centered interpretation of reality by lessening the focus on the transcendent divine order (Rowland 2018).

William of Ockham's (1287–1347) nomalism went even farther in opposing metaphysical reality. Ockham maintained that universals were not separate, real entities but rather just names or mental constructions. In his view, there were just individual items and universals were just practical classification schemes for related objects. A concentration on the individual and the observable resulted from this rejection of universals, which prepared the way for the emergence of empirical science and humanism in due course.

For the discussion of transhumanism as technognosticism, the victory of univocity and nominalism over philosophical realism has important ramification. As individuality gained traction and the transcendent divine order declined, people were viewed as the main agents of knowledge and advancement rather than as obliging participants in a divinely planned scheme. The Enlightenment principles that guide transhumanist ideas as well as contemporary science and technology owe much to this change.

The nominalist and univocal viewpoints are naturally extended by transhumanism, which emphasizes using technology to improve and transcend human constraints. Transhumanists support the quest of knowledge and technical invention as a way to get above the constraints imposed by biology and nature by accepting the notion that people are the main agents of their own growth. Transhumanism, then, is a kind of technognosticism that aims to use knowledge and cutting-edge technology to transcend the material world.

7. Assessing the legitimacy of Transhumanist goals

One could contend that the way transhumanists see reality and, by extension, humanity directly determines the legitimacy of their aspirations. Both a movement and an ideology, transhumanism aims to employ science, technology, and creative methods to improve and surpass human limits. These goals have as their foundations a certain conception of reality and the human condition.

That being stated, for the purposes of argument and clarity, I shall go into a simplified evaluation. Many times, but not always, transhumanists hold to a materialist and reductionist theory of reality, according to which all occurrences may be explained by the interactions of the physical elements that make up the universe. This knowledge permeates human nature as well, portraying humans as intricate biological machines whose physical, emotional, and cognitive characteristics may be reduced to brain networks, genetic codes, and physiological functions. Transhumanists argue, by adopting this materialist and reductionist viewpoint, that human nature is malleable and changeable by scientific and technological methods rather than fixed and unchangeable. The foundation of transhumanist objectives is this conviction that human nature is malleable. These aims include improving cognitive functions, extending longevity, and even combining with artificial intelligence to produce new forms of existence.

But this picture of reality and people has profound philosophical and ethical ramifications. It questions, to start, conventional religious and philosophical theories that stress the spiritual or transcendent elements of human nature, an outside reference point or anchor that bestows onto the human person a "non-natural" permanence and a deeper inherent worth. Transhumanism runs the danger of undercutting the moral, ethical, and spiritual aspects of the human experience by reducing people to simple biological machines.

The transhumanist quest of improved abilities and overcoming human constraints also presents moral questions regarding resource allocation, access to cutting-edge technology, and the possibility of making social and economic inequality already present worse. A society divided along lines of technical advancement may result if these technologies are only accessible to a privileged few, hence widening the gulf between the haves and have-nots.

Furthermore, by stressing the potential for technological advancement of humans, transhumanism might unintentionally foster a culture of perfectionism and irrational expectations in which people are always trying to better themselves at the price of accepting who they are and appreciating human variety. Transhumanist detractors contend that in the unrelenting quest of human improvement, the intrinsic worth and dignity of every person run the danger of being overlooked (Pauls 2006; Lipowicz 2020). They argue that a greater knowledge of the human condition and our interdependence with the environment around us has been sacrificed in favor of an overemphasis on individual agency and technical advancement brought about by the triumph of univocity and nominalism. Moreover, according to some, the technognostic approach undervalues the possible social, ethical, and environmental effects of unbridled technology advancement (Popp, Newell, and Jaffe 2010).

Whatever the case, transhumanist thought and its technognostic goals appear to have been greatly influenced by the victory of univocity and nominalism over metaphysical realism. These philosophical stances have prepared the way for the emergence of contemporary science, technology, and the transhumanist movement by refocusing attention from a transcendent divine order to the primacy of human activity and individualism. Nonetheless, we must continue to be conscious of the possible hazards and moral ramifications of transhumanism as it works toward the technognostic objective of overcoming human constraints via technological innovation. Of course, we can strive for a future in which the possible advantages of human enhancement are balanced with a profound respect for the intrinsic worth and dignity of every person and our interdependence with the environment; but, this can only be accomplished by having a careful, educated discussion about the philosophical and historical foundations of transhumanism.

8. Conclusion

Finally, mutuality, interdependence, solidarity, and empathy – traditional human values – are seriously threatened by transhumanism. These ideals, which are acknowledged by many philosophical and religious traditions as necessary for human flourishing and the common good, need to be carefully considered in view of the consequences of transhumanism. A lack of empathy and a contempt for the interdependence of people may arise from putting personal goals ahead of the welfare of the society. Thus, it is imperative to evaluate the consequences of transhumanism critically in order to guarantee that the quest of technical improvement is compatible with the maintenance of human mutuality, interdependence, solidarity, and sensitivity.

Of course, I am not talking here about therapeutic uses of technology but rather about "unnatural enhancements", therefore another worry is the idea that happiness comes with wisdom, which means living within bounds rather than exceeding them at all costs. It could turn out to be a risky fallacy to think that harnessing technology to get above our limitations will make us happy. Human experience indicates that in reaction to the constraints of nature and situation, qualities like courage, fidelity, fortitude, generosity, hope, moderation, and perseverance are developed.

Within the field of Christian spirituality, a deep trust in divine providence and a basic acceptance of human limitations coexist. Deeply based in humility, this viewpoint provides a comprehensive picture of human nature and upholds the inherent worth of the material universe and human body. The development of virtues like love, compassion, and service, which promote a strengthening of one's relationship with God through channels like prayer, worship, and meditation, is essential to this perspective.

In sharp contrast to this viewpoint is the transhumanist philosophy, which might be seen critically as a modern form of techno-Gnosticism. Driven by an unrelenting quest of knowledge and a wish to use technology to overcome human limitations, this ideology raises important concerns about how technology could promote human wellbeing. Recent research has demonstrated the growing worry that an overuse of technology might cause social isolation and weaken the foundation of meaningful human relationships, two factors essential to true human flourishing. When it takes its worst form, techno-gnosticism runs the danger of undermining fundamental human values and encouraging an individualistic, limited definition of well-being that puts productivity and efficiency ahead of interpersonal relationships and general health.

An expanded perspective from which to view transhumanism is offered by Christian theological anthropology, especially the idea of imago Dei. Because changing the human condition may have unintended implications, this method forces us to think about the ethical and moral aspects of human enhancement. Understanding that every person is unique and has intrinsic value, this paradigm helps to assess augmentation technologies more carefully by weighing prospective advantages against probable disadvantages.

Furthermore, a broader perspective of human flourishing that goes beyond simple physical or cognitive improvement is invited by the imago Dei viewpoint. It emphasizes how essential to a happy existence are virtues, deep relationships, and spiritual development. A critical evaluation of transhumanist goals is made possible by this thorough knowledge of human flourishing, which guarantees they do not unintentionally promote a perfectionist culture or ignore important aspects of human well-being.

And last, interacting with many theological and philosophical perspectives on reality can spark a more nuanced and inclusive discussion of the transhumanist goal. Recognizing the inherent drawbacks and blind spots of any one worldview makes it possible to have a more in-depth and productive conversation on the advantages and disadvantages of transhumanism, including its societal effects. Given these considerations, it becomes necessary to strike a compromise between the acceptance of technology and the preservation of basic human principles. Moreover, tackling the intricate ethical and moral conundrums raised by transhumanism, seen through the prism of contemporary techno-Gnosticism, requires promoting multidisciplinary communication and cooperation among theologians, philosophers, and scientists. A future that is more morally aware and human-centered is guided by such an approach, which also enhances the discussion.

References

Alcaraz, A. Ł. 2019. Cyborgs' Perception, Cognition, Society, Environment, and Ethics: Interview with Neil Harbisson and Moon Ribas, 14 October 2016, Ace Hotel, New York City. *Journal of Posthuman Studies*, 3(1): 60–73.

Braidotti, R. 2017. *Posthuman, all too human: The memoirs and aspirations of a posthumanist*. Tanner Lectures. Yale University.

Chesi, G.M. 2022. Classical Posthumanism. In: Herbrechter, S., Callus, I., Rossini, M., Grech, M., de Bruin-Molé, M., John Müller, C. (eds), *Palgrave Handbook of Critical Posthumanism*. Cham:Palgrave Macmillan. https://doi.org/10.1007/978--3-030--42681--1_30--1

Cord, F. 2022. Posthumanist Cultural Studies: Taking the Nonhuman Seriously. Open Cultural Studies, 6(1): 25–37. https://doi.org/10.1515/culture-2020--0138

De Sousa, R. 2000. Learning to be Natural. In: N. Roughley (ed.), *Being Humans: Anthropological Universality and Particularity in Transdisciplinary Perspectives*. Berlin/New York: De Gruyter, pp. 287–307.

Rowland, T. 2018. There Is Another Kingdom: On The Politics of Virtue. *Nova et vetera*, 16(4): 1337–1351.

Haig, A. R. 2015. Modernity, "Radical Orthodoxy", and Cornelius Van Til: A journey of rediscovery of participatory theism. In Colloquium, 47(2): 257–273.

Haraway, D. 2010. A Manifesto for Cyborgs: Science, Technology, and Socialist Feminism in the 1980s, 2190–2220. In: Vincent B. Leitch et al. (eds.), *The Norton Anthology of Theory and Criticism*. 2nd ed. Cambridge: Cambridge University Press.

Harbisson, N. 2019. Hearing colors: My life experience as a cyborg. In: Xavier Pavie (ed.), *Creativity, imagination and innovation: perspectives and inspirational stories*. London: World Scientific Publishing, pp. 117–125. https://doi.org/10.1142/9789813273009_0015.

Hull, D.L. 1986. On Human Nature. In: PSA: Proceedings of the Biennial Meeting of the Philosophy of Science Association, 1986(2): 3–13. doi:10.1086/psaprocbienmeetp. 1986.2.192787

Humanity+. 2016. The Transhumanist FAQ Version 3. https://hpluspedia.org/wiki/Transhumanist_FAQ_Version_3 (accessed: 12 Aug 2023).

Huxley, J. 1957. Transhumanism. In: New Bottles for New Wine. London: Chatto & Windus, pp. 13–17. http://www.transhumanism.org/index.php/WTA/more/huxley

King, K. L. 2003. What is Gnosticism?. Harvard University Press.

Lewis, C.S. 2014. That Hideous Strength: A Modern Fairy-Tale for Grown-ups. Project Gutenberg [online]. https://gutenberg.ca/ebooks/lewiscs-thathideousstrength/lewiscs-thathideousstrength-00-h.html (Accessed: 18 Aug 2023).

Lipowicz, M. 2020. Transhumanism and Christianity: A Ratzingerian Approach to the Concept of Biotechnological Human Enhancement. Religion and Theology, 27(1–2): 47–73.

Loy, D. R. 2019. *Nonduality: In Buddhism and beyond*. London: Simon and Schuster.

Marjanen, A. 2009. 'Gnosticism'. In: Susan Ashbrook Harvey, & David G. Hunter (eds), *The Oxford Handbook of Early Christian Studies* (2008; online ed., Oxford Academic, 2 Sept. 2009), https://doi.org/10.1093/oxfordhb/9780199271566.003.0011 (accessed 21 Sep 2023).

Milbank, J. 2018. Reformation 500: Any Cause for Celebration? *Open Theology*, 4(1): 607–629.

More, M. 1990. The Extropian Principles. *Extropy: The Journal of Transhumanist Thought*, 6(1): 16–18.

More, M. 1996. Transhumanism: Towards a Futurist Philosophy [online]. https://web.archive.org/web/20051029125153/http://www.maxmore.com/transhum.htm

Naumann, J. 2012. *Search for paradise: A patient's account of the artificial vision experiment*. Xlibris corporation.

Pauls, D. 2006. Transhumanism: 2000 Years in the Making. In: Theology and Human Nature. [online]. The Center for Bioethics and Culture Network. https://cbc-network.org/2006/11/transhumanism-2000-years-in-the-making/

Popp, D., Newell, R.G. & A. B. Jaffe. 2010. Energy, the environment, and technological change. *Handbook of the Economics of Innovation*, 2, 873–937.

Roughley, N. 2023. Human Nature. In: Edward N. Zalta& Uri Nodelman (eds.), *The Stanford Encyclopedia of Philosophy* (Winter 2023 Edition), https://plato.stanford.edu/archives/win2023/entries/human-nature (accessed: 23 Aug 2023).

Schwab, K. 2014. The Fourth Industrial Revolution: what it means, how to respond. [online, 14 Jan 2016], *World Economic Forum.* https://www.weforum.org/agenda/2016/01/the-fourth-industrial-revolution-what-it-means-and-how-to-respond/ (Accessed: 20 Aug 2023).

Shalet, D. 2019. Through the looking glass: Ghost in the Shell, transhumanism, and transcendence through the virtual. *Implicit Religion*, 21(4). https://doi.org/10.1558/imre.35338

Valčo, M. 2021. Transhumanism as a Challenge for the Christian Theological Understanding of 'Imago Dei'. In: R. Petkovšek and B. Žalec(eds.), *Transhumanism as a Challenge for Ethics and Religion.* Zürich: Lit Verlag, p. 111–118.

Zoltan, I. 2014a. The Transhumanist Future of Sex. Vice.com, October 20, 2014. https://www.vice.com/en/article/ypwn4k/the-transhumanist-future-of-sex (Accessed: 18 Aug 2023).

Zoltan, I. 2014b. Telepathic Melodies Are the Soundless Music of the Future. Vice.com, August 15, 2014. https://www.vice.com/en/article/vvb33b/telepathic-melodies-are-the-soundless-music-of-the-future (Accessed: 18 Aug 2023).

THE EXISTENTIAL, SPIRITUAL, AND PRACTICAL/PASTORAL DIMENSIONS OF MORTALITY: A COMPREHENSIVE EXPLORATION

Katarína Valčová

1. Introduction

This study will examine in brief the existential, spiritual, and practical/pastoral elements of mortality. My paper is situated at the intersection of pastoral practice, theological reflection, and philosophical study, trying to understand the complex interplay of thoughts, sentiments, and experiences related to the human awareness and touch with mortality.

By use of a mixed-methods approach, this work combines theoretical exegesis with qualitative studies carried out by other researchers. I've decided to interact with anything from scholarly books to stories from digital media to real-world case studies. This methodological pluralism promotes an interdisciplinary study of mortality and makes it possible to grasp it more fully. Comparative analysis is essential since it contrasts different viewpoints and experiences to show the variety and intricacy that are part of human experiences with death. This method makes it possible to examine subjective experiences and moral issues related to dying and death critically yet sympathetically.

My chapter primarily seeks to provide a comprehensive understanding of mortality that addresses the practical and pastoral ramifications while also acknowledging the existential anxiety and spiritual reflections it arouses. Practice of pastoral care depends critically on this equilibrium. Through a study of the existential issues of the meaning of life and the finality of death, the spiritual reflections on afterlife beliefs, and the practical elements of pastoral care and grief counseling, my research aims to offer a more thorough framework for comprehending and tackling the many facets of human mortality. In addition, the study seeks to advance the scholarly conversation on death and dying by refuting conventional wisdom and providing fresh perspectives on how people and society deal with the certainty of death. It also aims to provide educators, healthcare workers, and pastoral caregivers useful advice so they may help people and communities deal with death and bereavement with the understanding and compassion they need.

2. Life and Death/Death and Life: Some Remarks on Delineating the Boundary

It is difficult to define the essence of life, especially in the twenty-first century when the requirement of consciousness alone is seen inadequate for existence. As mentioned by Van Inwagen (1990) and Bedau (2014) in Luper's "Death" from The Stanford Encyclopedia of Philosophy (Luper, 2021) this intricacy is reflected in comprehending its cessation, death. Death, the end of life, necessitates a complex comprehension of the nature of life, including concerns regarding the suspension or reversibility of life and its connection to continuous existence. This sophisticated knowledge combines ethical issues with actual findings, therefore bridging the philosophical and practical domains.

Through their special capacity to evolve or maintain themselves by essential physiological processes, organisms show that they are "alive". This difference between being able to perform such activities and actively participating in them highlights a more fundamental ethical question: when does the termination of these activities indicate the end of life, and how should this transition be handled legally and ethically. The event resulting in the loss of vital processes is distinguished from the state of having lost such capacities by the "loss of life account" of death. As such, death can be seen as a state (being dead), a process (dying), or a sequence of discrete events throughout dying.

Moreover, defining the notion of death is not the same as defining its factual parameters. The method concentrating on brain stem death (Pallis, 1982) and the Uniform Determination of Death Act (National Conference of Commissioners, 1981) are two examples of criteria for death that perform important practical purposes even while a definition tries to capture the essence of death. In a field full with moral conundrums, particularly when decisions regarding organ donation or life-support removal are taken, they counsel medical professionals and legal professionals.

It is clear from this setting what moral ramifications there are for defining and determining death. Inspired by the Uniform Determination of Death Act (1981), American law holds that a person is dead when all of the brain's functions, including the brain stem, or the circulatory and respiratory systems cease irreversibly. Although such decisions have to follow medical guidelines, they also come into conflict with important ethical issues about the dignity of death and the sanctity of life. The method used in the United Kingdom, which concentrates on brain stem death, reflects a more precise standard, defined as the "permanent functional death of the brain stem" (Pallis 1982, in Luper, 2011). These standards, while being necessary in many practical contexts, raise more ethical concerns regarding the end of life and the obligations of those who make such decisions.

3. May Realizing One's Own Mortality Lead to a Better Life?

Death doula Alua Arthur explores the deep emotional and existential ramifications of human mortality in her thought-provoking TED talk (Arthur, 2023). The basic idea of "Death as a Contextual Framework" put forward by Arthur goes beyond the traditional understanding of death as the conclusion of life. Rather, she suggests that death is a prism through which we can view life and it enhances our existential experience. This viewpoint implies that accepting our mortality might be a trigger for existential clarity, in direct contrast to the usual emotional upheaval connected with death.

Arthur asks us to reevaluate how we view death. This concept personally really speaks to me, making one reevaluate life's goals and values in light of our impending death. Her contention that knowing one will die can be a motivating factor rather than a cause for fear provides a life-changing viewpoint on how we live.

Arthur introduces the novel position of end-of-life doulas as her talk goes on, holistic companions who provide emotional, spiritual, and practical care to those confronting the end of their lives. Known by several names, including death midwives or end-of-life coaches, these experts support compassionate death care. Their services represent a whole approach to end-of-life care; they include everything from arranging the bedside area to enabling conversations about death. Their commitment and depth of training are best shown by the INELDA (2023) approach, which emphasizes early grieving support, companionship throughout dying, and life exploration after diagnosis.

Arthur does a very sensitive and insightful job of combining existential thoughts with useful end-of-life care interventions. Her theoretical structure, "Death as a Contextual Framework", provides a paradigm change that changes our understanding of death from a terrifying conclusion to a significant component of our existential fabric. This reinterpretation presents death as a means to a greater comprehension and enlightenment, therefore challenging the common fears about it.

Furthermore, a major shift in our approach to deathcare has occurred with the inclusion of end-of-life doulas into the conversation about mortality. Beyond the conventional function of caregivers, these experts protect individual autonomy and respect final desires in life. Their method, which aligns with specific training like INELDA, highlights the usefulness of Arthur's speech.

The way that Arthur combined the existential and the pragmatic captures the complexity of our relationship with death. It forces us to face our own mortality with fresh purpose and gratitude for life rather than resignation. Her speech is evidence of how complexly philosophical ideas and practical concerns interact to shape our conception of death.

4. Contemplating Life's Meaning: A Response to Luper's narrow, subjective vision

Despite all of Alua Arthur's inspiration and stimulation, we haven't given the topic of life's meaning and how we should discuss it enough thought thus far. Referring to Luper (2014, 198), we come into a notion that suggests that the meaning of life is mostly self-determined:

"Your life is meaningful only if and to the degree that you successfully and freely pursue the goals to which you have committed your life". Meaning is what you give your own life; you adopt your goals and, more or less, attain them by yourself. You live for these accomplishments.

Although this worldview honors individual freedom, it may provide a limited and subjective understanding of existential meaning. According to Luper, people give their lives purpose by their accomplishments since they are self-referential agents. According to this perspective, the meaning of life is only a creation of own aspirations. Such a perspective may ignore universal or shared meanings that may be innate to human existence or generated from outside sources like spirituality, relationships, or community. " Stressing success as the essence of life runs the danger of marginalizing those who, for a variety of reasons, might not be able to reach their own objectives. This begs moral concerns about how inclusive Luper's (2014) thesis is. Can success alone provide meaning? What about people that run against roadblocks to their objectives? This strategy could unintentionally result in an exclusive conception of the meaning of life, implying that people who fail to reach their objectives are abandoned and may even become nihilists.

Luper's argument, as I have said before, mostly ignores the influence of outside forces in favor of internal sources of meaning. Human social and relational characteristics, cultural and spiritual influences, and even chance encounters can have a significant impact on how we view the meaning of life. The communal elements of meaning, in which people find value in their relationships, social positions, or group activities, refute the notion that meaning is a product of the individual. We also need to remember that goals and viewpoints change throughout life. Luper's perspective could not be able to explain this dynamism. People's hopes, goals, and sense of what matters in life can all alter dramatically as they mature. This flexibility implies that life meaning might not be as set in stone or as strongly related to particular accomplishments as Luper appears to suggest.

Pastorally speaking, there are important ramifications when life's purpose is tied to individual success alone. It may encourage a mentality that believes that one's value depends on achievement, which could result in feelings of inadequacy or failure when objectives are not achieved. Regardless of their accomplishments, the pastoral response I would like to advocate would rather highlight the intrinsic worth of every person. It would promote the search of virtue and spiritual development as well as finding purpose in relationships and the act of existence itself. Alternatively, metanarratives – like the creation and redemption stories that are part of religious faiths – can provide meaning.

Additionally, whilst Luper's thesis correctly emphasizes the role of personal action in deciding the trajectory of life, a more comprehensive perspective would take into account both personal agency and the larger background. This includes realizing how spiritual beliefs, cultural legacy, and community influence how one interprets the meaning of life. A balanced viewpoint proposes a more comprehensive method to comprehending life's purpose by recognizing the interaction between individual goals and the impact of outside forces. Luper's argument, then, would probably profit from a wider viewpoint even if it provides insightful information about the part that personal action and achievement play in giving life meaning. Personal accomplishments would be taken into account, but so would the roles of relationships, community, culture, spirituality, and most importantly, the idea of the intrinsic worth of the human experience. It would acknowledge the dynamic quality of life's purpose and the impact of outside forces as well as the way that personal objectives change. This comprehensive strategy is more in line with a pastoral viewpoint, which aims to develop an inclusive, sympathetic, and multidimensional sense of meaning and purpose in human life.

5. The Digitally-Mediated Lamentation: A Multi-Faceted Examination of Grief Narratives Among Children

Previously limited to private spaces, grief has found a moving release in the digital sphere, becoming a more shared and public experience. Digital media provide new outlets for expression and assistance, as seen by a YouTube video where kids relate their sadness after learning of their parent's terminal illness (Heart House Hospice, 2019). This story illustrates not just the emotional turmoil of loss but also the practicalities of life after loss, the quest for spiritual purpose, and the therapeutic potential of digital media in the modern world.

Important moral concerns are raised by the move to digital grief. One must carefully weigh privacy and the long-term effects of such exposure, for example, when children's grieving experiences are made public on websites like YouTube. It questions conventional wisdom that says sorrow is a personal experience and deepens our awareness of how, particularly for younger generations, grieving can be a shared, community process.

As shown in the movie, the moment of diagnosis is the first emotional turning point in the lives of these bereaved children. It is a psychologically shocking event that precedes the approaching loss (Heart House Hospice, 2019). This realization, which is sometimes felt as a significant incursion into the family sphere, forces one to face the erratic character of life.

Seeing the various emotional reactions of the siblings in the movie highlights the intricate complexities of bereavement in families. Even within a shared family setting, the individuality of mourning is demonstrated by the different ways that each kid processes the loss. This version emphasizes the need of providing individualized care for bereaved children, realizing that every child's experience with loss is unique and very personal.

The story tells how the kids, after their father passes away, are suddenly thrown into adult duties and must manage life's issues that their parent used to handle. As told, this abrupt change represents the loss of childhood innocence as well as the death of a loved one, both of which are expedited by the demands of their new world.

In a time when technology is everywhere, the narrator's search for help on Google, which takes them to Hart House, is a prime example of how digital platforms are becoming more and more important in offering bereaved families both practical and emotional support (Heart House Hospice, 2019). This episode is symptomatic of a larger trend in which new kinds of connection and support are provided by digital tools, which are becoming more and more important to the grieving process.

The story gains a religious dimension from the narrator's contemplation of his father's optimism in the face of terminal sickness and his conviction in parental watchfulness from heaven. These ideas raise concerns regarding the function of optimism and spiritual beliefs in the grieving process even if they might be consoling.

The story emphasizes online counseling as a way to demonstrate how technology democratizes access to mental health care and provides a special kind of pastoral care. This kind of digital interaction enables people – children in particular – to investigate their spiritual and emotional questions in a kind, encouraging setting.

As a "digital pulpit", the story thus presents YouTube as a contemporary forum for shared mourning experiences. This open sharing is a big change in the way society understands and processes grief from customary, private mourning rituals. It functions as a modern forum, allowing talks on loss and recovery that could otherwise stay in private settings. The story emphasizes the need of careful communication while taking into account the emotional condition of the communicator as well as the bereaved person when handling childhood bereavement. Highly regarded sources of educational resources include the Child Mind Institute (n.d. https://childmind.org/) and the National Alliance for Children's Grief (n.d. https://nacg.org/). Grief does not travel in a straight line and can reappear suddenly, therefore it is important to customize conversations about death to the child's age and emotional development. Grieving children need ongoing assistance, especially around emotionally charged occasions like holidays and anniversaries.

6. How to talk about death with children – various practical approaches to the problematic

Adults find it difficult to negotiate the emotional maze of death, and children find it even more confusing. It takes a sophisticated, sympathetic, and knowledgeable attitude to have discussions about mortality with the younger generation, as pastoral wisdom and academic study stress (Serani, 2016). "Speaking the truth" about death is morally required and supports genuine emotional expression as well as creating a setting that supports healthy grieving.

Parents have to negotiate a range of emotional reactions, from grief to rage, while discussing death with their kids. The grief process depends critically on giving these genuine responses room. Speaking clearly, it is better to use words like "dead" or "died" than euphemisms like "passed away" or "went to sleep". By demystifying death, such clarity promotes a healthy grieving process, as empirical research confirms (Serani, 2016). As one considers these recommendations, one realizes how careful handling mortality discussions with children must be. It goes beyond just giving them the facts to include helping them on an emotional journey while honoring their unique ability to comprehend and grieve loss.

Parents are also urged by Serani not to be afraid to admit their own ignorance of death. Such candour, particularly in the midst of deep loss, frank be a source of strength since it shows the youngster that uncertainty is a normal aspect of life. Choosing memorial songs or readings with children can also be a therapeutic exercise that gives them a sense of control and involvement during a trying time. Understanding that there is no one "correct" method to grieve, it is imperative to honor the variety of mourning styles (Serani, 2016).

Another level to the discussion is added by the intricacies of memorial ceremonics and funerals and their effects on children. Children must be made aware of what they may see, including the emotional climate and visual components like an urn or casket. The story goes on into the aftermath, preparing kids for times when they will really miss their loved one. In this regard, helping children through grieving becomes crucially dependent on parents' self-care. Children are keen observers; they recognize the behavioral clues given by adults. As well as being good for the parent, modeling appropriate coping strategies teaches the youngster how to control their own emotions (Serani, 2016).

Deborah Serani emphasizes how talking about mortality with children raises complex emotional, ethical, and practical issues. Though difficult, this project is essential and, when done with academic integrity and compassionate empathy, can deepen the child's and the parent's comprehension of this mysterious life event.

In addition to providing factual disclosure, physician and parent Dr. Kelly Fradin adds an important viewpoint to this conversation by highlighting that talking about death with children has psychological, emotional, and frequently spiritual aspects (Fradin, 2023). This method emphasizes how morally adults – be they parents, teachers, or medical professionals – have an obligation to compassionately and understandingly lead children through this difficult terrain.

Parents should critically evaluate their own emotional readiness before starting such important talks. Or are they too busy grieving to talk about such things? Getting support from friends, relatives, or neighborhood organizations is wise and appropriate when a parent's grief makes it difficult for them to meet their child's emotional needs. Instead of being negative, showing a child your own sentiments helps strengthen the emotional connection between you and them. It is a connection- and healing-process (Fradin, 2023).

Talking about dying with kids has ethical implications that need for a careful balancing act between emotional support and candor. Understanding the child's ability for comprehension and emotional processing, it is crucial to be both honest and kind in these conversations. Furthermore stressed by Fradin is the need of considering the developmental stage of the child. During the emotional turmoil of a family death, preverbal and toddler-aged children find stability in unambiguous statements and regular schedules. With their developing comprehension and curiosity, children three to eight years old may ask difficult questions that call for careful, age-appropriate answers. Even if they appear to turn inside or to their classmates for emotional comfort, individuals nine years of age and up still need substantial parental care (Fradin, 2023). The age-specific approaches emphasize how children's comprehension and coping skills are dynamic. It serves as a reminder that every child experiences death differently, thus our strategy should be based on their particular requirements and developmental stage.

Moreover, a thorough guide on how to talk about death with children may be found at the Australian website Raising Children Network (2023 https://raisingchildren.net.au/). This website emphasizes the need of respecting spiritual beliefs and cultural background in determining how a family handles talking about death. Eliminating euphemisms that could incite additional anxiety or misunderstanding can help to reduce possible miscommunication by using clear and explicit words like "death" or "died". Accompanying the child's interest in death with sensitivity and honesty, responses should be adapted to their emotional and cognitive development (Raising Children Network, 2023).

Like adults, children react emotionally to death in a variety of ways, from acceptance to sadness to worry. Knowing that kids might not be able to articulate their emotions completely emphasizes how crucial adult support is to helping them manage their emotions. For severe losses in particular, more resources could be required to properly address the psychological effects. The most crucial thing to keep in mind is that ethical issues, individual perspectives, and developmental appropriateness need to be included into our discussions on dying with children. Giving the youngster a comprehensive, caring, and transparent approach that is adapted to their emotional and psychological requirements should always be the goal.

7. Conclusion

In this work, existential issues, spiritual reflections, and pastoral pragmatics have been explored on a pastoral and intellectual trek into the maze-like aspects of human mortality. Our research has made clear how deeply ingrained and intricately human experiences and feelings are in the idea of mortality. It has not, subjectively, been an easy road. It is clear to me now that comprehending mortality is a very personal task as much as an intellectual one. It has made me reflect on our own mortality and how we deal with the certainty of death. Nevertheless, and this is maybe the most crucial aspect, our investigation has been not only about comprehending death but also about enhancing life, developing emotional intelligence and resilience, especially in youngsters when they face the facts of mortality.

In the digital realm, where we looked at how existential fears find both a haven and a battlefield on the Internet, we saw how intricately technology and our most basic human experiences interact. This feature of the research emphasizes the modern reality in which our contacts with important life events – including death – are frequently mediated by digital interfaces. Exploring the spiritual has revealed complex theological frameworks and eschatological paradigms that show how our earthly views of our life-journey and mortality are shaped by ideas about the afterlife. Not at all sideline, this spiritual question is essential to our comprehension of death and the grieving and healing processes that follow.

The dedication of this work to the pastoral and practical dimensions of death is what distinguishes it. In arguing for an updated pastoral care model, my investigation moves from academic discourse to a compassionate guide. This paradigm helps people – children especially – manage the emotional and psychological complexity that come with losing a loved one. This book, I hope, will act as a plea for an integrated approach to death, encouraging scholarly, theological, and pastoral carer cooperation. Particularly important in our digitalized society when real human connection and spiritual grounding are becoming more and more important, I support a multidimensional approach integrating existential awareness, spiritual understanding, and pastoral pragmatism. As it offers routes for emotional healing, spiritual development, and intellectual understanding, I think it is beneficial and essential to consider our common fears, hopes, and beliefs about mortality. We may go above received knowledge and oversimplified definitions by providing a sophisticated grasp of the existential and spiritual aspects of mortality. Our route is therefore to keep delving deeply into the intricacies of life and death, considering our own mortality as well as the mortality of those around us critically and morally. By doing this, we not only enhance our personal lives but also significantly advance the larger philosophical and ethical conversation on this most universal of human experiences.

Resources

Arthur, A. 2023. Why thinking about death helps you live a better life. https://www.youtube.com/watch?v=IkeuKPZxEhM (accessed 20 Sep 2023).

Bedau, M. A. 2014. The Nature of Life, 13–29. In: The Cambridge Companion to Life and Death. S. Luper (ed.). Cambridge: Cambridge University Press.

Child Mind Institute. N.d. https://childmind.org/ (accessed 20 Sep 2023).

Fradin, K. 2023. How to talk to your kids about Death: An age-by-age guide. https://www.todaysparent.com/family/family-life/how-to-talk-to-kids-about-death-2/ (Accessed 23 Sep 2023.

Heart House Hospice. 2019. Kids Share their Grief Experience. Help Us Understand Grief (H.U.U.G.) Program. https://www.youtube.com/watch?v=GAuxtrmYa2I (accessed 20 Sep 2023).

INELDA. 2023. What is an End-of-Life Doula? [online]. https://inelda.org/ (accessed 20 Sep 2023).

Luper, S. 2014. Life's Meaning, 198–213. In: The Cambridge Companion to Life and Death. S. Luper (ed.). Cambridge: Cambridge University Press.

Luper, S. 2021. Death. In: The Stanford Encyclopedia of Philosophy (Fall 2021 Edition), Edward N. Zalta (ed.), https://plato.stanford.edu/archives/fall2021/entries/death/ (accessed 20 Sep 2023).

National Alliance for Children's Grief. N.d. https://nacg.org/ (accessed 20 Sep 2023).

National Conference of Commissioners. 1981. Uniform Determination of Death Act (United States, 1981). https://lchc.ucsd.edu/cogn150/Readings/deathact.pdf (Accessed 22 Aug 2023).

Pallis, C. 1982. ABC of Brain Stem Death. *British Medical Journal*, 285: 1487–1490.

Raising Children Network. 2023. Death: how to talk about it with children [online]. https://raisingchildren.net.au/school-age/connecting-communicating/tough-topics/death-how-to-talk-about-it (accessed 24 Sep 2023).

Serani, D. 2016. The do´s and don´ts of talk with a child about death. *Psychology Today* [online]. https://www.psychologytoday.com/us/blog/two-takes-depression/201612/the-dos-and-donts-talking-child-about-death (Accessed 20 Aug 2023).

Van Inwagen, P. 1990. *Material Beings*. Ithaca: Cornell University Press.

Abstracts

Claudiu Marius Mesaroş

A Philosophical commentary on the Imago Dei in Gregory of Nyssa's De Hominis Opificio

One important question that can be explored for the benefit of contemporary transhumanism studies regards the ideal body for man. What is the paradigmatic or, if preferred, ideal description of the human body and nature? In his De Hominis Opificio, Gregory of Nyssa develops a philosophical, scientific, and theological concept of the human generic identity as Imago Dei starting from both the Biblical Genesis and from a large set of philosophical question regarding the localization of the soul in his relation to the body. The relation itself proves to be problematic and reveals only as action so that the name soul stands properly only for the activities that are common to soul and body. But the union is still unintelligible, therefore there is no place nor definition for the soul apart from the relation that it makes visible in actions. The impossibility to understand neither the substantial relation of body and soul nor the body or soul per se brings about a conclusion regarding the dynamic nature of human being: it is imago Dei in two extreme senses that only function as limits of an interval which finally must be apprehended as the interval of human action and creation.

Key words: *Imago Dei, philosophy of creation, allegory, mind-body, opposition*

Dong Tai Nguyen

The Opportunities and Challenges of Transhumanism: Insights from Confucian Philosophy and Anthropology

This paper explores the opportunities and problems presented by transhumanist philosophy by contrasting it with Confucian anthropology. Transhumanism is a movement that promotes using biotechnology to improve human potential and raises important ethical and human nature issues. We follow the development of it historically from the conception of human potential by Giovanni Pico della Mirandola to the expression of human transcendence by Julian Huxley. We investigate the consequences of transhumanism on human nature, ethics, and society norms via a Confucian perspective. Confucianism offers a special viewpoint on the moral conundrums of transhumanism, especially with relation to human dignity, the quest of immortality, and the harmony of technical advancement and ethical limitations. This comparison study shows that these two ideologies may be combined, emphasizing the need of moral direction in the age of unheard-of technical progress.

Key Words: *Confucianism, Confucian Anthropology, Human nature, Technological enhancement, Transhumanism*

Ha Thanh Pham and Hai Hoang Nguyen

Engaged Buddhism toward Transhumanism

Transhumanism is a social movement promoting genetic, wearable, and implantable technologies that artificially expedite the evolutionary process. However, accepting the transhumanist concept may differ due to the countries' cultural values and religious aspects. The philosophy of Buddhist traditions has specific levels of natural compatibility with transhumanist concepts. This article will examine transhumanism from the Buddhist perspective. First, we present some concepts Buddhism brought to humanity and the three most popular Mahayana schools in Vietnam: Meditation, Pure Land, and Tantric Buddhism. Engaged Buddhism in Vietnam, which Tran Nhan Tong developed, showed that the differences in practice principles of each school also bring about different perspectives on transhumanism. We consider some Buddhist principles of suffering and dependent origination from the point of view of neuroscience and biology. There are three kinds of suffering: physical, mental, and ignorance. The neuroscience and biological sciences are presented to clarify the above types of suffering. The principle of dependent origination and its consequence of no-self is proven in biology at the three levels of life: individual, cellular, and molecular. Some of the goals of transhumanism are to increase longevity, physical and mental enhancement, and well-being state viewed from the perspective of some of the most modern technologies. Gene modification and gene editing are essential among emerging technologies because this technology interferes with the evolutionary process. We will present genetic engineering as an example to clarify Buddhism's influence on humanity.

Key words: *Engaged Buddhism, Transhumanism, Buddhism in Vietnam, Human enhancement, Biotechnology*

Hoa Thi Kim Do and Duc Hong Nguyen

The Impact of The Fourth Industrial Revolution on Human Life: Perspectives from Vietnam

This thorough study assesses, with an emphasis on artificial intelligence (AI), how society views and affects the Fourth Industrial Revolution (4IR) technology. Using survey data from 2023 conducted in Vietnam, the study investigates public perceptions of how artificial intelligence (AI) affects human emotions, morals and ethics, religious convictions, and ways of living and acting. The results show complex viewpoints, which capture the revolutionary and complex effects of AI on society. It was shown that although most people agree that artificial intelligence (AI) has the power to change human emotions and behavior, worries about how it would affect moral principles, ethical standards, and religious views continue. The paper suggests, based on these findings, developing ethical literacy, valuing religious and cultural diversity, and putting in place all-encompassing plans to optimize the advantages and lessen the possible drawbacks of AI. We strongly advise educators, policymakers, and AI developers to take these results into account when integrating and regulating AI in society. Contributing to the current discussion on the social effects of AI, the paper emphasizes the need of advancing 4IR technologies in an ethical and socio-politically responsible manner.

Key words: *The Fourth Industrial Revolution, Transhumanism, Artificial Intelligence, Human enhancement, Vietnamese society*

Hoa Thi Kim Do

Ho Chi Minh's Thought on Human Development in Contrast to Transhumanism

The different viewpoints on human evolution and improvement between Ho Chi Minh's humanistic philosophy and the futurist ideology of transhumanism are compared in this study. Formulated in the sociopolitical setting of Vietnam's independence movement, Ho Chi Minh's humanism highlights moral qualities, group values, and holistic development, therefore highlighting the intrinsic worth of human existence within its natural cycle. On the other hand, transhumanists stress individual liberty and unrestricted improvement – possibly even immortality – by employing technology to overcome biological constraints. These ideas are contrasted to show significant ethical and social ramifications that force us to reconsider how we view society norms, human nature, and the future of humanity. The discussion of the future of mankind is furthered by the insightful understanding of the ethical issues entwined with ideas of human growth and improvement provided by the discourse between humanism and transhumanism.

Key words: *Ho Chi Minh, transhumanism, human development, human nature, humanity*

Hung Quang Nguyen

Confucian concep of man in the context of the Fourth Industrial Revolution: Vietnam's experience

Early Common Era introductions of Confucianism had a profound impact on Vietnamese culture and society, particularly when it was made the official religion of the Le and Nguyen dynasties (15th to early 20th centuries). Though Buddhism and indigenous faiths, together with the synthesis of Confucianism, Mahayana Buddhism, and local beliefs, have all played a significant role in forming Vietnamese traditional culture, Confucianism is perhaps still its mainstay. Confucianism is still a powerful force in modern Vietnam even though its influence declined after the colonial era and Marxism rose. In the context of the fourth industrial revolution in particular, this paper looks at traditional Confucian views on human nature and existence and how these views might change as Vietnamese society and its religious landscape react to contemporary scientific and technical breakthroughs. The study seeks to clarify the relationship between modernism and Confucianism, therefore exposing the continuous spiritual and cultural evolution of Vietnamese people in the face of the present world events.

Key words: *Vietnam, transhumanism, Vietnamese Confucianism, Buddhism, the fourth industrial revolution*

Ion Cordoneanu

An attempt at a metaphysical interpretation of posthumanism

We are in a full technological age and, according to Norbert Wiener, technology must become increasingly capable of formulating human purposes. This article highlights two perspectives on technology, one of the pillars of posthumanism. The former has been developed by Francis Fukuyama, according to whom biotechnology poses a significant threat through its potential to alter human nature, and humanity owes it to itself to develop institutions and laws that ensure the stability of the species. The latter view belongs to Yuval Noah Harari, who believes that liberalism, not only the political and economic paradigm of the twentieth century but the integrative anthropological vision, will be threatened by the new technological leap and that the beliefs about free will, the soul and the self will remain mere fiction. The aim of this article is to propose an interpretation from a metaphysical perspective of the technological age into which humanity is stepping, in an attempt to understand what place humanity is to assume in relation to technology. By the middle of the last century, Heidegger was formulating the question concerning modern technology. Based on his assumptions, we try to formulate a question concerning present-day technology, considering that, once it is in its world, the human being undergoes what we can call a metaphysical "mutation".

Key words: *Fukuyama, Harari, Heidegger, technology, human nature, free will*

Jozef Jenčík

Transhumanism, Power, and Anarchy: Embracing Collective Empowerment through Technologies

This paper explores the intersection of transhumanism, power dynamics, and anarchy, with a focus on the concept of collective empowerment in the context of technological progress. It challenges the conventional notion that increased physical agency through technology leads to power imbalances and argues for the potential of collective empowerment. By examining the philosophies of John Dewey and emphasizing the compatibility of democracy with both archy and anarchy, the paper explores the role of sovereignty in preserving existing inequalities and hindering technological progress. It highlights the importance of inclusive and participatory frameworks that dismantle the traditional power structures. Additionally, the paper examines the abuse of nascent participatory frameworks during crises and the paradoxical nature of collective feelings and duties. Through its analysis, this paper offers a nuanced perspective on how transhumanism, power, anarchy, and sovereignty intersect and presents pathways for embracing collective empowerment in the context of technological progress.

Key words: *Transhumanism, Power dynamics, Anarchy, Sovereignty, Collective empowerment, Technological progress, Inclusive frameworks*

Martin Kmec

Comenius's Anthropological Vision: Interpreting Human Nature in His Key Works and Their Modern Legacy

With a main emphasis on his masterwork, "Opera Didactica Omnia", and especially in "Great Didactics", this study offers an extensive examination of anthropological themes in John Amos Comenius's instructional writings. Through a study of Comenius's tractate "Centrum Securitatis", it also clarifies his religious and philosophical stance. This work clarifies Comenius's understanding of humanity by highlighting his special synthesis of philosophical, religious, and educational aspects. A debate on Comenius's beliefs' possible legacy and current significance follows this investigation. The relevance of Comenius's knowledge of human nature and abilities is assessed in the framework of contemporary philosophical and pedagogical discourse, especially his interpretation of the idea of "imago Dei" (the image of God). Reexamining and reinterpreting Comenius's foundational concepts, the paper seeks to add to the current discussion on human potential and educational philosophy.

Key words: *anthropology, human capacities, imago Dei, didactics, Centrum securitatis*

Martin Turčan

A Note on Anarcho-Transhumanism

The paper deals with the concept of anarcho-transhumanism from a theological perspective. The author tries to show some axiological parallels between the hypothetical world of transhuman anarchy and the story of Genesis 6. His focus is on the essential values of anarcho-transhumanism – i.e. (1) human perfection and (2) human freedom (plus (3) human knowledge) – and gives a theological warning that if we are to choose either anarchy or dystopia in the future transhuman reality, as anarcho-transhumanists claim, then we should be worried about the very concept of transhumanism. The reason is a rather pessimistic anthropology of the Bible, well-illustrated by the story of Genesis 6 where the mentioned values (which should be amplified in the hypothetical anarcho-transhumanist world) do not interact positively.

Key words: *transhumanism, anarchism, freedom, human perfection, Genesis 6, Nephilim*

Mendo Castro Henriques

'Transhumanism', a category mistake: insights from Bruno Latour

This article exposes transhumanist goals to an evaluation based on the analytical framework of the philosopher and anthropologist Bruno Latour (1947–2022). Latour never wrote explicitly about transhumanism, but his work helps to clarify it as a category mistake. He calls us to envisage the uncertain boundaries between the human and the non-human; thus, we can free ourselves from the conventional image of modernity in which transhumanism and a great deal of humanism, too, are encapsulated. The article uses mainly three of Latour's books, namely: We have never been moderns (NBM, 1991) Rejoicing (R, 2000), and An Inquiry into Modes of Existence (AIME, 2012) [French original edition year]. It focuses on how Latour evolved from the concept of social construction to the anthropological and philosophical concept of instauration, which he even applied to read Alan Turing. In the process, he enables us to point out that transhumanism incurs in a category mistake because it deals with human beings as a known nature and thus exasperates humanity's unresolved dualities

Key Words: *Transhumanism, Modernity, Science, Religion, Humanities, being-as-other*

Noemi Bravená

Humanity as Imago Dei in the Theology of Dietrich Bonhoeffer

Theological anthropology of Dietrich Bonhoeffer is examined in this work along with its relevance to transhumanist notion of human perfection and accountability. Based in Christian theology, Bonhoeffer emphasizes a contrast between human limitations and divine perfection by presenting humanity as 'Imago Dei' (the image of God). The paper makes the case that transhumanism can be critically seen via the prism of Bonhoeffer's beliefs on human liberty, the partition of the world, and human nature as intrinsically "better". The goal of scientific improvement and immortality is contrasted with the transition from a condition of imperfection to spiritual connection with God via trust in Jesus Christ. The essence of human perfection, the boundaries of human enhancement, and the ethical consequences of technology in human evolution are among the existential and ethical issues brought up by transhumanism. In the age of transhumanism, it concludes, Bonhoeffer's theology offers an essential foundation for comprehending the moral and spiritual aspects of human progress.

Key words: *Bonhoeffer, Imago Dei, Christian anthropology, transhumanism, human perfection, ethics, technology, freedom.*

Noemi Bravená and Helena Hejlová

Transhumanism as a New Topic in Education

The notion of human enhancement and its interfacing with technologies to improve physical and cognitive abilities is new to education, which pertains to the primary question addressed in this paper: Where can we find room for integrating the topic of transhumanism into the national curriculum of primary schools? The main contribution of this paper is the formulation of issues and questions that highlight a deficit in the state curriculum concerning digital literacy connected with technological, ethical, and transcendent human education. The concept of transformative education, which provides an appropriate platform for contemplating the purpose of education as a sturdy foundation for the development of all topics, including those related to new technologies, is discussed.

Key words: *Transhumanism, education, transformative education, transcendence, digital competence, ethical competence, responsibility, freedom, human reduction*

Wolfgang Palaver

The Desire to Be like God: Addressing Temptations Coming Along with AI

This article delves into the complex interplay between religion and technology, particularly as it relates to Artificial Intelligence (AI). It explores the anthropological roots of humanity's fascination and trepidation towards AI, attributing these emotions to an inherent desire that surpasses our current existence. The first section highlights the role of religion in shaping perspectives on technology, both in advocacy and criticism. The second section examines the risks posed by weak AI, such as the challenges to democracy presented by social media and certain algorithmic applications. The third section shifts focus to strong AI, discussing the human aspiration to create human-like robots and the trend of transforming ourselves into machine-like automatons. Through René Girard's mimetic theory, the article illuminates the potential for conflict inherent in creating human-like robots and the dangers of striving for godlike autonomy, which could lead to technological subjugation and the demise of humanity as we know it. Finally, drawing on Romano Guardini's insights, the article suggests a path towards using technology without succumbing to enslavement, advocating for a form of technological asceticism that empowers us to remain masters of our creations. The paper offers a nuanced understanding of the ethical, anthropological, and philosophical implications of AI in the context of human desire and technological advancement.

Key Words: *Anthropological Desire, Artificial Intelligence Ethics, Mimetic Theory, Technological Asceticism, Human-Automation Interface, Democracy and Digital Algorithms*

Bojan Žalec

New Age and Romanticism, Transhumanism and Enlightenment: The Importance of Transcendence and Authenticity

The author explains that the New Age can be understood as a form of neo-Romanticism, and transhumanism as a form of neo-Enlightenment. In addition, transhumanism can also be understood as a form of exclusive humanism in the Charles Taylor's sense. The author argues that extreme transhumanism is dangerous. He cites two reasons for this. First, extreme transhumanism "abolishes" transcendence. Thus, it repeats the fatal attempt of the Enlightenment. In this way, like the Enlightenment, it opens the door to violence, inhumanity and catastrophe. Second, there is no foundation in the horizon of transhumanism for the value of authenticity, which is a key value of modern Western social and political grammar. Therefore, transhumanism poses a threat to this grammar.

Key words: *New Age, transhumanism, Romanticism, Enlightenment, transcendence, authenticity, exclusive humanism, danger of transhumanism*

Piotr Orłowski

Imago Dei and Transhumanism: Theological Worries

Within the classical discourse on humanity as the image of God (Imago Dei), certain interpretations suggest an inadvertent endorsement of transhumanist ideologies. These interpretations postulate that, according to thinkers like Thomas Aquinas, the essence of Imago Dei lies in human intellectual nature, leading to the assumption that enhancing intellectual capabilities through disembodiment aligns with the divine image. This paper critiques such interpretations as overly reductionist, failing to incorporate the broader anthropological framework of Aquinas' thought. The analysis commences with an exploration of a specific inquiry in Summa Theologiae, where St. Thomas deliberates on who reflects God's image more profoundly: angels or humans. The paper posits that the transhumanist endeavor, rather than advancing the human state 'in the image of God,' veers towards an aspiration to be 'like God' – a fundamentally different and theologically significant distinction.

Key words: *intellect, exemplarism, transhumanism, singularity, Thomism*

Michal Valčo – Radoslav Hanus

Contingency, Relationality, and Narrativity: Three Constitutive Aspects of Human Identity

The deep interactions among narrativity, relationality, and contingency as essential components of the human identity are examined in this work. In their existential ontology as well as its ethical and spiritual aspects, it suggests that humans are essentially contingent. Relationality, in which the self is understood in the framework of its relationships and interactions with others, is closely related to this contingency. Proposed as the unifying factor that unites these elements and shapes identity by the ongoing creation and reconstruction of individual and group narratives is narrative. By means of a multidisciplinary methodology, this study explores the ways in which these three elements combine to provide a thorough comprehension of human identity. In order to highlight the intricate dynamics underlying the human experience, the paper looks at narrative identity in the framework of human contingency and relationality. This strong anthropological framework also provides important perspectives on how to tackle the problems raised by transhumanism. It offers another viewpoint that challenges the fragmented and frequently reductionist picture of humanity put out by Transhumanist ideologies by stressing the fundamental worth and connectivity of human beings. This viewpoint emphasizes not only the need of human agency and dignity but also the moral ramifications of technical developments on society and human identity.

Key Words: *Contingency, human identity, narrativity, relationality, imago Dei*

Michal Valčo

Transhumanism as a Techno-Gnostic Challenge to Theological Anthropology

Theological and philosophical foundations of transhumanism, a movement that promotes using technology to improve human potential and go beyond biological constraints, are examined in this paper. Using the idea of Gnosticism, which holds that the human body is something intrinsically limiting, low, and repulsive and that salvation (or: liberation, elevation, fulfillment) comes through secret knowledge or gnosis, I contend that transhumanism – more especially, some of its more extreme strands – can be considered a type of techno-Gnosticism. Similar to Gnostics, transhumanists use technology to manipulate reality and gain knowledge in order to escape the bounds of the material world. In this work, I examine how this viewpoint affects our knowledge of human nature and contend that it begs significant concerns regarding the connection between technology and human well-being. In the conclusion, I argue that even as transhumanism presents exciting opportunities for human improvement, it also entails serious dangers and difficulties that need to be properly taken into account in any endeavor to achieve a transhumanist future.

Key Words: *Transhumanism, Gnosticism, Techno-Gnosticism, Human Nature, Imago Dei*

Katarína Valčová

The Existential, Spiritual, and Practical/Pastoral Dimensions of Mortality: A Comprehensive Exploration

In this study, we investigate the important subject of human mortality. This voyage leads us throughout the many terrains of existential philosophy, introspection, and pragmatic conversation. We start by looking at the nuanced emotional experiences of children who are grieving, focusing especially on the significant contributions that pastoral care and digital settings play. Our research centers on the interaction of these components in forming modern coping strategies. After this, the study turns its attention to the philosophical dimensions of mortality, providing a thorough examination of the pervasive existential fear that people experience in view of the transience of existence. Using a wide variety of materials, such as literary masterpieces and newly developed digital technologies, the study explores the ageless human need for immortality. This pursuit is outlined as a complex coping mechanism that finds resonance in the larger society and goes beyond personal attempts to face mortality. The essay also enhances its story with a discussion of doable strategies for starting discussions about death with kids. The practical techniques included give an otherwise theoretical discussion a concrete aspect. A whole story is presented by the study by fusing existential, pastoral, and psychological viewpoints. It catches the variety of ways that people and communities face, negotiate, and finally accept the unavoidable fact of death.

Key Words: *Death, mortality, grief, coping mechanisms, pastoral approach, speaking about death with children*

Hang Thi Thu Vu

The Effects of Technology on Happiness: A Vietnamese Perspective

This research examines, with an emphasis on Vietnam, how technology progress affects happiness and well-being. It looks at the ways that technology affects social contacts, recreational activities, and service and information access among other aspects of Vietnamese life. Also included are possible drawbacks of technology, such addiction, social isolation, and information overload. With its extensive analysis of the body of literature, the study provides a complete picture of the state of knowledge in this field. It contains results of a qualitative research on local views and opinions regarding the place of technology in daily life carried out in Vietnam. These revelations advance knowledge of how technology affects happiness in Vietnam and add to more general conversations on how technology affects human well-being. Particular relevance of the results is found in nations with comparable socioeconomic and cultural backgrounds. In the end, this study tries to start a more sophisticated and critical discussion on happiness and technology. It seeks to guide projects and policy creation that make good use of technology to promote happier and more contented lives.

Key Words: *Technological Impact, Vietnam, Happiness and Well-being, Social Interaction, Digital Overload*

Winfried Löffler

The Plasticities of Human Nature: From Trivial to Horrendous

This paper critically examines the concept of 'human nature' and its inherent plasticities, navigating the terrain between traditional existentialist concerns and contemporary transhumanist ideas. It begins by addressing the precarious nature of defining human nature, highlighting the potential risks of essentialist and authoritarian misuse, and the need to recognize human evolutionary change. A moderate definition of 'human nature' is proposed, emphasizing the sum of typical properties, structures, and capabilities of humans. Insights from classical philosophy, particularly the Aristotelian-Scholastic tradition, are explored to illustrate the inherent flexibility and potential for development in human nature. Contemporary perspectives on human evolution, genetic variation, and medical technologies are also discussed, underscoring the dynamic nature of human existence. The paper concludes with a critical analysis of transhumanism, acknowledging its ethical concerns and the potential risks associated with technological and genetic interventions in human nature. In sum, the paper advocates a balanced approach to understanding human nature, one that embraces its plasticities while also considering the ethical implications of altering it.

Key Words: *Human Nature, Transhumanism, Evolutionary Biology, Ethical Implications, Classical Philosophy, Habitus, Natural Law, Genetic Intervention*

Hans Conrad Zander
Von der Religiosität der Katzen
24 Sonntagsweisheiten
Mit weisem Spott füllt Hans Conrad Zander Ihre sonntägliche Leere. Sie wundern sich über: „Die Unterhose über Grönland" „Das Vermächtnis des Hilfsgeistlichen Alfred Birch", „Von der Lust ein Fremder zu sein", „Warum ich Adolf Hitler gut verstehen kann", „Ode an die Geschirrspülmaschine", und zahlreiche andere Sonntagsweisheiten – bekannt aus dem WDR. In der „Theologie der Wiederholung" erfahren Sie, warum Sie dieses Buch immer wieder lesen müssen. Sie brauchen die Sonntagsweisheiten von Hans Conrad Zander.
Bd. 1, 3. Aufl. 2012, 136 S., 7,90 €, gb.,
ISBN 978-3-88660-516-3

Hans Conrad Zander
Von der rechten Art, den Glauben zu verlieren
Eine Überzeugung, ja den Glauben zu verlieren, gehört zu den Risiken des modernen Lebens. Jedem kann dies widerfahren. In solcher Drangsal hilft Hans Conrad Zander mit „praktischen Ratschlägen". Er hilft, den Glauben gelassen zu verlieren und warnt Sie vor der größten Gefahr: der Gefahr, gleich einen neuen anzunehmen. Zum Verständnis Ihrer Selbst und der Welt brauchen Sie das Werk von Hans Conrad Zander.
Bd. 2, 3. Aufl. 2009, 64 S., 7,90 €, gb.,
ISBN 978-3-88660-999-4

Hans Conrad Zander
Lob der Dummheit
15 Reportagen mit Sinn
Leben unter Dieben in Köln, unter amerikanischen Intelligenzforschern, unter Krokodilfängern im australischen Busch: Hans Conrad Zander berichtet davon in 15 ausgewählten Reportagen. Eine davon ist mit dem Kisch-Preis ausgezeichnet worden. „Zu Unrecht", wie der Autor selber urteilt. Denn so spannend sich jeder dieser Berichte liest, so wenig ist darin die Spur eines „rasenden Reporters" zu finden. Statt der Zeit hinterher zu jagen, hat Hans Conrad Zander sie angehalten und sich in seine Geschichten mit einer Aufmerksamkeit hineinbegeben, die das Lesen zu einem doppelten Vergnügen macht.
Bd. 3, 2. Aufl. 2011, 248 S., 9,90 €, gb.,
ISBN 978-3-8258-5593-2

Hans Conrad Zander
Die emanzipierte Nonne
Gottes unbequeme Freunde
Heiraten? „Nie ist es mir gelungen", schreibt Theresia von Avila, „meinen Verstand jemandem unterzuordnen, dem es daran fehlt. Welche Gnade, wenn Gott einer Frau die Tyrannei eines Ehemanns erspart." – Worte einer spanischen Nonne des 16. Jahrhunderts, der „Grossen Theresia".
So eigenwillig sind sie alle, die Heiligen, die Hans Conrad Zander in diesem Buch vorstellt: Neun Männer und Frauen, die sich im Leben an nichts gehalten haben als an das Wort des heiligen Augustinus: „Liebe Gott und tue, was du willst."
Bd. 4, 3. Aufl. 2011, 224 S., 9,90 €, gb.,
ISBN 978-3-8258-6053-0

Hans Conrad Zander
Napoleon in der Badewanne
Das Beste aus Zanders Großer Universal-Geschichte
„Napoleon in der Badewanne", Papst Pius V. beim Schokoladetest im Vatikan", „Sarah Bernhardt als Erzengel Raffael", „Francis Drake auf der Lauer hinter einem grossen Kaktus in Panama", „Ludwig XIV. beim Zähneziehen in Versailles": Aus Hans Conrad Zanders legendären Beiträgen zur Sendereihe „Zeitzeichen" des Westdeutschen Rundfunks wählt dieses Buch die 24 besten aus. Klassische Bildung als reines Lesevergnügen gemäss der antiken Maxime: „Zuerst unterhalten, dann belehren".
Bd. 5, 2005, 200 S., 9,90 €, gb., ISBN 978-3-8258-6054-7

Hans Conrad Zander
Von der frommen Kunst, beleidigt zu sein
Eine christliche Handreichung an den Islam
„Warum", fragte ich die Marokkaner, die schon seit Stunden mit mir am Tisch saßen und über Gott und die Welt schwatzten, „warum ist eigentlich der Mond das Symbol des Islam?" Sekunden später rannte ich quer durch Marrakesch um mein Leben. Ich hatte nicht bedacht, daß das französische Wort „lune", anders als das deutsche Wort „Mond", einen ironischen Unterton hat. „Lunatique" heißt „verrückt". In Marrakesch bin ich mit dem Leben davongekommen. Ich wage nicht, mir auszumalen, wie es mir in Kabul oder in Teheran ergangen wäre.
Bd. 6, 3. Aufl. 2013, 48 S., 5,90 €, br.,
ISBN 978-3-8258-9411-5